T0215759

HYDROPHTHALMIA

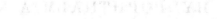

HYDROPHTHALMIA
OR
CONGENITAL GLAUCOMA
Its Causes, Treatment, and Outlook

by

J. RINGLAND ANDERSON

M.C., M.D., B.S. (Melb.), F.R.C.S. (Edin.), F.R.A.C.S.,
D.O.M.S. (Lond.)

Ophthalmic Surgeon to the Alfred Hospital, Melbourne

WITH A FOREWORD BY
SIR JOHN HERBERT PARSONS
C.B.E., D.Sc., F.R.C.S., F.R,S.

CAMBRIDGE
Published for the
British Journal of Ophthalmology
AT THE UNIVERSITY PRESS
1939

CAMBRIDGE UNIVERSITY PRESS
Cambridge, New York, Melbourne, Madrid, Cape Town,
Singapore, São Paulo, Delhi, Mexico City

Cambridge University Press
The Edinburgh Building, Cambridge CB2 8RU, UK

Published in the United States of America by Cambridge University Press, New York

www.cambridge.org
Information on this title: www.cambridge.org/9781107625518

First published 1939
First paperback edition 2013

A catalogue record for this publication is available from the British Library

ISBN 978-1-107-62551-8 Paperback

To

MY WIFE

CONTENTS

Chapter VII. PROGNOSIS (*contd.*)

Tables at back

Analysis of Early Specimens

Analysis of Specimens over 2½ years and under eleven

Analysis of Specimens over eleven years

available for download from www.cambridge.org/9781107625518

ILLUSTRATIONS

FOREWORD

In a foreword to Dr Ringland Anderson's book on *Detachment of the Retina*, I expressed the hope that others would follow his good example and provide other such monographs. It is a matter for congratulation that he himself has now written one on *Hydrophthalmia*, a disease better known under the picturesque but otherwise unsatisfactory name Buphthalmia. The last monograph on this subject was published in 1897 by Dr Edmund L. Gros, under the title *Étude sur l'Hydrophthalmie ou Glaucome infantile*, and was an excellent résumé of our knowledge up to that date. The present is a much more extensive treatise and will long remain authoritative. In dealing with a disease of such obscure aetiology, in which, however, congenital malformations are a prominent factor, the scientific approach must be by way of pathology and comparative anatomy. In both of these respects the treatment here is exhaustive, and beautifully illustrated. Dr Anderson has taken advantage of his special opportunities to obtain specimens from Australian fauna—ornithorhyncus, echidna, pseudochirus, dasyurus—and to describe the condition of the angle of the anterior chamber in them and in tarsius. This is in itself a valuable contribution to comparative anatomy. The remarkable association of hydrophthalmia with neurofibromatosis, facial naevi and other angiomatous conditions is fully discussed.

To the practising ophthalmic surgeon the most important part of the book is the description of all the different methods of operative treatment which have been tried, with a thorough analysis of the results obtained by various surgeons. One cannot help regretting that the survey shows no signs of indicating in the treatment of hydrophthalmia any such hopeful improvements in operative technique as were beginning to bear fruit when Dr Anderson's book on *Detachment of the Retina* was published, and which have proved so successful.

J. HERBERT PARSONS

INTRODUCTION

CONSULTING ROOM, MELBOURNE, 1933.

Father of a 9-year-old boy blind from congenital glaucoma. Grahame had a trephine operation on each eye when he was a year old. Would he have had a better chance without such treatment?

Surgeon. I do not know.

Father. Do any untreated patients with this disease retain sufficient vision to enable them to earn their living for a few years?

Surgeon. I do not know.

Father. If he marries will his children be affected?

Surgeon. I do not know.

The following pages are the result of an attempt to answer these questions: Through the generosity of Messrs G. J. and E. B. Coles, it was possible to send out 874 Questionnaire forms to 346 oculists throughout the world. A summary of the data obtained will be found later in this book.

The author is grateful to the following surgeons for supplying valuable material: Humphrey Neame, London; E. O. Marks, Brisbane; W. R. Fairclough, Auckland, and J. M. Wheeler, New York. The author is indebted to Professor A. W. Mulock Houwer and Captain v. Blaauboer for the specimens from Tarsius. The following pathologists have most willingly aided in its investigation: Drs Rupert Willis, R. B. Maynard and Adelaide Gault. Dr Kevin O'Day kindly allowed the author to examine his sections of *Dasyurus* and *Pseudochirus*. The microphotographs are by Mr Lewis Booth of the Alfred Hospital and Mr H. Marriott of the Department of Anatomy, Melbourne University. The author would express his appreciation of the generosity of those who permitted the use of plates from older works. To Miss Jean McNab and Miss Elizabeth Agar the author would offer his warmest thanks for hours spent in typing and translation.

If it had not been for the enthusiasm and the outstanding ability of Miss Diana Mann, B.Sc., this book would not have been written. For three years her eagerness to understand some of the mysteries of congenital glaucoma has led her through many hundred pages of foreign works, through the examination of several hundred slides and through the almost endless arduous tasks that are known only by those who carry out a work of this kind. For these labours the author is deeply grateful.

Sir John Parsons, Mr R. R. James and Mr H. B. Stallard have helped in the production of this work and to them and to the Directors of the *British Journal of Ophthalmology* the author would acknowledge his indebtedness.

CHAPTER I

GENERAL: AETIOLOGY

DEFINITION

The condition to be described is that of an eye which has become enlarged under the influence of increased intra-ocular pressure. As the ability of the ocular tissues to stretch is practically limited to the period of childhood, and as glaucoma in the first few years of life is almost always associated with ocular distension, the term "Congenital Glaucoma" appears suitable for this condition. By congenital glaucoma we mean a state of raised tension due to an intra-uterine defect and manifest during the first few years of life.

The definition excludes from the scope of this work true cases of infantile staphyloma, which show evidence of perforation, in which the iris is incorporated with the cornea. Of course, the hypertension that is the cause of enlargement in congenital glaucoma may not be in evidence at the time of examination. The state of raised tension may have passed, but before doing so it sets up a series of degenerative changes and interferes with the nutrition of the various tissues to such an extent that ultimate blindness is almost inevitable.

Glaucoma in children, as in adults, may be primary or secondary. The term primary is reserved for cases of obscure origin, and simply implies ignorance as to the cause. It is hoped that in time the term may become obsolete. This study is mainly concerned with primary infantile glaucoma.

Some cases of glaucoma in children are obviously due to certain malformations, of which the most common are aniridia and microphthalmia. In aniridia, glaucoma is undoubtedly often caused by the union of the iris root and the posterior surface of the cornea. In microphthalmia the narrowness of the circumlental space plays a part. As the finer changes which may hinder the function of the drainage channels are beyond our knowledge at present, our conceptions are largely hypothetical.

TITLE

Of the many different names given in the past to the condition under discussion, "Hydrophthalmia" and "Buphthalmia" have been most widely used. A. Fuchs (1924) reserved the term "buphthalmos" for the condition in which an anterior staphyloma arises in infancy and "hydrophthalmos" for "primary infantile (congenital) glaucoma".

The term buphthalmia, though picturesque and of ancient origin, should be excluded, for in these days of scientific exactitude long-continued usage does not warrant the perpetuation of a term that is clinically inaccurate. Ambroise Paré (1517–90) wrote "Œil de bœuf (βοῦς ὀφθαλμός) est une maladie d'œil quand il est gros et éminent, sortant hors la teste, comme on voit les bœufs les avoir". The eye of the bull does not suggest the failing vision or the raised tension, which are essential features. This term has been applied more suitably to the condition of megalocornea or megalophthalmia. The dual application of this term, and the following multiplicity of synonyms, make it desirable for us to adhere to the one or two most suitable titles. Amongst the terms used for congenital glaucoma and for megalocornea are the following: keratoglobus, keratomegalia, cornea globus, cornea bulbosa, hydrophthalmos congenitus anterior, hydrops camera anterior, and others. The terms keratoglobus turbidus and keratoglobus pellucidus have been used to distinguish congenital glaucoma from megalocornea.

In this work we shall use only the terms congenital glaucoma and hydrophthalmia, which will be considered as synonymous. It is suggested that all others be discarded.[1]

RETROSPECT

In the opinion of Julia Bell (1932) the early writers, Hippocrates, Galen, Celsus, and others, did not clearly describe as an entity the condition now known as hydrophthalmia.

Saint-'Yves, in 1722, described the various forms of ocular enlargement in a chapter entitled "De la grosseur démesurée du Globe de l'Œil". They were grouped as

(a) the naturally large eye;

(b) exophthalmos due to causes other than increase in the size of the globe;

(c) an increase in the size of the globe with too great an abundance of the aqueous humour constituting a hydropsy of the globe (Bell).

---

[1] After consultation with two classical scholars, it appears that the widely used endings -ophthalmos and -ophthalmus are incorrect, the word for the morbid state being hydrophthalmia. In medical terminology, hydro- is prefixed to names of parts of the body to denote that such part is dropsical. According to the Sydenham Society *Lexicon*, the meaning of this term is "expansion of the whole eye with increase of its fluid contents". Quoted by *Shorter Oxford Dictionary*.

Terson (1925) considered that the first reference to hypertension in hydrophthalmia was made by Beger in his thesis presented at Tübingen in 1744.

Von Muralt (1869) emphasised the fact that this condition was a form of glaucoma. He and von Graefe considered that the enlargement of the cornea was primary and that hypertension followed the atrophy of the corneal nerves. Raab (1876), Gallenga (1885) and Mauthner (1882) were the earliest observers to state that the glaucoma was secondary to a uveal inflammation. Manz (1883) and Grahamer (1884) found no signs of inflammation.

The earliest series of cases with detailed histological reports appears to have been that of Schiess-Gemuseus (1884). Then followed Gallenga (1885), Dürr and Schlegtendal (1889), Cross (1896), von Hippel (1897), Collins (1900), Reis (1905) and Seefelder (1906).

Even after hypertension was recognised as a factor producing enlargement, there was much confusion between pathological "hydrophthalmia" and the physiologically large eye or cornea now known as "megalophthalmia" or "megalocornea". This considerably delayed a true understanding of the disease. The definitions given by Kestenbaum (1919) are now generally recognised.

SUMMARY OF QUESTIONNAIRE

As a result of sending out forms to oculists in most countries, information was collected concerning 205 eyes of 116 patients. 874 forms were sent to 346 oculists living in thirty-two different countries. Of these 111 completed forms were returned from thirty-one oculists in fifteen countries. Six doctors wrote to say that they had not treated a single patient with congenital glaucoma. One—Colonel R. E. Wright of Madras—sent notes of twenty-nine patients, and Zeeman of Holland reported twenty-four patients. The staff of the Royal London Ophthalmic Hospital sent reports of ten cases, and Lindner of Vienna described seven. One oculist reported five cases, one four cases, four reported two cases each, seven reported one case each.

Reports of	9 cases	came from	Australia
,,	7	,, ,,	Austria
,,	2	,, ,,	Belgium
,,	1 case	,,	Canada
,,	5 cases	,,	Czecho-Slovakia
,,	2	,, ,,	Finland
,,	1 case	,,	France

Reports of 6 cases came from Germany

,,	15	,, ,,	Great Britain
,,	24	,, ,,	Holland
,,	7	,, ,,	Hungary
,,	29	,, ,,	India
,,	1 case	,,	Italy
,,	1	,, ,,	New Zealand
,,	6 cases	,,	U.S.A.

Of these cases 147 eyes of ninety patients were operated on. Several have been omitted as they were possibly examples of juvenile glaucoma or interstitial keratitis. The total number of the remainder was 139 eyes of eighty-four patients. They received approximately 243 operations.

24 eyes received only 1 operation

24	,,	,,	2 operations
16	,,	,,	3 ,,
9	,,	,,	4 ,,
4	,,	,,	more than 4 operations

An analysis of the type of operation used shows a great preference for the operation of sclerectomy, and particularly by means of a trephine, viz. ninety-five eyes of fifty-six patients.

Trephine	was performed	126	times on	95	eyes
Anterior sclerotomy	,,	27	,,	17	,,
Cyclodialysis	,,	31	,,	24	,,
Paracentesis (one or a series)	,,	9	,,	9	,,
Iridencleisis	,,	8	,,	8	,,
Herbert's sclerotomy	,,	5	,,	2	,,
Iridectomy	,,	11	,,	8	,,

Thirty-one eyes were enucleated. As a rule this followed an injury such as a bump against a chair or other obstacle.

AETIOLOGY

Incidence. The rareness of the disease is seen from the following reports. In Seefelder's clinic (1906) only forty-six examples were found amongst 129,520 patients from 1891 to 1905, percentage 0·035. In the Tübingen clinic from 1875 to 1903, 0·079 % of the patients had the disease. Gallenga considered that the majority of these patients came from hilly or marshy country. Seefelder's patients came chiefly from plain country. Kaminsky (1913) found this disease in 0·041 % of Breslau patients, and Jaensch (1927) in the same centre found twenty-three cases (0·032 %) amongst 72,681 admittances from 1916 to 1925. Carvill (1932) found the incidence to be 0·01 % amongst 31,648 patients with ophthalmic disorders. In another American series, amongst almost a quarter of a million patients, the incidence was 0·011 % compared with that of 0·78 % for patients with glaucoma of all types (Lehrfeld and Reber, 1937).

The relative frequency of this disease may become greater now that blindness due to ophthalmia neonatorum has almost ceased and the treatment of other acquired conditions in early life has become more effective. Hydrophthalmia is one of the chief causes of blindness amongst children, and is the most common of the developmental causes. Dürr and Schlegtendal (1889) stated that in 1885 the Clinic for the Blind contained ninety-nine pupils, of whom nine were blind from congenital glaucoma. Priestley Smith (1896) found 5 % of the inmates of a blind school with congenital glaucoma. During the first twenty-five years of this century it caused 13·5 % of the admissions to the Institute for Blind Children in Lausanne (Gonin, 1925). Lamb (1925) reported that 5·3 % of the pupils in the Missouri School for the Blind had become blind from this disease.

During the years 1919–24, 4·75 % of the admissions to the German Institutes for the blind were the result of glaucoma. Of this percentage half, or sixty persons, suffered from the congenital form. Hübner (1926) and Hirsch (1902) found that 2·4 % of the inmates of blind institutes were affected by this disease.

Bilateral incidence. In approximately two out of every three patients with hydrophthalmia both eyes are affected. This is similar to the finding for retinal detachment. In

de Grosz's series, 64 % were bilateral
Zahn's   ,,   70 %   ,,
Seefelder's   ,,   67 %   ,,
Jaensch's   ,,   60 %   ,,

Of the ninety-four cases of hydrophthalmia reported in answer to the questionnaire recently issued by us, 86 % were bilateral. The right eye was affected in four of the eight unilateral cases.

There may be a difference in the time of onset and in the degree of the disorder in the two eyes.

Bell found that relatively few unilateral cases were hereditary. In the hereditary group of fifty-eight cases, approximately 10 % were unilateral, and in the non-hereditary group of 268 cases, 35 % were unilateral.

Information is too meagre to enable us to decide whether or not the former are mainly primarily inherent affections and the latter secondary to infection or local injury.

Kiehle and Pugmire (1934) found unilateral hydrophthalmia in different degrees in opposite eyes in identical twins. The affected eye of one was trephined successfully and that of the other, being blind, was excised. Bilateral hydrophthalmia was found by Gault (1937) in identical twins aged 6½ years. They were practically blind. An iridectomy had been performed on one eye. All these had been treated with eserine. Duncan (1937) examined female twins, aged seven months, who had bilateral hydrophthalmia and almost complete retinal detachments. Several months later one died and an intra-ocular neuro-epithelioma with widespread dissemination was found.

Influence of sex. The predominance of males amongst hydrophthalmic patients is as unexplained as it is marked. While adult glaucoma affects three females to two males, the following figures have been given for congenital glaucoma:

de Grosz (1932)	116 patients,	62 % males
Zahn (1904)	73 ,,	58·9 % ,,
Kunzmann (1899)	37 ,,	70 % ,,
Seefelder (1906)	47 ,,	67 % ,,
Lamb (1925)	28 ,,	71 % ,,
Lehrfeld & Reber (1937) 28	,,	71 % ,,

Haag (1915) and Lawford (1907) found the sexes affected equally by juvenile glaucoma. Löhlein (1913), in his study of 1640 cases of glaucoma under thirty years of age, found a slight predominance of males.

Bell wrote: "Sex incidence for purely hereditary cases does not differ significantly from that calculated from 304 due to all causes, which is of interest in view of the fact that hereditary disease does on the whole tend to become manifest in men more frequently than in women."

In the predominance of the male sex, hydrophthalmia resembles juvenile glaucoma and differs from the senile form which is more common amongst females (Lehrfeld and Reber, 1937).

Time of origin. It is difficult to determine the time of origin of the glaucomatous process. When we consider the degree of distension that is sometimes present at birth, we realise that hypertension must have developed soon after the anterior chamber first appeared and the activity of the filtration process began. The time of this is probably about the middle of the sixth month. Seefelder (1920) considered that the fourth month was the probable time of origin of hydrophthalmia in his specimen associated with an iris coloboma, a retinal detachment and an orbital cyst. Lagrange (1925) described the angle in his eighth specimen as being foetal in type, resembling that found in the sixth month of intra-uterine life.

In Christel's specimen (1912) the posterior part of the lens was covered with epithelial cells and the lens fibres were incompletely developed. Schlemm's canal was absent. The lens was absent in Schlaefke's specimen (1913) and in Seefelder's specimen II and III (1906). Spielberg's specimen (1911) was enlarged at birth even though the child was premature. These findings suggest an early origin.

Age of onset. While the defect producing hydrophthalmia is usually congenital, the disease may not become evident for some time after birth. Different criteria have been adopted by different people in determining the age of onset. Seefelder relies on the first appearance of acute signs. The common statement that the eyes were large at birth he did disregard as certain evidence that the disease was congenital, especially if the acute symptoms appeared later. He did not contradict the view that intra-uterine glaucoma might occur with the later development of acute symptoms, but he considered such findings to be rare in his series. Few would agree with his belief that hydrophthalmia may arise at any stage of juvenile life and lead to excessive ocular distension.

Here, as in many other sections of this work, the need for careful study of eyes in early life is felt. Until this is done we will remain unable to decide whether the so-called onset is truly such or an exacerbation. Many of the late onsets are probably recrudescences of intra-uterine developments. In these the same changes in Schlemm's canal are reported by Reis (1920), Seefelder, and others, as are found in those cases where the parents recognised the disease early.

Cross (1891) considered that in one of his series the onset was very late. The patient was a machinist, who had always been shortsighted (R. −19·0 D., L. −23·5 D.) and who had observed failing sight only during her twenty-fourth year. The corneae were enlarged (R.

14·0 mm., L. 13·5 mm.), the tension raised and no cupping was detected. It is difficult to know whether this patient had congenital glaucoma in her myopic and somewhat enlarged eyes. There is, however, little support for the theory that she developed hydro-phthalmia when twenty-four years old.

Of Seefelder's forty-seven cases the onset was given as at birth in nine cases and during the first year in twenty-four; in Zahn's fifty-seven cases the figures were twenty-four and twenty-eight, in Grosz's forty-five cases twenty-seven and six, and in Golomb's twenty-seven cases fourteen and eleven. So in 81·3 % the onset was probably before the end of the first year.

If we summarise the information contained in Seefelder's, Dett-mering's, Stölting's, Fleischer's and the questionnaire series, we obtain the following:

> At or before birth in 102 cases, that is 40 % of those with reliable information.
>
> At 6/12 months or under in 86, that is 34 % of those with reliable information.
>
> At 1 year or under in 30, that is 12 % of those with reliable information.
>
> At 6 years or under in 28, that is 11 % of those with reliable information.
>
> At over 6 years in 5, that is 2 % of those with reliable information.
>
> No, or unreliable, information in 80.

Thus in 87 % of these cases the condition was recognised under the age of one year. On the other hand, five patients were more than six years old before their eyes became affected. This brings us to the relationship of hydrophthalmia to juvenile glaucoma.

Relationship to juvenile glaucoma. No absolute distinctions can be made to separate juvenile glaucoma from hydrophthalmia on the one hand and senile glaucoma on the other. It is probable that at one end of the scale, that is, in early life, an innate defect in structure is the cause of hypertension and that degeneration is merely a secondary phenomenon. At the other end of the scale raised tension is due almost entirely to various degenerative changes associated with old age, and inherited defects play a minor part. There is an inter-mediate group in which both factors appear to be pathogenic in varying degrees.

Probably thirty or thirty-five years might be taken as an upper age limit for juvenile cases. In deciding the lower limit, between juvenile glaucoma and hydrophthalmia, we have taken as a criterion the absence or presence of the most characteristic sign of congenital glaucoma, viz. distension of the eyeball. Thus glaucoma due to a congenital defect may be classed as juvenile if it fails to develop until the eye is no longer distensible.

The ocular disorder then, that we are to consider, is that which is due to a rise in tension occurring at so early an age that the coats of the globe distend. It is necessary now to ask two questions. First, is raised tension always found in the condition we are calling congenital glaucoma? Just as the answer to a similar question relating to glaucoma of later life is in the negative, so it is here. The association with normal tension is certainly much rarer in the adult group. Such a finding does not disprove the pathogenic influence of hypertension, but simply suggests that it is transient, though with permanent and characteristic results. It is easier to understand the occurrence of normal tension or even hypotension in a distended eye than in one that cannot distend because of the inelasticity that comes with age. One can imagine the results of distension counteracting its causes. Yet, though the tension may return to normal, degenerative changes are set in motion which may persist and produce results that make the actual causes of raised tension difficult to recognise. This has led to considerable confusion in interpreting the late lesions found in an affected globe.

The second question is, can distension develop as the result of raised tension in later life? It is known that areas of local distension, staphylomata, can arise as a result of inflammation where a weakened area bulges in response to even normal tension. But can uniform distension occur as a result of hypertension in the mature eye in the absence of the weakening effect on the sclera of inflammation? This question is very difficult to answer. Certain cases observed by Colonel Wright suggest that, at any rate in Indian races, such distension is possible up to the age of twenty-five. Thiele (1930) referred to other instances of a late onset. On the other hand, the majority of observations made in Europe indicate that the cornea and sclera are not distensible after about seven years of age. Probably a considerable proportion of such late cases have suffered from interstitial keratitis.

Thus among the forty-five cases of hydrophthalmia (reported by de Grosz) the disease was evident in twenty-seven at birth or during the first week of life, in six during the first year, in eight during the third year and in two at eight years. A study of most of the reputed instances of a late onset has unconvincing results. As examples let

us consider the two with the latest onsets in the forty-five cases.
It is said of these that hydrophthalmia was not present till the age
of fourteen. One case, Derby's (1882), was a man aged twenty,
whose sight and that of three other children of a blind father
failed at about fourteen years of age. The condition was undoubtedly hydrophthalmia in this patient, but the age of onset
is not definitely stated. The second case is one reported by Grahamer
(1884), and is an example of an inaccurate reference. The author's
account is of a girl who was examined at the age of fourteen years.
The left eye at birth, however, had been larger than normal, and of bluish
appearance. The right eye was emmetropic and of normal tension.

Thirdly, it might be asked what degree of tension can exist in
childhood without scleral stretching? This again we cannot answer.
It is possible that in some cases congenital defects produce a low
degree of hypertension without distension, so that the process is not
evident until aggravated by disease or at puberty. This might explain
the occasional finding of congenital and juvenile glaucoma respectively
in the two eyes of one individual, or in two members of one family.

There are certain similarities between congenital glaucoma and
juvenile glaucoma that help to confirm the affinity between the two
conditions. In both forms, congenital anomalies are common. These
include persistent hyaloid arteries, persistent pupillary membrane,
anomalies of the retinal vessels, lamellar cataracts, aniridia, colobomata, and other deformities of the globe and very high myopia.

As we shall see later, there is ample evidence in the majority of cases
to prove the dependence of congenital glaucoma upon anomalies.
Schmidt-Rimpler (1877) considered that 50 % of cases with juvenile
glaucoma have a defective canal of Schlemm. Löhlein postulated
a milder degree of defect than that required to produce the congenital
form of glaucoma. Verhoeff examined histologically the eyes of two
patients with juvenile glaucoma and found a defective form of filtration angle as in hydrophthalmia. He considered these two forms of
glaucoma to represent differences in degree of the same condition.

Löhlein (1913) found that

> 38·8 % of cases of juvenile glaucoma were recognised between
> 15 and 20 years.
> 21·3 % of cases of juvenile glaucoma were recognised between
> 20 and 25 years.
> 1·3 % of cases of juvenile glaucoma were recognised under the
> age of 5 years.

Some observers consider that there is a period, perhaps the first decade, in which glaucoma may appear either as hydrophthalmia or without ocular enlargement. Possibly a proportion of these cases have suffered from interstitial keratitis.

"Typical juvenile glaucoma as a rule gives a worse prognosis than typical senile glaucoma" (Gjessing, 1931). Juvenile glaucoma occupies an intermediate position not only regarding its age of onset but also its sex incidence, its association with other ocular defect, and its rapid and relentless course.

Influence of heredity. Heredity appears to play a greater part in the congenital and the juvenile forms of glaucoma than in the senile type.

The anterior chamber tends to be deeper than normal in the former two, and shallow in the latter. "The anterior chamber is greatly deepened in buphthalmos" (Elliot). Amongst Bell's pedigrees of hereditary glaucoma there are thirty-two references to the depth of the anterior chamber. Twenty-one eyes had deep or very deep anterior chambers. In thirteen of the twenty-one eyes, glaucoma developed before the age of nineteen. The association of early onset and deep anterior chambers is one of the interesting features in a pedigree reported by Calhoun (1914). Of the patients in this pedigree, six eyes had corneal measurements of 12·0 mm., the others of less than this. This pedigree exemplifies the devastation wrought by juvenile glaucoma, as well as a degree of anticipation.

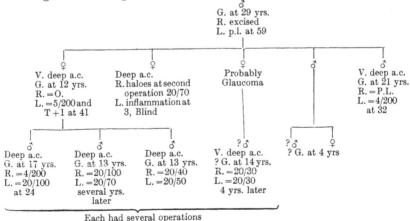

One may contrast with this pedigree one reported by Lawford (1907). Four males in a sibship of ten developed glaucoma probably late in life. Their ages at the time of examination were sixty-six, sixty-seven, seventy-two and seventy-seven.

The deep anterior chamber may perhaps be explained by the greater plasticity of the tissues in youth, which allows the shape to be modified through raised pressure. It suggests that the primary cause in youthful cases differs from that in most senile ones, where shallowness of the anterior chamber is the rule in glaucoma.

While the inheritance of hydrophthalmia is generally recessive, hereditary glaucoma in the adult appears to be dominant. Amongst the sixty-eight pedigrees collected by Bell, three or more successive generations were affected in 29 %. In Fleischer's and Plocher's pedigrees five successive generations were affected. Shumway (1931) reported a family with four successive generations affected by juvenile glaucoma. The affected members developed the disease before the sixteenth year and with the exception of the youngest all were blind by twenty years of age regardless of operative and other treatment. It appears that one-half of the descendants in five generations of a family reported by Courtney and Hill (1931) have juvenile glaucoma.

The form of glaucoma occurring in one family as a rule does not vary, so that there is usually either inflammatory or simple glaucoma. From this one draws the conclusion that the two forms are due to different causes. Exceptionally, both forms may alternate (Nettleship, 1909). It is to be assumed that a local or general disposition to glaucoma is inherited, and the appearance of the disease depends on other factors either inherited or acquired.

It has been very difficult to prove any racial tendency, though for long there has been an impression that the Jewish race is more susceptible to glaucoma than Gentiles are. One must remember the recent observation of a Jewish oculist: "Every Jew with glaucoma is registered at several hospitals and several private consultation rooms. Gentiles ask for advice of one person only" (Brav, 1931).

Heredity in congenital glaucoma. In 1909, Nettleship stressed the need for more data relating to the heredity of glaucoma. There is still too little to justify definite conclusions. The relatively late age of onset and the death of many patients soon after development of glaucoma make the collection of the necessary material difficult.

Especially it is difficult to estimate the effect of heredity in the case of congenital glaucoma, owing to the infrequent marriage and parenthood of the afflicted.

"The available material provides no guide as to whether the marriage of a man or woman who has an arrested buphthalmos is justified, or whether such a parentage carries grave menace to the offspring" (Bell).

Though Seefelder in his investigation of forty-seven cases of congenital glaucoma found no evidence at all of direct inheritance, Zahn found fourteen hereditary cases among his series of seventy-three, and Golomb four among thirty-two.

Jüngken (1842) found a family of seven children who were all hydrophthalmic, and Johnson (1898) reported a family of five, the three youngest of whom had hydrophthalmia. In neither family were other affected relatives mentioned. In Angelucci's family (1894) three brothers were affected. Amongst the eighty-five cases reported in the questionnaire, including Zeeman's twenty-four patients, there were twelve instances of a familial tendency, that is, 14 %.

4 had 1 brother affected.

3 had 1 sister affected.

2 had 1 brother and 1 sister affected.

1 had 2 sisters affected.

2 had 1 sister and another member of sibship affected.

The father of one of these had a retinal detachment in one eye and a lamellar cataract in the other (Fairclough, 1937).

One of the striking features of the published pedigrees of congenital glaucoma, if we exclude those cases in which a parent was affected, is the infrequent affection of more than one sibship. Zahn (1904), however, reported three exceptions, and Fleischer (1918) one to this rule.

In Fleischer's and in two of Zahn's pedigrees, cousins of the afflicted family were affected, whilst in the third of Zahn's pedigrees a grandfather of an affected child of nine months was reported to have become blind in early life, from dropsy of the eyes. Bell stresses the point that Zahn was one of the few observers who really sought the hereditary factor in these pedigrees, and he found three. Again, Sourdille (1925) reported a child blind of infantile glaucoma whose paternal aunt had lost both eyes through rupture following hydrophthalmia. These cases are important as proving true heredity, since the appearance of the disease in several members of a sibship might be due merely to some common factor in their environment, or to some associated disease, for example interstitial keratitis.

In a study of the literature it was found that the affected child was the last child in eleven of twenty families of three or more

children. As half of these affected children were aged less than one
year little importance can be attached to this point. There was only
one instance of the first child being affected. In three families the
second child was affected.

Of thirty-five families, of two children and more, referred to in
the literature, at least two miscarriages were reported in seven. In
eleven of these families more than one child died in infancy.

The parents' health was referred to in thirty-eight cases and in
nine of these it might be classed as poor. Ill-health of the patient
was recorded in sixteen of a series of thirty-one cases.

Argyll Robertson (1891), Venneman (1891) and von Ammon (1847)
observed the presence of hydrophthalmia in both mother and children.
In Argyll Robertson's pedigree, the three children of an affected
mother had hydrophthalmia. The condition was bilateral in all except
one daughter, who had one normal eye. The father had developed
sympathetic ophthalmia in early life. Delord operated on a child
whose father had been operated on by Galezowski. Wallenberg (1910)
reported the occurrence of congenital glaucoma in four generations.

When congenital glaucoma is transmitted, it is probably as a simple
recessive, that is, it will not develop unless two conductors of the
disease marry, when approximately 25 % of their children will be
affected. The affected members and two out of three of the apparently
normal members of the family will in their turn be conductors.
Evidence of this recessive heredity is the infrequent affection of
more than one sibship in the published pedigrees, its tendency to be
familial, and the occasional consanguinity of the parents.

Recessive heredity is not disproved by the occasional occurrence
of hydrophthalmia in successive generations. This may be due to
the marriage of an affected person and a conductor. An example of
recessive heredity is Vogt's observations of hydrophthalmia in rabbits
(1919). In one litter of rabbits, four were found to have marked hydrophthalmia, two of these were mated, and of the litter of three all
were found to have bilateral hydrophthalmia when a few weeks old.

Although males are more frequently affected than females there is
no evidence to suggest that the inheritance of either hydrophthalmia
or juvenile glaucoma is sex-linked.

Influence of consanguinity. Close relationship of the parents has
been described by Laqueur (1897) in five of thirteen children, by
Zahn (1904) in 10 % and by Seefelder in only one of forty-seven
patients. In a series of twenty-eight families collected from the litera-

ture the parents were related in three. In a series of sixteen families no relationship of grandparents was found. The parents of cases 42, 43 and 44 of Zahn's series were brother and sister. In case 4 of Reis's series two affected brothers were the children of cousins. The parents of case I of Dürr and Schlegtendal's series were first cousins and two of her brothers were similarly affected. Kaminsky (1913) did not find any blood relationship amongst thirty-four patients and Jaensch (1927) found one instance in his series of thirty-nine patients. The parents of a child referred to by Spratt (1913) were second cousins. Cogan (1935) referred to a family of four hydrophthalmic children with parents who were cousins.

This is of some importance as suggesting recessive inheritance of hydrophthalmia. A rare recessive gene is most likely to be found in both partners in a marriage if they have ancestors in common from whom it is inherited.

Anticipation. The phenomenon of anticipation has been used to account for many congenital defects, including glaucoma. That early onset is rare in primary glaucoma is shown by one series of 3021 cases, of which 0·5 % developed between ten and nineteen years of age and 3 % between twenty and twenty-nine. In a series of 196 hereditary cases these percentages are increased to 27 and 25 % respectively.

"The mean age of onset in definitely hereditary cases is twenty years earlier than that for the general series of cases" (Bell).

Graefe studied the condition in at least three generations, and noted an earlier age of onset as time went on. Werner (1929) found the mother and three children in a family of six with juvenile glaucoma. The ages of onset were approximately twenty-nine, seventeen, nineteen, sixteen years. Calhoun (1914) noted anticipation in eight cases in three generations. Lawford quoted many interesting pedigrees. The ages of onset in one were seventy-one in the first generation, forty to forty-eight in the second, and twenty-five to thirty in the third. In another, forty was the age of onset in the first generation, twenty-eight and twenty-five in the second, and the five cases in the third were between seventeen and twenty-eight years of age. Lawford refers to similar pedigrees described by Mules, Story and Priestley Smith. Gilbert (1912) described a married couple with ordinary senile congestive glaucoma, and found several descendants with the juvenile form. Germann (1909) reported a man with the senile form and a son and two daughters with juvenile glaucoma.

These last cases are interesting in that they link up the senile and juvenile types of glaucoma. On the other hand, there are few examples linking juvenile glaucoma with hydrophthalmia. In sixty-eight pedigrees of hereditary glaucoma collected by Bell, only two instances were found. The youngest of four sisters in a family reported by Löhlein (1913) had marked hydrophthalmia, and the other three had glaucoma, which appeared at the ages of fifteen, seventeen and ten respectively. In a pedigree reported by Derby (1882), a glaucomatous father, who had been blind for twenty-five years, had in a family of eleven children three blind with glaucoma, and one with hydrophthalmia. The condition arose in the eldest before he was twenty. He had large corneae and deep anterior chambers. The second had hydrophthalmia in the right eye, the left had ruptured earlier. The age of onset for the remaining two was "about fourteen". Hirschberg (1913) watched a girl for years with the congenital form in one eye and the infantile form in the other.

SUMMARY

1. Congenital glaucoma and hydrophthalmia are preferred as titles to all others. The use of the remainder should be abandoned. All the forms of this disease may be considered to be secondary and the isolation of a so-called primary or single group is unwise.

2. The incidence in various German clinics varies from 0·032 to 0·079 %. The percentage of those in Institutes for the Blind varies (from 2·4 to 13·5 %) according to the total proportion of children in the institute concerned.

3. Approximately two-thirds of the patients are males. A similar proportion have both eyes affected, though when hereditary cases only are considered this may be up to 90 %.

4. The age of onset of the great majority is at, or very soon after, birth.

5. No hard and fast line divides the congenital, juvenile and adult forms of glaucoma. The difference depends largely on a varying degree of innate defect and of factors that tend to promote hypertension. As a rule the more severe the anomaly the earlier will be the onset of glaucoma.

6. Heredity plays an important rôle in the development of glaucoma. Consanguinity appears to be of little significance.

REFERENCES

DEFINITION, TITLE, RETROSPECT

1869 VON MURALT. Inaug. Dissert. Zürich. Quoted by Dürr and Schlegtendal.

1876 RAAB. *Klin. Monatsbl. f. Augenheilk.* p. 22. Quoted by Dürr and Schlegtendal.

1882 MAUTHNER. *Glaucomtheorien und Secundärglaukom*, p. 250. Quoted by Dürr and Schlegtendal.

1883 MANZ, W. *Bericht über die Naturforschersammlung im Freiburg.* Quoted by Dürr and Schlegtendal.

1884 GRAHAMER. *Arch. f. Ophthal.* 30, 265.

1884 SCHIESS-GEMUSEUS. *Arch. f. Ophthal.* 30, pt. 3, p. 202.

1885 GALLENGA, R. *Ann. di Ottal.* 14, 322. Quoted by Dürr and Schlegtendal.

1889 DÜRR and SCHLEGTENDAL. *Arch. f. Ophthal.* 35, pt. 2, p. 88.

1896 CROSS, F. R. *Trans. Ophthal. Soc. U.K.* 16, 340.

1897 VON HIPPEL, E. *Arch. f. Augenheilk.* 35, 355; *Arch. f. Ophthal.* 44, 539.

1900 COLLINS, E. T. *Lancet*, 1, 1.

1905 REIS, W. *Arch. f. Ophthal.* 60, 1.

1906 SEEFELDER, R. *Arch. f. Ophthal.* 63, 481.

1919 KESTENBAUM, A. *Klin. Monatsbl. f. Augenheilk.* 62, 736.

1924 FUCHS, A. *Atlas of the Histopathology of the Eye.* Vienna: F. Deuticke, 1924 and 1927.

1925 TERSON, M. A. *Bull. et Mém. Soc. franç. d'Ophtal.* 38, 220.

1932 BELL, J. *The Treasury of Human Inheritance*, 2, pt. 5, 443.

AETIOLOGY

1842 JÜNGKEN, J. *Die Lehre von den Augenkrankheiten.* Berlin. Quoted by Lagrange.

1847 VON AMMON, A. *Klin. Darstellung der Krankheiten.* Quoted by Bell.

1877 SCHMIDT-RIMPLER, H. *Graefe-Saemisch Handbuch*, 5, 1.

1882 DERBY, H. C. *Arch. of Ophthal.* 11, 37.

1884 GRAHAMER. *Arch. f. Ophthal.* 30, 3.

1889 DÜRR and SCHLEGTENDAL. *Arch. f. Ophthal.* 35, 88.

1891 CROSS, F. R. *Trans. Ophthal. Soc. U.K.* 11, 231.

1891 ARGYLL ROBERTSON. *Trans. Ophthal. Soc. U.K.* 11, 239.

1891 VENNEMAN, E. *Ann. d'Ocul.* 128, 137.

1894 ANGELUCCI. *Arch. di Ottal.* 10 and 12, 333.

1896 PRIESTLEY SMITH. *Trans. Ophthal. Soc. U.K.* 16, 349.

1897 LAQUEUR, L. *Zeitschr. f. prakt. Ärzte*, No. 21. Quoted by Reis.

1898 JOHNSON, W. B. *Trans. Amer. Ophthal. Soc.* 8, 308.

1899 KUNZMANN. Inaug. Dissert. Zürich. Quoted by Lagrange and others.

1902 HIRSCH, L. *Entstehung und Verhütung der Blindheit.* Quoted by Jaensch.

1904 ZAHN, E. Inaug. Dissert. Tübingen. Quoted by Jaensch.

1906 SEEFELDER, R. *Arch. f. Ophthal.* 63, 481.

1907 LAWFORD, J. B. *Roy. Lond. Ophthal. Hosp. Reps.* 17, 57.

1909 NETTLESHIP, E. *Trans. Ophthal. Soc. U.K.* 29, 152.

1909 GERMANN, D. *Klin. Monatsbl. f. Augenheilk.* July.

1910 WALLENBERG. *Klin. Monatsbl. f. Augenheilk.* 48, 495.

1911 SPIELBERG, C. *Klin. Monatsbl. f. Augenheilk.* 49, 313.

1912 CHRISTEL, P. *Arch. f. Augenheilk.* **71**, 247.
1912 GILBERT, W. *Arch. f. Ophthal.* **82**, 389.
1913 KAMINSKY. Inaug. Dissert. Breslau. Quoted by Lagrange.
1913 SCHLAEFKE, W. *Arch. f. Ophthal.* **86**, 106.
1913 SPRATT, C. N. *Jl. Amer. Med. Ass.* **61**, 2, 1110.
1913 LÖHLEIN, W. *Arch. f. Ophthal.* **85**, 393.
1913 HIRSCHBERG, J. Heidelberg Congress.
1914 CALHOUN, F. P. *Jl. Amer. Med. Ass.* July.
1915 HAAG, C. *Klin. Monatsbl. f. Augenheilk.* **54**, 133.
1918 FLEISCHER, B. *Klin. Monatsbl. f. Augenheilk.* **61**, 152.
1919 VOGT, A. *Klin. Monatsbl. f. Augenheilk.* **63**, 233.
1920 SEEFELDER, R. *Arch. f. Ophthal.* **103**, 1.
1920 REIS, W. *Arch. d'Ophtal.* **40**, 577.
1925 LAMB, H. P. *Amer. Jl. Ophthal.* **8**, 784.
1925 SOURDILLE, M. E. *Bull. et Mém. Soc. franç. d'Ophtal.* **38**, 220.
1925 GONIN, J. *Bull. et Mém. Soc. franç. d'Ophtal.* **38**, 614.
1925 LAGRANGE, F. *Bull. et Mém. Soc. franç. d'Ophtal.* **38**, 3.
1926 HÜBNER. *Zeitschr. f. Augenheilk.* **58**, 358. Quoted by Jaensch.
1927 JAENSCH, P. A. *Arch. f. Ophthal.* **118**, 1, 77.
1929 WERNER, S. *Acta Ophthal.* **7**, 162.
1930 THIELE, R. *Kurzes Handbuch der Ophthal.* **4**, 828.
1931 GJESSING, H. *Arch. of Ophthal.* **6**, 494.
1931 BRAV, A. *Amer. Jl. Ophthal.* **48**, 14.
1931 COURTNEY and HILL. *Jl. Amer. Med. Ass.* **97**, 2, 1602.
1931 SHUMWAY, E. *Jl. Amer. Med. Ass.* **97**, 2, 1608.
1932 CARVILL, M. *Trans. Amer. Ophthal. Soc.* **30**, 71.
1932 DE GROSZ, E. *Arch. d'Ophtal.* **49**, 625.
1934 KIEHLE and PUGMIRE. *Arch. of Ophthal.* **12**, 751.
1935 COGAN, D. *Amer. Jl. Ophthal.* **18**, 557.
1935 WRIGHT, R. E. Personal Communications.
1937 FAIRCLOUGH, W. A. Personal Communication.
1937 GAULT, E. L. Personal Communications.
1937 LEHRFELD and REBER. *Arch. of Ophthal.* **18**, 713.
1937 DUNCAN, W. J. L. Personal Communications.

CHAPTER II

DIFFERENTIAL DIAGNOSIS

Myopia. There are certain fundamental differences between myopia and congenital glaucoma that make confusion between the two unlikely. In congenital glaucoma the cornea and adjacent sclera distend first and then the posterior portion of the sclera. In myopia the post-equatorial region is first affected and the cornea, as a rule, not at all. The former condition is characterised by congestive attacks, raised tension and a cupping of the optic disc, whilst none of these changes occurs in myopia. It is of interest to compare the illustrations showing the two different types of distension as seen in cross-sections of eyes with congenital glaucoma and myopia (see Figs. 1 to 8). The difference between the two conditions is great, but it is difficult to estimate the importance of each when both are found in the same globe. Nettleship (1888) found that almost two-thirds of his young patients with glaucoma were myopic. He revived a question raised by von Graefe twenty years earlier: does myopia predispose to glaucoma, or are both dependent on some related local cause? Löhlein held that myopia may follow glaucoma and that both may have a common cause. Ischreyt (1909) was not convinced of this relationship.

Würdemann (1934) reported six cases of glaucoma in patients under thirty years of age. In five he found progressive myopia and in one a reduction of hypermetropia. Capetta and Motolese (1936) investigated a group of seventeen patients with juvenile glaucoma. They found that

10 eyes were hypermetropic
11   ,,   mildly myopic $\left.\begin{array}{l} \\ \\ \end{array}\right\}$ 47 %
4   ,,   markedly myopic
and 7   ,,   emmetropic

Twelve of the patients were male.

Brückner and Franceschetti (1931) discussed the findings in twenty-five children with a form of myopia which they considered to be different from the type that increases during school life. These children with "infantile myopia" were at the beginning of school age, *i.e.* about six or seven years, and showed myopia of from 3 to 25 dioptres and a myopic astigmatism ranging from 1 to 4 dioptres.

Certain features suggested kinship with hydrophthalmia. They were (1) the majority of the patients were male, viz. two-thirds in comparison with five-eighths in hydrophthalmia; (2) the small temporal conus seldom exceeded a third of the diameter of the optic disc. In hydrophthalmia 23 % of Dettmering's cases showed a conus.

Other features of the myopic fundi were (1) absent pigment epithelium in the posterior pole and particularly between the disc and the macula; (2) a dark spot at the macula due to an increase in the pigment; (3) a reduction in the retinal reflex and the light streak on the vessels. The visual acuity of these eyes was subnormal, but the visual fields and dark adaptation were normal. As a rule the parents and other children were not myopic. The rate of progress of myopia, which varied greatly, did not appear to be associated with near work. One patient showed an increase of 11 dioptres in twenty-one years and another child showed no increase over a period of eighteen years. Brückner and Franceschetti (1931) held the view that the myopia was axial, for no indicial changes were found. They considered that the pigment changes were not due to the stretching of the coats of the eyeball and that they were in some way related to the origin of the myopia.

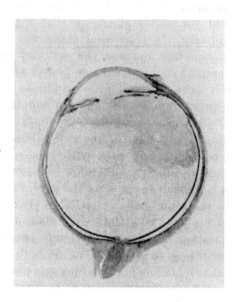

Fig. 1. Normal eye. ×2.

If we study the "other" eyes of the cases of unilateral hydrophthalmia we find an undue preponderance of myopia. This suggests that such eyes were mildly glaucomatous. Some of the cases classed as unilateral by the authors concerned are excluded here, as both eyes showed some slight evidence of distension or of hypertension. Certain ones may have been merely large normal eyes, but they have been included in the section dealing with mild or spontaneously arrested hydrophthalmia. See under Prognosis.

In the series of Fleischer (1918), Stölting (1908), Dettmering (1932),

Seefelder (1906) and the questionnaire there are twenty-nine unilateral cases. Amongst the "unaffected" eyes of these there are:

2 myopic eyes: Fleischer 4 L. (Cornea 11·5 mm.: −15·0 D.S.),

Stölting 4 R. (Cornea 11·0 mm.:

−6·0 D.S.), also reported by Dettmering 15 R.

Dettmering's case 1 L. may belong to this group. (Cornea 11·0 mm., showing faint grey opacities. Anterior chamber and optic disc normal. Vision when aged 20 years = 0·2 − 0·3 and −14 D.S.)

22 normal eyes.

4 not described.

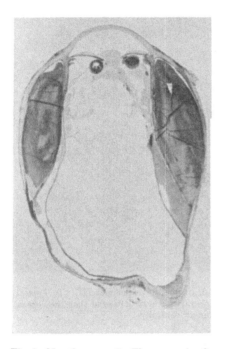

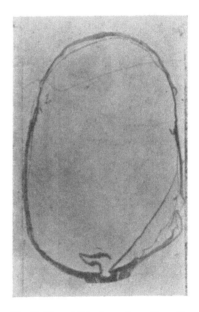

Fig. 2. Myopic eye. ×2. The cornea is of normal thickness, but the posterior half of the sclera abnormally thin. Aphakia and choroidal haemorrhage are evident.

Fig. 3. Unpublished specimen I. ×2. The staphylomatous condition was probably secondary and due to a perforating ulcer during measles.

In addition there were eight that were possibly examples of large normal eyes. (Fleischer 2 R., 3 R., 5 L., Seefelder 19 R., questionnaire 22 L., 25 L., Zeeman (1918) 7 R., 17 L.) There is a sufficiently great incidence of myopia to suggest that hypertension had been influential in producing the bulbar distension and the altered refraction. Both the mother and the brother of Seefelder's case 35 were highly myopic.

Tears in Descemet's Membrane in Myopia

Faber (1905) was the first to describe these tears in myopia. In 1906 instances were reported by Fleischer, Stephenson, Bickerton and Casey Wood. Coats (1907) wrote that such tears were very rarely found, and when present he suspected a glaucomatous element,

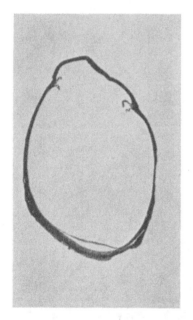

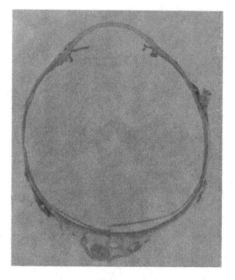

Fig. 4. Unpublished specimen II. × 2. The youngest recorded specimen with neurofibromatosis.

Fig. 5. Unpublished specimen III. × 2. Typical peripheral synechia. Observe that the cornea is thinner centrally.

instead of uncomplicated myopia. A consideration of these tears in congenital glaucoma will be found in a later chapter. The state of the refraction in hydrophthalmic eyes is discussed in Chapter IV, Part I.

Coats (1907) reported four myopic eyes with tears in Descemet's membrane. One of these (case 14) was undoubtedly hydrophthalmic. He stated that the occlusion of the angle was distinctly of "the buphthalmic type". The general form of the angle was obtuse but a triangular spur of iris ran forward on to the back of the cornea causing occlusion. The spaces of Fontana were practically non-

existent and the whole region was much condensed, the canal of
Schlemm being only doubtfully traceable. True glaucomatous cupping
was present. In Faber's second case and in Stephenson's case an
unusually high degree of astigmatism, in Fleischer's second case very
deep anterior chambers and in the case of Bickerton and Stephenson
the somewhat enlarged corneae suggested some other factor in addition
to myopia.

It is uncertain whether the myopia found in hereditary glaucoma
is entirely secondary to it, or whether the relationship is a correlated
inheritance similar to that between myopia and other anomalies

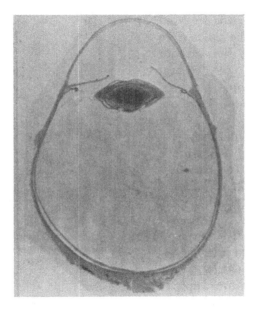

Fig. 6. Unpublished specimen IV. × 2. Typical example with wide open angle. The cornea
   is thinnest peripherally. Though the posterior part of the globe is equal in size to that
   of Specimen III the cornea is much more distended.

which cannot be classed as exciting causes, *e.g.* hemeralopia and
medullated nerve bundles. Löhlein, Plocher, Fleischer, and others,
believe that the myopia in juvenile glaucoma results from the glaucomatous condition.

(High-grade myopia appears to be transmitted as a recessive.
Jablonski found $16.5 \pm 3.4\%$ high myopes among the children of
non-myopic parents which does not disagree with the theoretical
expectation of 25 %. As might be expected the children of two

parents with high-grade myopia are affected. Since myopia is a very common disease consanguinity can play only a subordinate part, though Stilling stressed its significance in high-grade myopia.)

One cannot agree with the view put forward by Stilling, that high myopia is of the same nature as hydrophthalmia. There is marked contrast between the characteristic forms of distension that occur and the sequelae of the two conditions. In hydrophthalmia, the stretching is most marked in the anterior part of the globe, and leads to rapid destruction of the tissue close to the angle of the anterior chamber and to corneal changes. In myopia, however, the most distended parts are those posterior to the ora serrata, and the most obvious changes are those near the posterior pole. The measurements made by Reis, Seefelder, Ischreyt, and Takaskima are of interest. As an example of the comparative measurements, the following figures are valuable (Seefelder, 1906). The first set of figures apply to

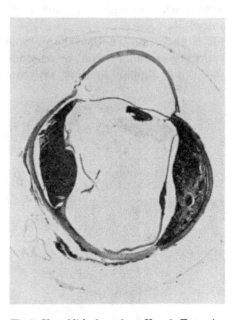

Fig. 7. Unpublished specimen V. × 2. Extensive sub-choroidal haemorrhage. Loaf-shape is due to the failure of the equatorial fibres at the limbus to distend.

a myopic eye, those in brackets to a hydrophthalmic eye of approximately the same size:

Sagittal diameter—cornea to staphyloma, 35·0 ⎫
Sagittal diameter—cornea to optic disc, 32·0 ⎬ (36·0) mm.
Horizontal diameter, 27·5 (29·0) mm.
Vertical diameter, 26·0 (27·5) mm.
Vertical corneal diameter, 10·5 (14·0) mm.
Horizontal corneal diameter, 11·5 (15·5) mm.

Distance from the limbus to the tendon:

    (a) of the external rectus muscle, 8·0 (12·5) mm.
    (b) of the internal rectus muscle, 6·0 (10·0) mm.

Distance of the inferior oblique muscle from the optic nerve, 15·5 (9·5) mm.

Distance of the superior oblique muscle from the optic nerve, 18·5 (11·0) mm.

Width of line of insertion:

Of the external rectus muscle, 9·5 (13·0) mm.

Of the superior oblique muscle, 10·0 (15·5) mm.

Thiele summarised the main characteristics of these types of distension as follows:

HYDROPHTHALMIA	HIGH MYOPIA
1. Diameter of cornea. Increased.	Unchanged.
2. Radius of corneal curvature. Increased.	Within normal limits. The exceptions noted by Fleischer are probably abortive hydrophthalmia.
3. Tears in Descemet's membrane and corneal opacities.	Very rare.
4. Widening and extension of the limbus.	Formation of posterior staphyloma and degeneration near macula and round optic disc.
5. Distance between limbus and muscle insertions greatly increased.	Distance between posterior pole and muscle insertions greatly increased.
6. Stretching and thinning of anterior sclera.	Stretching and thinning of posterior sclera.
7. Raised intra-ocular tension or signs of past hypertension.	Normal tension.

Raised tension in myopic eyes is not as uncommon a finding as was once supposed. Fuchs wrote that strongly myopic eyes are to be regarded as having almost complete immunity against glaucoma. Glaucoma is possibly more difficult to recognise in high myopia, and cupping of the disc may not appear as early as in hypermetropia. 30 % of Gilbert's patients (1912) with the senile form of simple glaucoma at the Munich clinic were myopes. Only 23 % of those with congestive glaucoma were emmetropes. Lange (1912) found that 43·3 % of his patients with simple glaucoma were myopic. Löhlein (1912–13) found only 15 % of his patients with senile glaucoma to be myopic. In these estimates the varying relative frequency of myopia in different countries must be considered. The figures would probably be lower in English-speaking countries.

It is of interest to note, however, that myopia is found even more frequently in juvenile glaucoma. It was present in 31 % of Haag's cases. Löhlein (1913) and Keerl (1920) considered that 50 % of patients with juvenile glaucoma were myopic.

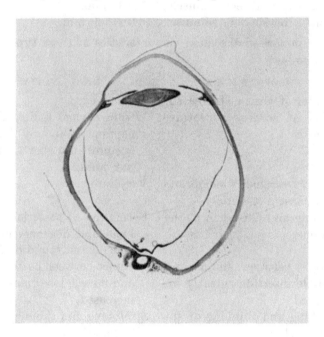

Fig. 8. Unpublished specimen VI. × 2. Very distended eyeball removed at age of ten years.

Anterior staphyloma. An anterior staphyloma is a protuberant corneal cicatrix, in which the prolapsed iris is incorporated. Corneal perforation, usually from ulceration, sometimes from an injury, is an essential feature, and may take place before birth. It is primarily the ectatic nature of the resulting scar that gives the bulging appearance of the cornea and not as in hydrophthalmia the enlargement of a normal cornea under raised intra-ocular pressure. Hypertension may, however, develop in a case of staphyloma as a result of the irido-corneal adhesions.

Partial staphylomata are usually conical. The so-called total staphylomata, which are usually hemispherical, always show a peripheral zone of more or less normal corneal tissue. The protuberant scar is derived mainly from iris tissue and so differs from the condition known as keratectasia in which the protrusion is purely of corneal tissue.

The absence of perforation makes us class as hydrophthalmic certain cases of ocular enlargement which at first sight resemble staphylomata in that there is a central union of iris and cornea. Here the enlargement is due simply to hypertension, though the cornea is probably weaker than normal, and so may be more readily distended. In other cases hypertension acting on a defective cornea may ultimately cause perforation (see Juler's case). It may be impossible to distinguish clinically between such a case and one where a corneal ulcer has led to pre-natal perforation with iris prolapse, producing a staphyloma and the almost inevitable secondary hypertension and further enlargement (Fig. 3). Cases of congenital staphyloma are rare, and since their origin is obscure and they almost always show evidence of hypertension we will include them later in the discussion of the pathology of congenital glaucoma. Strictly, we may describe as hydrophthalmic only those cases where raised intraocular pressure due to a congenital lesion has caused some degree of distension.

Keratectasia. Protrusion of the cornea, without previous perforation or an adherent iris, is known as keratectasia. As a rule this condition is due to failure of the cornea that is weakened by inflammation or ulceration, to withstand normal intra-ocular pressure. After interstitial keratitis the whole cornea may protrude, and if the protrusion is excessive Descemet's membrane may rupture as in hydrophthalmia and, indeed, the conditions may so nearly resemble hydrophthalmia that an accurate diagnosis is difficult (Parsons, 1931).

Keratoconus. This is a form of keratectasia in which the centre of the cornea bulges and becomes conical. Though tears in Descemet's membrane are frequently found, this condition is not likely to be confused with hydrophthalmia. An obvious structural difference exists. In congenital glaucoma the cornea and neighbouring sclera are greatly enlarged and the cornea flattened, while in keratoconus only the central part of the cornea is affected, and it becomes thin and prominent and as a rule surrounded by a pigmented ring.

Congenital glaucoma is nearly always found in the first half of the first decade, and amongst males. Keratoconus develops as a rule in the second decade, and in Australia, at least, the majority of the patients are country girls.

Megalocornea. There are various considerations that make the recognition of megalocornea difficult. If we are to rely on corneal measurements, are we to take into consideration the sizes of the eyeball, of the head, and of the body itself? There is no satisfactory way of measuring the eyeball during life. Radiography of the orbit and of the eyeball by one of the bone-free methods may help in this respect. Without some such means it is impossible during life to decide whether a cornea of known size is relatively too large or too small for its eyeball. Probably it is the relationship of the two that is the important factor.

If we rely simply on appearance, errors in diagnosis may arise from the position of the eyeball in the orbit, the relationship of the palpebral aperture, and certain other factors. Just as with congenital cataract, so in families affected with megalocornea, the parents and neighbours often diagnose the condition from the appearance. In Kayser's family the affected children were said to have "Calwer augen", Calw being the district in Württemberg in which the family lived.

It is wisest, therefore, for us at present to rely simply on corneal measurements. In endeavours to establish the normal size, Priestley Smith and Peters each made measurements of approximately 1000 eyes. In the latter series we find an average value of $11 \cdot 67 \pm 0 \cdot 01$ mm.; thirty eyeballs measured $12 \cdot 50$ mm. and five measured $12 \cdot 75$ mm. 49 % of the corneae measured either $11 \cdot 50$ or $11 \cdot 75$ mm. It may be considered that any cornea measuring $13 \cdot 0$ mm. or more is almost certainly anomalous. If it can be ascertained that corneae measuring $12 \cdot 0$ to $12 \cdot 75$ mm. are large relatively to the size of the eyeball, they may be regarded as megalocorneae.

An extensive investigation was carried out by Friede (1933) recently. During the period 1921–32 he made measurements of 10,940 eyes and amongst his conclusions were the following: (1) that the range of variation in the horizontal diameter is $13 \cdot 5$ to $7 \cdot 0$ mm., (2) that if we include the largest and the smallest corneal diameters measured by other observers then the range of variation is from $18 \cdot 0$ to $5 \cdot 0$ mm., *i.e.* $13 \cdot 0$ mm. altogether, (3) that the distribution is such that a corneal diameter of $11 \cdot 6$ mm. is the most frequent, and (4) that the frequency of large and small corneae, in which the two sides often differ, decreases steadily towards the ends of the range of variation. The vertical diameter of the normal cornea is $11 \cdot 0$ mm. Friede described as transition forms of microcornea those with a horizontal diameter of 11·0 mm. and a vertical diameter of 10·7 to 10·5 mm.

Friede considered his results justified the following classification:

1. Normal corneae   11·0 to 12·0 mm. horizontal diameter.
2. Microcorneae   5·0 to 11·0 mm. horizontal diameter.
3. Physiologically large 12·1 to 13·0 or 13·5 mm. horizontal diameter.
   or Macrocorneae
4. Megalocorneae   11·0 to 18·0 mm. horizontal diameter.

Groups 2 and 3 are essentially distinguishable, but the transition forms are difficult to recognise. Macrocornea is a large cornea (12·1 to 13·5 mm.) associated with an apparently equal enlargement of all other parts of the eye. "Megalocornea is a surface variation of the cornea and sclera in the sense that the surface of the cornea is enlarged and that of the sclera reduced." There may thus be very large and also very small megalocorneae with a diameter of less than 13·0 mm.

For a long time megalocornea was held to be "hydrophthalmus sanatus". Axenfeld, for example (1905, 1911), described cases as such even in the complete absence of signs of hypertension. This view became untenable when in 1913 Kayser's pedigree with seventeen cases of megalocornea appeared. Confirmation was provided in 1921 by Grönholm's pedigree with thirteen cases. In 1932 Kayser summarised the appearance of the eyes in these two pedigrees as follows: "None of the sixty eyes has any sign of arrested hydrophthalmia, and similarly there is none among the other members of the family. That a disease could appear in one family thirty-four times and in another thirty-six times in abortive forms with most minimal characteristics, and not once in a definite form, is unthinkable."

Grönholm (1921) wrote: "the big gleaming beautiful eyes dominate the face and lend it a remarkable appearance." Kayser added that the eyes have a peculiar lustre which is not seen in hydrophthalmic eyes. This is due to the spherical condition of the cornea which when studied from the front or from the side produces a characteristic picture (see Fig. 9). Horner's original title "megalocornea globosa" appears suitable when one considers only the appearance of these eyes. In Kayser's articles (1932, 1936) there are illustrations of a typical megalocornea (Fig. 10). For the sake of contrast he described a case of "hydrophthalmus sanatus". The patient had been under observation for twenty years and during the period of observation the disease had been at a standstill with good vision and with regular and not inverse astigmatism. The radius of the cornea was approximately the same but the anterior chamber was shallower and deep cupping and tears in Descemet's membrane were present.

Even though one of the characteristics of hydrophthalmia certainly is a tendency to remain quiet for a time and then flare up, it is highly improbable that the hydrophthalmic process could lead to the great increase in the corneal diameter that is found at times, viz. 16–18 mm., and then disappear so completely that none of the signs of hydrophthalmia persisted. One would expect the corneo-scleral angle to be enlarged but in megalocornea this is normal and one would not expect

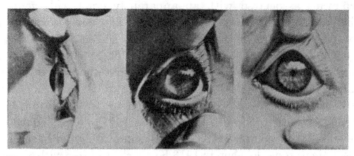

Fig. 9. Megalocornea (left and centre) to show typical lustrous appearance. Compare with hydrophthalmus sanatus (right). (Kayser, 1932.)

characteristic corneal tears to vanish. Zahn reported an exacerbation of hydrophthalmia at the age of forty-eight. Reference to periodic rises in tension will be made later.

Before proceeding further, it will be wise to consider the points in which congenital glaucoma and megalocornea differ. Since the papers by Kayser (1914), Seefelder (1916) and Kestenbaum (1919), there can be no doubt that we are considering two separate conditions, though intermediate states are found which cause confusion.

Seefelder prepared a paper, describing megalocornea as an entity, for the suddenly cancelled conference to be held in St Petersburg in 1914. He preferred the title "Gigantophthalmos". von Muralt in his Inaugural Dissertation (Zürich) in 1869 stated that "cornea globosa semper lucida" was different from hydrophthalmia. Twenty years later Horner (1889), that great Swiss pioneer of ophthalmology, described two distinct forms, keratoglobus pellucidus or pure megalocornea and keratoglobus turbidus. He and Michel considered that a familial tendency, an enlarged clear cornea without loss of function and a tendency to cataract in later life, were the characteristics of the former condition. Little notice was taken of these views, and during the next thirty years a very confused state existed in which the two conditions remained undifferentiated. Axenfeld, Fuchs, von Hippel, Römer, Reis, Warlomont, Epinatjew and others, were inclined to think that the two conditions were different manifestations of one disease. In 1913, Treacher Collins reported "a case of buphthalmos, with full vision and without any cupping of the optic disc". In 1920, he wrote that the stretching of the corneae in this case could not be attributed to hypertension, and he entitled the condition "megalocornea". In Fuchs's *Textbook of Ophthalmology*, 1923, we read: "It is impossible, however, to draw any sharp dividing line between the two forms." Even as late as 1924, de Schweinitz considered megalocornea, hydrophthalmia, keratoglobus and buphthalmia as synonymous.

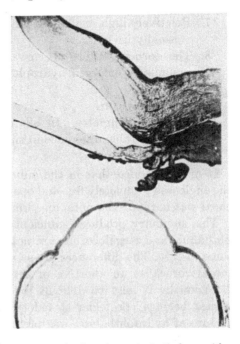

Fig. 10. Angle and anterior half of eye with megalocornea. (Kayser, 1936.)

Doggart (1930) considered that there was probably no hard and fast line between the two conditions. In 1931, Parsons mentioned no differentiation between megalophthalmia and buphthalmia. Vail (1931) preferred to use the title "anterior megalophthalmos" for hydrophthalmia. Mathewson (1930) when describing a father and two sons with this condition used the term "megalocornea".

Seefelder (1916) gave ten reasons why he did not consider megalocornea to be the result of raised tension:

1. The absence of corneal opacities and particularly of tears in Descemet's membrane.
2. Though the anterior portion of the eye is enlarged, the limbus is not widened.

3. The corneo-sclerotic groove is normally defined.
4. The normal appearance of the sclera even in the region of the anterior chamber, where it would appear much more stretched.
5. The absence of any excavation of the optic disc.
6. The absence of functional disturbance.
7. Relatively high regular astigmatism. In hydrophthalmia it is usually irregular.
8. The corneal radius of curvature is less than normal. In similarly enlarged hydrophthalmic eyes it is usually much greater.
9. Normal tension.
10. Bilateral symmetry. In bilateral hydrophthalmia, usually a considerable difference in size is found.

It may be added that in the only histological examination made the angle was completely free and open, and the entrance to Schlemm's canal was normal. The optic disc was quite uncupped.

This summary produces sufficient evidence to prove that hydrophthalmia and megalocornea are not different manifestations of the same disease. The differences are so marked that we cannot consider megalocornea as an abortive or arrested form of hydrophthalmia. Occasionally it may be difficult to decide to which class a certain cornea belongs. Seefelder stated that in one patient the complete picture of hydrophthalmia was present in one eye, and in the other only such changes as would undoubtedly have led him to make a diagnosis of megalocornea if "the whole state of affairs had not shown that it was abortive hydrophthalmos".

Megalocornea is a matter of a completely healthy eye in a healthy person, whereas hydrophthalmia is a defective and a diseased organ which very often appears in weakly nervous children, who at the same time show other constitutional weakness.

Thiele writes: "Undoubtedly many eyes with an enlarged cornea were formerly described as megalophthalmic on account of the absence of typical glaucoma symptoms. With modern methods of investigation it is possible in most cases to discover those fine tears in Descemet's membrane, which show the effect of an expansion from within, that can be brought about only by raised tension." Further aid in differentiation is available from a careful study of the patient's pedigree. Stähli (1914), when reporting four cases of undoubted

megalocornea, gave certain additional reasons for his belief in this
condition as an entity: first, that hyperplasia of other organs, *e.g.*,
macrodactylia occurs; second, that in large pedigrees of megalocornea
no instances of hydrophthalmia occur; third, that numerous stages
between megalocornea and normal sized corneae occur which cannot
all be glaucomatous in origin; and fourth, that the mere finding of
an enlarged cornea is insufficient reason to justify a belief in raised
intra-ocular pressure as a cause.

Schieck (1931) considered that a small number of cases of megalocornea represent abortive hydrophthalmia. Most of the evidence, however, is of little value, for it consists of the absence of certain signs of
hydrophthalmia, such as reduction of the corneo-scleral angle and
splits in Descemet's membrane in cases of undoubted hypertension,
and the presence of fine band-like corneal opacities in an apparently
typical megalocornea (Axenfeld). In some instances in the literature,
insufficient data are supplied to permit definite diagnoses, *e.g.* Zorab's
patient with hydrophthalmia in one eye and megalocornea in the
other (1920). Killick (1913) reported a patient in whom one eye was
blind from progressive congenital glaucoma. The other eye had a
normal disc and normal vision, and yet the diagnosis of stationary
congenital glaucoma was made.

Law (1931) reported under the title of "Megalophthalmos" a globe
that was almost certainly hydrophthalmic. Many vertical ruptures
of Descemet's membrane were present as well as a scar on the right
temple which was attributed to birth injury.

Failure to separate these two conditions has produced some of the
conflicting statements regarding the outlook in hydrophthalmia and
its tendency to spontaneous cures. For example, Fischer (1896)
reported a patient with so-called "stationary buphthalmos" which
in the absence of tension and cupping we must consider to be megalocornea; particularly as after the extraction of the patient's cataracts
at the age of fifty-three, the vision was 6/5 and the fields only slightly
contracted.

In megalocornea there is no sign of progression; the visual loss
so common in later life is due as a rule to lenticular opacities.
The condition has been found without signs of hypertension in a
patient as old as eighty-five years of age. One characteristic of hydrophthalmia is the progressive nature of the degenerative changes
present.

Kestenbaum (1919) wrote that megalocornea was different from hydrophthalmia clinically, in its prognosis, and in its pathogenesis. The distinguishing features were:

(a) Unimpaired function.

(b) Clarity of cornea, and in particular absence of tears in Descemet's membrane.

(c) Absence of hypertension and glaucoma cupping.

He summarised other points of differentiation as follows:

MEGALOCORNEA	"BUPHTHALMOS"
1. Vast majority males.	5 males to 3 females.
2. Almost always bilateral.	35 % unilateral.
3. Enlargement almost always symmetrical.	Usually unsymmetrical.
4. Almost always hereditary.	Rarely so.
5. Normal corneal convexity.	Decreased.
(42·0 to 45·2 dioptres, Kayser.	37 dioptres.
40·0 to 44·5 dioptres, Stähli.)	
6. Embryotoxon very frequent.	Not observed.
7. No ill-effects during puberty. (Reis.)	Usually present.

The clinical characteristics of megalocornea may be considered under the following headings:

1. Cornea. The main characteristic and the most striking feature of this condition is the enlarged but otherwise healthy cornea. Its diameter may vary from 12·5 to 18·0 mm., the average measurement being 14·8 mm. Corneal opacities unless due to injury or secondary ulceration are absent. No tears in Descemet's membrane are present. Kayser found the centre of the cornea reduced in thickness but the periphery thicker than normal. Melanosis corneae or Krukenberg's spindle may be present. Kayser described the development of a spindle in the left eye of his third case at the age of twenty-three years. Two years later a similar change occurred in the right eye. It is important to note that this lesion is, therefore, not necessarily congenital in origin as has been suggested. The pigment varied in amount and disposition from time to time and was evidently not as fixed in the endothelial cells as Hanssen's (1923) anatomical examination suggested. His was the only histological report till Kayser in 1936 examined one eye from the patient referred to. He found no pigment on the cornea or the central area of the iris. This was attributed to the patient having spent the last few weeks of his life on his back. Profuse pigment was present in the angle and on the periphery of the iris.

An arcus senilis or its equivalent juvenile form has been frequently described. Vail (1931) found twenty-four instances in his collection of sixty-nine cases. Kayser (1932) pointed out that no case of embryotoxon in a new-born patient had been reported. The youngest instance was in a child of his, aged ten years. Nerve fibres have been described as being unusually distinct in megalocornea.

The corneal radius of curvature may be less than normal. In similarly enlarged hydrophthalmic eyes it is usually much greater—radius of anterior curvature of cornea: lowest 7·0 mm., highest 8·5 mm., average 7·5 mm. (31 observations). Normal, average 7·5 mm.

Kayser (1932) held that in megalocornea the radius remained normal or only slightly less than normal in a very remarkably constant fashion.

2. Refraction. A relatively high degree of regular astigmatism is commonly found. Vail summarised the refractive errors as follows:

Emmetropia, 17 cases. Hypermetropia and hypermetropic astigmatism, 29. Myopia and myopic astigmatism, 44. Mixed astigmatism, 2. Total, 92. Of these, astigmatism was with the rule in 24 cases, and against it in 7.

3. Corneo-scleral junction. Though the anterior portion of the eye is enlarged the limbus is not widened as it is in hydrophthalmia. The corneo-scleral groove is normally defined.

4. The sclera appears normal, even near the limbus, where it appears so stretched in hydrophthalmia.

5. The anterior chamber is usually deep. The absence of this striking feature in large physiological globes (cornea up to 14·0 mm. and more) aids in the differentiation from megalocornea. It is deep in advanced cases of hydrophthalmia.

6. The iris is stretched and its stroma appears atrophic and, as a result of weakening of the dilatator muscle, miosis is usually present. In Kayser's specimen the ciliary body and the iris root were displaced posteriorly but the scleral spur was of average length. The iris showed no definite changes, but in the angle there was a great deal of amorphous pigment which had drifted into it and had been taken up by the cells. The retinal pigment evidently tends to disintegrate as in stretched myopic eyes. Kayser considered that this form of pigment proliferation was not common in megalocornea.

Iridodonesis is usually present.

Vail (1931), when discussing the changes in the iris, stated that the atrophy begins in the periphery and appears to spread centrally, affecting the dilatator and not the sphincter muscle. One result of this is miosis and another the production of the "target" reflex, in which the circular bands represent the pupil, the sphincter, atrophic iris, the angle, the ciliary body, and the ora serrata. Some authors consider this to be a pathognomonic sign.

As the scleral aperture is enlarged up to 18 mm. it is not surprising that changes in the iris are found, for this structure spreads across the aperture. The iridodonesis, and the scattering of the iris pigment that leads to the appearance of Krukenberg's spindle, are probably due to this stretching.

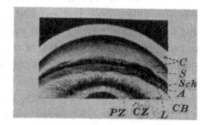

Fig. 11. Gonioscope view of angle in a case of megalocornea. *PZ*, pupillary zone of iris. *CZ*, ciliary zone of iris. *L*, last roll of the iris. *CB*, ciliary body band. *A*, black line sharply dividing the ciliary body from *Sch*, Schlemm's zone. *S*, scleral band. *C*, cornea. (Troncoso and Givner, 1936.)

Gonioscopy and transillumination have revealed a tendency for the iris to show most signs of atrophy from stretching in the ciliary zone. In this area the iris may be reduced to radial fibres showing black against a red background on transillumination. Gonioscopy has revealed a black line between the band representing Schlemm's canal and the ciliary body band. Schlemm's band may be covered with pigment and numerous granules may be found in the meshes of the trabeculae (Troncoso). (Figs. 11, 12, 13.)

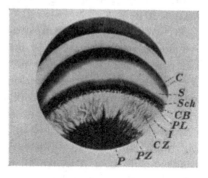

Fig. 12. Gonioscopic view of the angle of a normal eye showing iris processes (*PL*) appearing at the edge of the iris. They are rarely so numerous. (Troncoso and Givner, 1936.)

7. The **lens** may be partially dislocated as a result of the stretching of the zonule. It may become cataractous and the results of extraction have been well summarised by Vail. Remains of pupillary membrane are not uncommonly found on the lens capsule.

8. Other ocular tissues are normal. That the optic disc should be so is of particular interest.

9. The complete absence of signs of glaucoma. This state is discussed later.

10. Ocular tension. Hypotension is frequently found, *e.g.* the tension was under 10·0 mm. of Hg in five of Vail's series; Peters refers to 14·0 mm., 19·0 mm. and a third patient with hypotension; Kayser found three in a series of nine with low tension, and in Troncoso and Givner's patient it was 8·0 mm. (Schiötz). With the stretching and overgrowth near the angle one would expect to find larger channels for the escape of fluid, and as Troncoso and others have suggested atrophy of the ciliary processes might lessen the formation of aqueous.

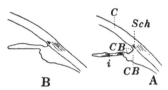

Fig. 13. A. Schematic section of the angle in megalocornea. *i*, iris; *CB*, ciliary body; *Sch*, Schlemm's canal; *C*, cornea. B. Section of normal angle for comparison. (Troncoso and Givner, 1936.)

When hypertension is found with megalocornea it occurs late in life (see case 10 of Kayser's pedigree). It may be associated either with obstruction at Schlemm's canal by pigment, or sclerosis of the meshwork or with subluxation of the lens.

11. Vision. There is a minimum of interference with function unless secondary degenerative changes, *e.g.* cataract, occur.

The other characteristics of megalocornea will be grouped as follows:

INCIDENCE

1. Bilateral occurrence. Megalocornea is bilateral and almost always symmetrical.

2. Age. The youngest patient described so far was aged three years and the oldest eighty-five years. Vail found forty-three over twenty years. It seems probable, however, that the condition is always recognisable at birth, as in the "Calwer augen" reported by Kayser. It may be because there is no pain or loss of function as in hydrophthalmia that megalocornea in young infants has not been brought to the notice of doctors.

3. Sex. It occurs almost exclusively amongst males, possibly 8 % are females. The proportion is in keeping with that in colour-blindness and other conditions generally described as sex-linked. Of six affected females all had an affected parent, and two had an affected father and a mother of affected stock (Bell, 1932).

INHERITANCE

Approximately eighty patients with megalocornea have been described in the literature, and three-quarters of these are in pedigrees (Kayser). The inheritance is manifested as a recessive sex-linked character which is transmitted through unaffected females to males.

This is seen typically in Kayser's pedigree (1919). In it sixteen members of five generations were affected, and with one exception the transmission was through unaffected females.

Kayser held that in the rare instances of direct inheritance of hydrophthalmia the sexes appear to be equally affected. It is not of the gynophore type in which men are affected by female carriers as in the case of megalocornea.

Women can only be expected to show an anomaly of sex-linked heredity if a conductor marries an affected person. This is most apt to occur when relations marry. It was found twice in Grönholm's pedigree (1921), in which eleven males and two females of three generations were affected.

Megalocornea may also be transmitted as a dominant. In Gredig's pedigree (1926) eleven males and two or three females in four generations were affected. The transmission was by four or perhaps five affected males, and by only one female. Dominance is also suggested by two pedigrees reported by Friede (1923). In these, megalocornea appeared in two and three generations respectively. In both pedigrees the anomaly was transmitted by affected females.

Koby and others have commented on the dominant sex-linked inheritance of Krukenberg's spindle and its occurrence with megalocornea. Franceschetti observed both conditions in two brothers. Stähli found both in an uncle and his nephew.

It cannot yet be determined whether these cases are not simply, as Stähli suggested, variation phenomena falling quite outside the normal distribution (13·0 mm.) (Franceschetti, 1930). If the offspring of parents with large corneae are investigated, a relatively large number of people with large corneae will be found, so that a regression to the parents occurs. Only a small proportion of the offspring will tend again towards the median of the population. It was formerly held that this—Galton's regression—was always in the same numerical proportion to the average size of the population, that is, one-third. Mendel's experiments in crossing, however, show that this is not so. Johannsen also has shown that there is no regression in pure lines.

Regression is therefore a sign that the population investigated differs genotypically. If then in the inheritance of the size of the cornea a regression to the parent size occurs, it means that both large and small corneae are inheritable. Such large corneae have been called macrocorneae. From the small amount of material available, it cannot be determined whether a line can be drawn between this form of dominant macrocornea and the sex-linked megalocornea (Franceschetti).

The pedigrees of Kayser and Grönholm undoubtedly suggest that megalocornea is an anomaly, and that cases do not merely belong to the extreme end of the normal range of corneal measurements. It seems likely that we have here a foetal type of eye in which the cornea has retained its large size relative to the eyeball. Though Stähli considered that megalocornea might be a simple variation phenomenon without associated anomalies, yet Franceschetti and others found the latter to be numerous, e.g. ectopia pupillae, dislocated lens, iridodonesis, persistent pupillary membrane, Krukenberg's spindle and embryotoxon.

Theories of origin

This is not the place to consider fully the theories that have been put forward to explain megalocornea. A brief summary of the views, however, is of value.

1. Von Hippel (1900) considered that foetal corneal disease and ulcus corneae internum might produce an enlarged cornea in which complete transparency might return. If part of the course of this infection were postnatal, its nature would possibly be recognised. The final result of this condition, whether intra-uterine or not, would be either megalocornea, or, if secondary glaucoma developed, hydrophthalmia.

2. Schmidt-Rimpler (1908) classed megalocornea, keratoglobus, and cornea globosa as one condition, and if in such cases cupping of the disc was found, he considered the cause to be past and transient hypertension.

3. Seefelder considered that megalocornea or gigantophthalmos—the title he preferred—was a manifestation of gigantism or overgrowth of the entire eyeball. Bondi (1898) expressed the same idea. He stated that in one patient one eye (15·5 mm.) was larger than its almost normal fellow (13·0 mm.). This theory, however, is unlikely, as the radius of corneal curvature remains normal, and lenses when removed intracapsularly and the posterior segment of the globe appear to be

normal. Pathological examination alone can settle this problem. Kayser (1936) has made the only examination of an undoubted case of this kind. It is probable, however, that Best's specimen (1929) with a corneal diameter of 14 mm. and a radius of curvature of 7·0 mm. was an example of megalocornea. At forty-eight years of age the vision was 5/15 in each eye, the discs normal and no tears were found in Descemet's membrane. In the eye that was examined histologically Schlemm's canal was present, and though the ciliary body was very atrophic, no stretching of the anterior portion of the globe was present. The pigment epithelium of the iris and the sphincter were not completely differentiated and the iris, clinically, appeared to be almost devoid of structure.

Seefelder, Stähli, Wright (1926), and Soriano (1919), held that an excessively large cornea generally indicated an abnormal size of the whole eye. Wright found one eyeball in life to be 27·0 by 27·0 mm., and he considered that the nucleus of the lens he extracted was unusually large. Kayser and Friede opposed this view.

Kayser (1920) stated that the normal lens has a cross-section of 8·67 mm. and thickness of 4·3 mm. and that in a megalocornea of 15·0 mm. the dimensions should be 11·2 × 4·5 mm., and in one of 18 mm. they should be 13·4 × 6·6 mm. Such large lenses have not been found by surgeons when extracting cataracts. As Haab's patient, before operation, had 1·5 dioptres of hypermetropia, and afterwards 10·5 D., one believes that the lens was probably normal. Such findings suggest that the influence of the lens or the retina has less effect on the growth of the cornea than some writers think. Kayser found a normal retina and a normal lens in his case and considered that neither could have been an incentive to extra corneal growth.

If megalocornea is a form of ocular gigantism one may ask: does a peculiar form of growth of the lens or its isolation within its capsule separate it from the ties with the other ocular tissue and free it from the factors making for excessive growth?

Kayser disagreed with Stähli who believed that megalocornea was a variation. Kayser considered that it was beyond the range of physiology and unlike the very large physiological cornea. "The cornea sits like a hemisphere on the bulbus and the increased refraction of the margins gives the special lustre of 'big beautiful eyes'." Horner's title "cornea globosa" was very suitable. "A giant who had a cornea of 18 mm. would have to be 2·65 m. tall, whereas the tallest man known was 2·14 m."

It must be remembered that the radius of corneal curvature and the corneal thickness are not increased. In Gertz's cases the radii were 7·9 and 8·5 mm. and the corneal base was 18 mm. As Kayser pointed out, since the diameter of a sphere of 8·4 mm. radius is 16·8 mm., the scleral aperture, which is 18·0 mm., can only be closed if the peripheral part of the cornea flattens while the centre retains the normal curvature. If the corneal enlargement were proportional in the above case, the cornea would have a radius of curvature of 10·0 mm., which would produce an impossible refractive condition. Vail measured the centre of one cornea with the slit-lamp and found it to be of normal thickness. Therefore in megalocornea not even the cornea is enlarged proportionately in all its dimensions.

Seefelder (1933), when supporting the idea that the other tissues in megalocornea are probably not enlarged, stated that the anterior chamber is usually deeper than is necessary to correspond to proportional enlargement. One eye, for example, with a corneal base of 14·5 mm. had an anterior chamber 8·0 mm. deep, whereas a depth of 3·5 mm. would have been proportional.

As Seefelder also pointed out, the surface of the iris and the zonule are increased but their total mass is not. The iris therefore appears thin and atrophic, the pattern is radial and the crypts shrunken. Diascleral illumination may show the radial spaces red up to the scleral root. Vail has stressed the importance of the weakness of the dilatator fibres with a normal sphincter and a consequent miosis.

If the enlargement of the globe were even approximately proportional one could not expect a wide divergence in the refraction of eyes with equal-sized corneae, the same radius of curvature, and a normal lens. The following are three examples chosen by Seefelder:

Seefelder's case: Cornea 14·4 mm., Radius 7·6 mm., Refraction − 3 D.
Stähli's case: ,,   14·5 mm.,   ,,   8·0 mm.,   ,,   + 3 D.
Soriano's case: ,,   15·0 mm.,   ,,   7·6 mm.,   ,,   − 13 D.

Kayser claimed that megalophthalmia could exist only when the corneal curve had a radius of 10·0 mm., and that the lens should be proportionately enlarged. These changes are not found. Iridodonesis is a frequent sign, and its presence suggests a small lens. Numerous lenses have been removed intracapsularly, and were found to be of normal size. Seefelder, Berg and others excluded enlargement of the whole eye by careful refraction after extraction of the lens.

It was uncertain whether the whole eyeball or merely the cornea is enlarged in megalocornea, until the only histological examination recorded was made by Kayser (1933, 1936). His measurements were:

Cornea	14·0 × 14·5 mm.	Normal 11·0 × 11·6 mm.
Depth of A.C.	7·5 mm.	
Vertical diameter of globe	24·0 mm.	
Horizontal diameter of globe	24·5 mm.	
Sagittal diameter of globe	27·0 mm.	
Diameter of lens	9·2 mm.	
Thickness of lens	4·0 mm.	

Therefore the globe was of normal size and the enlarged cornea was an example of isolated gigantism. This lack of proportion probably occurs in the great majority of globes that show a megalocornea. Kayser believed that the eyes in his pedigree and in those of Grönholm, Goertz, and Berg would show a similar state. Such a finding illustrates Waardenberg's contention that many hereditary factors underlie ocular development and that for the transmission of the correlation between corneal refraction and corneal size a combination of five polymer entities are essential. The hereditary absence of the size-restriction factor would explain megalocornea (Waardenburg, 1933).

Troncoso and Givner (1936) reported that by gonioscopy of an eye with typical megalocornea they found considerable stretching of the iris and the ciliary body. This, however, was not in keeping with the theory of over-development of the whole globe, for the size and relations of the structures of the angle were not proportional to the enlargement of the cornea. These observers estimated the horizontal and the vertical meridians to be 25·0 mm. (normal 24·13 and 23·48 mm.), but 13 dioptres of myopia were present.

Stähli postulated an hereditary hyperplasia of the cornea, followed by pigmented corneal changes, iris atrophy, and luxation of the lens.

4. Reis (1920) and Friede suggested that megalocornea was atavistic in origin. A theory probably suggested by the well-known facts that the anterior segments of the eyes of infants and lower animals are relatively larger than in the mature state of the human eyeball. Such a theory assumes that megalophthalmia is not present, but simple megalocornea. Treacher Collins (1921) has written: "The cornea in man's eye is smaller relatively to the size of the globe than in any other mammal. In all mammals below man the diameter of the cornea

measures more than half the antero-posterior diameter of the globe; in the chimpanzee it is about half; in man alone it is considerably less than half." Or again: "From the sixth month of foetal life, when the anterior chamber is first formed, to the end of the second year, the growth of the cornea is rapid; during that time it doubles its size; at the sixth month of foetal life the diameter is 5·5 to 6·0 mm.... During the whole of foetal life, and at birth, the diameters of the cornea measure more than half those of the eyeball, whilst in the fully developed eye they are less than half."

5. Usher (1920), in an interesting paper, suggested that environmental conditions play an important part in the production of enlarged corneae in goldfish. Five fish with bulging corneae were reported, which, on examination, showed eyes that were normal except for the great size of the corneae and the depth of the anterior chamber. They differed from the "popeye goldfish", in which the whole eyeball is enlarged, and from other forms of fish which show exophthalmos. The goldfish in question lived under conditions that favoured the production of thyroid hyperplasias, but no explanation was given for the limitation of the abnormal growth to the cornea.

6. The association of calcium deficiency with over-growth of tissues is sufficiently common in general pathology to suggest some influence of such a state in ocular hyperplasias. This view is strengthened by the common occurrence of megalocornea in arachnodactyly, viz. half of twenty-five cases reported. Gnad (1931) found microphakia (5·25 × 6·5 mm.) with megalocornea of 13·5 mm. diameter. However, the serum-calcium was normal and no skeletal changes were present in the case of Troncoso and Givner. The characteristics of calcium deficiency are partial diaphysial gigantism, thin fine fingers and toes, mask-like facies, winged scapulae, coarse straight hair, and ocular signs (Drysdale and Herringham, 1907; Ormond and Williams, 1924; Collins, 1920; Riser, 1936).

There is little need for surprise at finding a simple corneal enlargement, for, in the animal kingdom, a relatively large cornea is the rule to which there are, of course, certain exceptions. If we accept 24·0 mm. as the normal antero-posterior axis of the human eye and alter the sizes of animals' eyes to this dimension we find by calculation that the great majority will possess a corneal diameter greater than that of a man. Of sixty-three eyes, with corneae varying from 4·5 to 33·0 mm. in diameter, Friede (1933) found that 92 % had a cornea wider than that of man (11·56 mm.). He found no evidence that as a result there was an associated megalophthalmia. The following criteria were used:

(*a*) The size of the eyeball. The domestic cat for example has a cornea that is greater than that of man, viz. 17.0×16.0 mm., and yet its globe is only $20.6 \times 20.5 \times 20.2$ mm.

(*b*) The thickness of the cornea.

	CORNEAL DIAMETER (ARC)	CORNEAL THICKNESS	
		CENTRAL	PERIPH.
Man	11·5 mm.	0·9 mm.	1·3 mm.
Tarsius	19·0 mm.	0·3 mm.	0·35 mm.
Domestic cat	17·0 mm.	0·9 mm.	0·5 mm.
Hyena	19·0 mm.	0·4 mm.	0·9 mm.

(*c*) The depth of the anterior chamber.

	CORNEAL DIAMETER (ARC)	ANTERIOR CHAMBER
Man	11·5 × 11·2 mm.	3·5 mm.
Tarsius	19·0 × 19·0 mm.	5·1 mm.
Racoon (prowler)	12·9 × 12·0 mm.	5·5 mm.

Night prowlers with large corneae have deep anterior chambers, *e.g.* puma, cornea 20.9×20.9 mm. and anterior chamber 5·4 mm.

Ungulates with large corneae have shallow anterior chambers.

(*d*) The radius of curvature of the cornea. This radius, in megalo-cornea, is not regular like that of a sphere and it is rarely so in the animal kingdom.

(*e*) The size of the lens. Quite commonly the lens is larger and its zonule stronger in the eyes of animals with large corneae, but this is not a constant finding.

(*f*) The size of the optic disc. Though in many animals the disc appears to vary in size with the cornea there is no constant relation-ship, *e.g.*

	CORNEAL DIAMETER	SAGITTAL AXIS	WIDTH OF OPTIC DISC
Man	11·56 mm.	24·0 mm.	3·6 mm.
Gibbon	11·0 mm.	18·4 mm.	2·9 mm.
Seal	25·0 mm.	38·0 mm.	2·1 mm.
Wild bear	18·0 mm.	26·9 mm.	4·4 mm.

Therefore we find as a rule in animals with large corneae that the other parts of the eye are smaller in proportion to the cornea than is the case in man. (Figs. 14 and 15.)

Megalophthalmia

It is doubtful whether in addition there is a condition that should be described as macrophthalmia or megalophthalmia.

If it exists it is much rarer. Kayser, Seefelder and others consider that its existence is unlikely. Berg discussed this condition. In it the various tissues which are enlarged appear to maintain their normal proportions, as they do in Friede's group 3—macrocorneae.

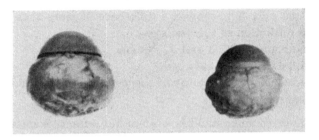

Fig. 14. Eyes of adult and young Tarsius. Side view to show size of cornea. Life size.

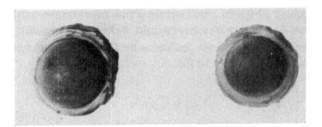

Fig. 15. Front view of eyes of Tarsius to show circular shape of cornea. Life size.

Hartlieb (1931) drew attention to a patient who, though a female, appeared to have unilateral megalocornea, or as he suspected, gigantophthalmia. The diameter of the left cornea was 14·0 mm., right cornea 11·5; the radius of curvature in the horizontal meridian was 8·1, right cornea was 7·9. The corneal refraction was 41·7 D., 42·7 D. on the right. The left iris appeared to be a little broader than the right. The cornea, lens and vitreous were free from opacities and no cupping of the disc was found. The tension was 17 mm. Hg on both sides. The left eye was emmetropic and the right eye had 1·25 dioptres of myopia. The visual fields were normal. The left eye showed 17·0 mm. of exophthalmos and the right 15·0 mm. The patient stated that her father's mother had a similar eye. The following findings suggested enlargement of the globe:

1. The increased curvature of the cornea in addition to its enlarged surface. Waardenburg found that the normal corneal refraction was an inherited characteristic with high-grade stability and very slight range of modification, *i.e.* the corneal refraction was almost without exception the same in both eyes in any one individual. It bore no relation to the total refraction of the eye. Of a hundred cases with anisometropia only 5 % showed a difference of more than 0·5 D. in the corneal refraction of the two eyes.

2. Emmetropia and 5/5 and $J_{0·1}$ vision.

3. Iris appeared to be enlarged.

4. The absence of embryotoxon suggested that the condition was not a typical megalocornea.

It is difficult to understand how a normal refractive state could be maintained with such an increase in corneal area and curvature and an enlarged iris without some enlargement of the posterior ocular tissues. Proportional enlargement would have meant an antero-posterior axis of 29·0 mm., and surely some interference with function or with intra-ocular appearance would have been present. Further light may be thrown on these problems by Roentgenometry as carried out by Katz and Ledoux (1935).

SUMMARY

1. There is seldom room for confusion in the diagnosis of congenital glaucoma.

2. The claim that it is identical with myopia cannot be substantiated. Hypertension may, however, occasionally play a part in the production of myopia in early life. This is suggested by the undue preponderance of myopia in the "unaffected" eye in unilateral hydrophthalmia and the presence of "tears" in Descemet's membrane in myopia.

3. The incidence of glaucoma amongst young myopes is discussed.

4. Anterior staphyloma is a cicatricial bulging of the cornea and the prolapsed iris which follows a corneal perforation, that may be congenital. It may produce secondary hypertension, and may closely resemble a hydrophthalmic condition in which there is a congenital central union of iris and cornea.

5. Keratectasia is a bulging or stretching of the cornea alone, due to a special corneal weakness, it is not necessarily connected with raised intra-ocular pressure.

6. The condition known as megalocornea is discussed at length, and its existence as an entity established. It is hereditary, and is not associated with glaucoma, but is possibly a reversion to a more primitive mammalian condition.

It appears to be established beyond doubt that megalocornea is a simple developmental anomaly affecting the cornea, and that though the iris and ciliary body may be stretched the other ocular tissues are normal.

7. The occurrence of a true megalophthalmia is unproved.

8. *Conclusion.* There are several conditions which bear points of resemblance to hydrophthalmia; though a typical case of hydrophthalmia cannot be mistaken, a very mild case may resemble megalocornea or simple myopia; a severe keratectasia may simulate hydrophthalmia, and an anterior staphyloma may lead to hypertension and is therefore considered together with congenital glaucoma in the study of its pathology. Ocular enlargement, mainly affecting the anterior segment, and hypertension with its sequelae (cupped disc, loss of function) serve to distinguish hydrophthalmia from other conditions. When these characteristics are not sufficiently pronounced to furnish a differential diagnosis, a study of heredity or of the condition of the other eye may help; at any rate the hydrophthalmia if present must fortunately be of so mild a degree that the surgeon need not interfere.

REFERENCES

MYOPIA: DIFFERENTIAL DIAGNOSIS

1888 NETTLESHIP, E. *Roy. Lond. Ophthal. Hosp. Reps.* **12**, 220.

1905 FABER, E. Inaug. Dissert. Tübingen. Quoted by Coats.

1906 SEEFELDER, R. *Arch. f. Ophthal.* **63**, 481.

1907 COATS, G. *Trans. Ophthal. Soc. U.K.* **27**, 48.

1908 STÖLTING. *Arch. f. Ophthal.* **67**, 171.

1909 ISCHREYT, G. *Arch. f. Augenheilk.* **84**, 165.

1912 GILBERT, W. *Ber. d. deutsch. Ophthal. Gesell. Heidelberg*, **38**, 333. Quoted by Elliot.

1912 LANGE, O. *Klin. Monatsbl. f. Augenheilk.* **50**, 540.

1912 LÖHLEIN, W. *Ber. d. deutsch. Ophthal. Gesell. Heidelberg*, **38**, 142. Quoted by Elliot.

1913 LÖHLEIN, W. *Ber. d. deutsch. Ophthal. Gesell. Heidelberg*, **39**, 97. Quoted by Elliot. *Arch. f. Ophthal.* **85**, 393.

1918 ZEEMAN, W. P. C. *Klin. Monatsbl. f. Augenheilk.* **60**, 400.

1918 Fleischer, B. *Klin. Monatsbl. f. Augenheilk.* **61**, 152.
1920 Keerl. Inaug. Dissert. Leipzig. Quoted by Waardenburg, *Bibliographia Genetica*, 7, 336.
1931 Brückner and Franceschetti. *Arch. f. Augenheilk.* **105**, 1.
1932 Dettmering, M. Inaug. Dissert. Göttingen.
1934 Würdemann, H. V. *Trans. Western Ophthal. Soc.* 1st Annual Meeting, p. 67; Abst. *Amer. Jl. Ophthal.* **18**, 1174.
1936 Capetta and Motolese. *Boll. d'Ocul.* **15**.

Megalocornea

1889 Horner, F. *Gerhart's Handbuch der Kinderkrankheiten*, 7.
1896 Fischer, E. C. *Trans. Ophthal. Soc. U.K.* **16**, 350.
1905 Axenfeld, Th. *Klin. Monatsbl. f. Augenheilk.* **43**, 157.
1911 Axenfeld, Th. *Klin. Monatsbl. f. Augenheilk.* **49**, 505.
1913 Killick, C. *Trans. Ophthal. Soc. U.K.* **33**, 194.
1913 Collins, E. T. *Trans. Ophthal. Soc. U.K.* **33**, 193.
1913 Kayser, B. *Klin. Monatsbl. f. Augenheilk.* **51**, 2, 246.
1914 Kayser, B. *Klin. Monatsbl. f. Augenheilk.* **52**, 226.
1914 Stähli, J. *Klin. Monatsbl. f. Augenheilk.* **52**, pt. 2, 83.
1916 Seefelder, R. *Klin. Monatsbl. f. Augenheilk.* **56**, 227.
1919 Kestenbaum, A. *Klin. Monatsbl. f. Augenheilk.* **62**, 734.
1920 Zorab, A. *Trans. Ophthal. Soc. U.K.* **40**, 139.
1921 Grönholm, U. *Klin. Monatsbl. f. Augenheilk.* **67**, 1.
1923 Fuchs, E. *Textbook of Ophthal.* 4th ed. p. 472.
1923 Hanssen, R. *Klin. Monatsbl. f. Augenheilk.* **71**, 399.
1924 de Schweinitz, G. E. *Diseases of the Eye*, 10th ed. Philadelphia: Saunders.
1930 Doggart, J. H. *Brit. Jl. Ophthal.* **14**, 229.
1930 Mathewson, G. H. *Amer. Jl. Ophthal.* **13**, 318.
1931 Gnad, F. *Klin. Monatsbl. f. Augenheilk.* **87**, 33.
1931 Law, F. W. *Proc. Roy. Soc. Med.* Oct.
1931 Parsons, J. H. *Diseases of the Eye.* London: Churchill.
1931 Schieck, F. *Kurzes Handbuch der Ophthal.* **4**, 237.
1931 Vail, D. T. *Arch. of Ophthal.* **6**, 39.
1932 Kayser, B. *Klin. Monatsbl. f. Augenheilk.* **89**, 770.
1933 Friede, R. *Klin. Monatsbl. f. Augenheilk.* **91**, 767; *Arch. f. Ophthal.* **131**, 1.
1936 Kayser, B. *Klin. Monatsbl. f. Augenheilk.* **96**, 721.

Incidence

1932 Bell, J. *The Treasury of Human Inheritance*, **2**, pt. 5, 443.

Inheritance of Megalocornea

1919 Kayser, B. *Klin. Monatsbl. f. Augenheilk.* **62**, 349.
1921 Grönholm, V. *Klin. Monatsbl. f. Augenheilk.* **67**, 1.
1923 Friede, R. *Arch. f. Ophthal.* **3**, 393.
1926 Gredig, C. *Arch. der Julius Klaus Stiftung, Zürich.* Quoted by Franceschetti, *Kurzes Handbuch der Ophthal.* **1**, 730.
1930 Franceschetti, A. *Kurzes Handbuch der Ophthal.* **1**, 727.

THEORIES OF ORIGIN OF MEGALOCORNEA

1898 BONDI, M. *Wien. Med. Presse*, **39**, 1041. Quoted by Kestenbaum.

1900 VON HIPPEL, E. *Graefe-Saemisch Handbuch*, **1**, 102.

1907 DRYSDALE and HERRINGHAM. *Quarterly Jl. of Med.* 1907–8, **1**.

1908 SCHMIDT-RIMPLER. *Graefe-Saemisch Handbuch*, pt. 2.

1919 SORIANO, F. *Klin. Monatsbl. f. Augenheilk.* **63**, 763.

1920 COLLINS, E. T. *Trans. Ophthal. Soc. U.K.* **40**, 132.

1920 KAYSER, B. *Klin. Monatsbl. f. Augenheilk.* **64**, 292.

1920 REIS, W. *Arch. d'Ophtal.* Oct. **37**, 577.

1920 USHER, C. H. *Trans. Ophthal. Soc. U.K.* **40**, 120.

1921 COLLINS, E. T. *Trans. Ophthal. Soc. U.K.* **41**, 10.

1924 ORMOND and WILLIAMS. *Guy's Hosp. Reps.* **74**, 385.

1926 WRIGHT, R. E. *Brit. Jl. Ophthal.* **6**, 35.

1929 BEST, F. *Klin. Monatsbl. f. Augenheilk.* **82**, 525.

1931 GNAD, F. *Klin. Monatsbl. f. Augenheilk.* **87**, 33.

1933 FRIEDE, R. *Klin. Monatsbl. f. Augenheilk.* **91**, 767; *Arch. f. Ophthal.* **131**, 1.

1933 KAYSER, B. *Klin. Monatsbl. f. Augenheilk.* **91**, 343.

1933 SEEFELDER, R. *Zentralbl. f. die ges. Augenheilk.* **29**, 1.

1933 WAARDENBURG, J. P. Quoted by Kayser. *Klin. Monatsbl. f. Augenheilk.* **91**, 343.

1936 KAYSER, B. *Klin. Monatsbl. f. Augenheilk.* **96**, 721.

1936 RISER, R. O. *Amer. Jl. Ophthal.* **19**, 155.

1936 TRONCOSO and GIVNER. *Amer. Jl. Ophthal.* **19**, 549.

MEGALOPHTHALMIA

1931 HARTLIEB, R. *Klin. Monatsbl. f. Augenheilk.* **87**, 54.

1935 KATZ and LEDOUX. *Amer. Jl. Ophthal.* **18**, 914.

CHAPTER III

THE STRUCTURE AND DEVELOPMENT OF THE INVOLVED TISSUES: THEIR EMBRYOLOGY AND COMPARATIVE ANATOMY

THE DEVELOPMENT OF INVOLVED TISSUES

As an introduction to a study of congenital glaucoma, it is essential to consider the structural changes that occur during embryonic and early life in the anterior ocular tissues. There are two periods of relatively rapid ocular growth after birth, separated by a time when little change is found. The first period is during the first few years of life, and during this time it is the area in front of the muscle insertions that grows. This period and the tissues affected during it correspond with the time and site of the main development of hydrophthalmia.

The second period is from about puberty until the early twenties. During this time the tissues of the posterior segment are mainly affected, but the distance between the fovea and the optic disc remains the same as at birth. It is during this later period that the other common form of distension, viz. myopia, occurs, and the tissues growing then are those principally affected. If, later in life when growth is finished, hypertension occurs, the only part that can distend is the weakest part, viz. the lamina cribrosa. Medullation is complete during the first three weeks, and probably the lamina cribrosa is fully grown by then.

The sclera. In all species the anterior part of the sclera appears first and progresses farthest during embryonic life (Mann). The first sign of condensation of the outer sclera is found at the 48·0 mm. stage in that part which will later overlap the angle of the anterior chamber. At this stage condensation of the deep corneal layers is relatively advanced and a deep band runs towards the equator. Scleral condensation is more advanced by the 65·0 mm. stage, but the sclera is still thinner than the cornea.

The greater likelihood of scleral distension during the first two decades is suggested in the following paragraph. "At birth the sclera is immature and is lacking particularly in elastic fibres and until the beginning of the third decade it is particularly poor in this tissue. From then on, until the age of sixty years, this increases greatly" (Krekler, 1923).

The cornea. One may consider that a cornea is present when, at the 18·0 mm. stage, a narrow slit appears in the mesodermal lamina that lies between the surface epiblast and the anterior surface of the lens (Mann). This space will become the anterior chamber and by the 26·0 mm. stage it will be lined by endothelial cells.

"In the human foetus, before the iris is formed, and before there is any anterior chamber, two parallel rows of cells are seen lying interposed between the cornea and the anterior capsule of the lens. The anterior chamber is developed as a space between these two rows of cells, the anterior of which becomes the lining endothelium of Descemet's membrane, and the posterior the endothelium on the surface of the iris and of the pupillary membrane" (Collins). In congenital anterior staphyloma it is possible for the corneo-sclerotic junction to become displaced posteriorly with regard to the uvea, and yet for the various parts of each tissue to maintain normal relations or approximately so. Probably in pre-natal life the connection between the uvea and the external structures including the ciliary muscle is less firm than in adult life. A similar loose connection is found in many lower animals, especially in birds (Parsons, 1904).

Collins (1899) found in ten microphthalmic eyes that the angle did not extend beyond the transparent cornea—a condition usually peculiar to the eyes of lower animals in which at the edge of the transparent cornea a well-defined ligamentum pectinatum begins.

It is of interest to recall that the lids adhere during the third month and re-open during the seventh month. What influence in the development of hydrophthalmia the withdrawal of this protection and support may have is uncertain.

The size of the cornea. At birth the cornea is relatively large, its horizontal diameter being three-fifths of the antero-posterior axis of the globe, viz. 10·0 mm. It attains its full size at the age of two years approximately. According to Kayser (1926) the average diameter of the cornea

> at the age of 0 years = 9·44 mm., the average range of variation
> = 2·6 mm.,
> at the age of 6/12 years = 10·82 mm., the average range between
> 2/25 and 1 year = 1·87 mm.,

at the age of 1 year = 11·39 mm., the average range between 1 and 6 years = 1·77 mm.,

at the age of 5 years = 11·5 mm.

Priestley Smith found the mean horizontal diameter between the ages of five and ninety years was 11·6 mm. and that variations beyond 11·0 and 12·0 mm. were present in about 50 %. He also found that the average size did not vary with the refraction of the eye, and that though there was no constant relationship between size of globe and corneal diameter, yet as a rule small and large corneae were found with small and large globes respectively.

Man's cornea when compared with that of other mammals is very small in proportion to the size of the globe. In all other mammals but man and the higher apes the corneal diameter is more than half the antero-posterior diameter of the globe. See megalocornea and eyes of *Tarsius*. (Figs. 14, 15.)

Corneal curvature. By the fifth month of intra-uterine life the corneal curve has become apparent. At birth the cornea is more curved at the periphery than centrally. This is the reverse of the adult state. Gullstrand held that the normal cornea could best be described as consisting of a central optical zone that was practically spherical, and was decentred outwards and usually downwards. Its extent was about 4·0 mm. horizontally and a little less vertically. Around this is the peripheral part which shows marked flattening, which is more pronounced nasally than temporally, and usually more above than below. The corneal curvature is greater in the newborn than in the adult. The average radius according to Gullstrand is 7·7 mm. Steiger found that it varied between 7·5 and 8·1 mm. (see Parsons, 1904), and Tscherning's range was from 7·0 to 8·5 mm. A. Cucchia (1925) found the radius of curvature of the cornea to increase in proportion to the increase in the size of the body. At 3/12 the radius of curvature of the cornea = 3·1 mm. At 6/12 the radius of curvature of the cornea = 4·4 mm.

    ,, 8/12   ,,   ,,   ,,   ,,   = 5·1 mm.

    ,, 10/12   ,,   ,,   ,,   ,,   = 8·5 mm.

According to von Reuss in a five to six-year-old child the radius is 7·36 average, in a twelve-year-old child 7·45 mm., and by puberty the adult state is reached.

Though the corneal diameter of the high myope is usually within normal limits, yet the corneal curvature as a rule is greater.

Numerous alterations in position are observed when studying the relations that various structures near the angle bear to each other at different stages of embryonic life. It is difficult to know which of the processes is primary. There is a forward growth of the ectodermal iris and the ciliary body and, later, a tendency for the ciliary processes to move outwards towards the sclera. There is a forward movement of Schlemm's canal and the scleral spur in relation to the iris and the ciliary muscle, and also an apparent deepening of the angle of the anterior chamber.

The deepening of the angle of the anterior chamber (see Figs. 16 to 28). This extension of the angle is associated with a relative increase in the size of the cornea to the globe. It is observed in the development of the human embryo and in the evolution of man. It may be studied by comparing the varying relationship of the angle to three structures, viz. Schlemm's canal, the origin of the ciliary muscle and the circulus arteriosus iridis. Ida Mann has emphasised the constant relationship to each other that these structures maintain and the manner in which the angle appears to move backwards and the margin of the optic cup forwards. In the adult the ciliary muscle arises from the scleral spur just in front of the bottom of the angle and behind Schlemm's canal. The circulus arteriosus iridis is level with or even slightly behind the deepest part of the angle. As Collins pointed out, a vertical line drawn through the centre of Schlemm's canal in man would pass into the angle and almost through the circulus arteriosus iridis of the iris and only a few of the ciliary processes would lie to its inner side. At the end of the seventh month of intra-uterine life of the human foetus and in monkeys this line would pass into the extreme angle and leave the greater part of the ciliary processes external to it (Figs. 22, 29.) In the fourth month, and in carnivora and ungulata, this line would pass external to the angle, which ends where Descemet's membrane begins to split up. The circular artery and a large part of the ciliary processes would be on its inner side.

The development and the retrogression of the associated mesoderm. In a consideration of congenital glaucoma the greatest importance must be attached to the development and the retrogression of the thin layer of mesoderm that separates the anterior surface of the lens from the surface ectoderm. This layer is clearly seen at 16·0 mm. In the 48·0 mm. stage signs of forward growth of the ectodermal iris can be observed.

The transient nature of so much of this tissue and of its complicated blood supply is of great interest. It is peculiar to mammals (Mann), and interference with its normal course may account for coloboma, aniridia, anterior synechia and congenital glaucoma.

There are many divergent views concerning the time of origin of the anterior chamber. Possibly it is during the third to the fifth month, which is considerably later than was thought at first. The space that appears at the 20·0 mm. stage is probably the result of fixation and sectioning, though Mann at one time considered this to be the beginning of the anterior chamber. She considered that the anterior layer of mesoderm at this stage could be considered to be the rudimentary cornea. In an attempt to eliminate errors due to faulty fixation Speciale-Cirincione (1917) used frozen sections and first found an anterior chamber at the beginning of the eighth month. The misleading nature of the majority of sections is shown by the presence of spaces under the lens capsule, between the walls of the optic vesicle and elsewhere. Direct transference of specimens into 60 or 70% alcohol can produce anterior chambers of any depth at almost any stage (Seefelder). Seefelder and Wolfrum (1906) found no sign of the anterior chamber until the end of the fifth month, Fig. 16). This figure also shows the first signs of Schlemm's

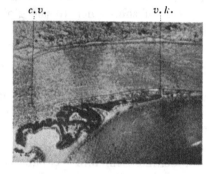

Fig. 16. Foetal eye at the end of the fifth month. The earliest signs of the periphery of the anterior chamber and of Schlemm's canal (*c.v.*) are visible. Associated mesoderm separates the lens and the pigmented epithelium from Descemet's endothelium. There is no scleral spur. *v.k.* = anterior chamber. (Seefelder and Wolfrum, 1906.)

canal situated very far posteriorly. Even in the next month they found the lens and the cornea in contact centrally (Fig. 17).

The cells on the deep aspect of the rudimentary cornea become arranged in a definite row and form Descemet's endothelium. The latter appears first in the periphery but does not grow in from the periphery. "The centre of the cornea is from the first the thinnest part" (Mann). Descemet's membrane is not laid down until the 76·0 mm. stage. As early as the 25·0 mm. stage signs of condensation are visible in the deepest part of the cornea. They spread to the periphery and unite with similar tissues in the sclera. The collagenous fibrils increase and the nuclei lessen, so that by the seventh month the cornea histologically resembles the adult state. In passing it is of interest to recall that the collagenous fibrils appear earlier in the anterior than in the posterior part of the sclera. The elastic tissue that is mixed with the collagen in the sclera increased rapidly during the first two months of life (Krekeler). These facts probably influence the varying distensibility of the globe that is suggested from a study of the shapes of different hydrophthalmic eyes. The age of onset is probably the main factor that determines the shape.

If we study a section of a foetal eye at the three to four months' stage (70·5–100·0 mm.) we observe that though the anterior portion of the sclera is thinner than the posterior part it is denser in structure and that the uvea tends to increase in width towards the cornea. A closer study reveals two developments of the greatest importance: (a) Bundles of connective tissue fibres running equatorially on the inner surface of the sclera close to the cornea. The anterior portion of these will become the scleral spur. They form a marked contrast with the vast majority of the scleral fibres, which run meridionally. The laying down of more equatorial fibres determines the shape of the scleral channel

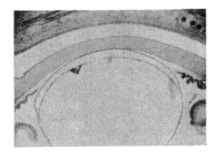

Fig. 17. Foetal eye at the beginning of the sixth month. The lens and cornea are in contact centrally. There is a faint pupillary membrane. The uveal meshwork is present. (Seefelder and Wolfrum.)

and consequently the canal of Schlemm. These fibres remove the dissimilarity in structure between this foetal band and the adjacent sclera. Immediately behind the spur is another band of condensation that tends to become obscured towards the end of intra-uterine life. It may be called the foetal scleral band to show its transient visibility. It is Virchow's "Skleralwulst-Formation". (b) Mesodermal cells lying between this connective tissue and the corneal endothelium. Those that are most superficial become the meridional fibres of the ciliary muscle (fourth month). The sclero-corneal trabeculae develop from those that lie between the developing scleral spur and the margin of the corneal endothelium (fifth month). The cells lying deep to these become the uveal meshwork. In an embryo of 183·0 mm. (almost six months) Fischer (1933) described the nuclei of the primitive scleral spur as round and irregularly arranged and those of the ciliary muscle and the sclero-corneal trabeculae as elongated and directed meridionally.

By the 65·0 mm. stage (almost three months) the top of the iris is level with the angle of the chamber, though the ciliary region is undifferentiated. At this stage the mesoderm is densely cellular and sharply limited anteriorly. It becomes more open in structure and spaces develop in it in subsequent stages. Schlemm's canal is visible (Mann), and, lying deeply in the mesoderm, it is level with the apex of the angle. It is of value to note that Fischer found a lumen in only some sections of a 105·0 mm. embryo (fifteen weeks), and that Seefelder and Wolfrum found a lumen in places only, at the end of the fourth month.

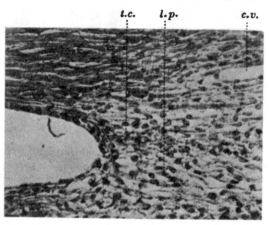

Fig. 18. Foetal eye at the beginning of the sixth month. High power. Uveal meshwork fills the angle. Sclero-corneal trabeculae run backwards towards scleral spur and ciliary muscle. (Seefelder and Wolfrum.)

The primitive structure of the uveal meshwork is of interest, for it already differs from that of the trabeculae. The cells are chiefly spindle-shaped and lie irregularly. They are rich in protoplasm but little fibrillar substance lies between them. Though the ciliary muscle and the trabeculae contain elastic tissue at an early stage this meshwork is free from it (Fig. 18).

By the fifth month the foremost end of Schlemm's canal lies in front of the apex of the angle. The anterior chamber begins to contain aqueous about this time. "In many specimens, even up to the sixth month, the anterior chamber appears empty, extremely narrow and compressed" (Mann). The strongly developed meridional fibres of the ciliary muscle are directly continuous with the more clearly defined scleral projection. The latter is well behind the angle and cannot be considered as a spur until at least the end of the seventh month. Sondermann (1930–31) described a vessel which runs from the pupillary membrane into the angle and finally appears in the marginal

layers of the sclera—the vena irido-scleralis. As a result of obstruction a sinus-like enlargement of this vein occurs at the inner surface of the sclera and later spreads backwards, so that sclera lies also on its inner surface. Sondermann considers that this occurs about the fourth month, and that it is the origin of the projection which later will become the scleral spur.

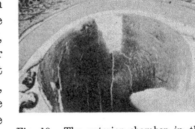

Fig. 19. The anterior chamber in the middle of the sixth month. (Seefelder and Wolfrum.)

Seefelder and Wolfrum found that uveal meshwork was present early in the sixth month (Fig. 18). Hitherto it was part of an un-differentiated cellular mass already referred to, which is found between the sclera and the pigmented epithelial layer at the end of Descemet's endothelium even in the second and third months.

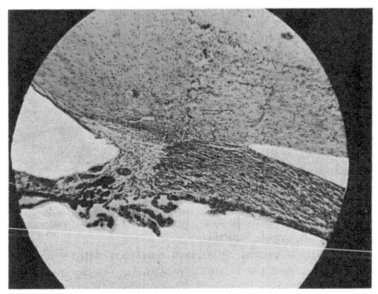

Fig. 20. × 55. Angle and ciliary region at six months. Observe (1) posterior position of Schlemm's canal and spur; (2) profuse uveal meshwork; (3) early circular fibres of ciliary muscle.

By the seventh month Schlemm's canal is farther forwards but not entirely in front of the angle. The spur now lies behind the angle, which is filled by loose open tissue. The iris is well grown and the circular muscle fibres in the ciliary muscle have appeared. The iris until this stage has lagged behind the rest of the eye. At the fifth month it is almost covered by the limbus as in aniridia. In the eighth month the pupil becomes smaller, probably because of the development of the sphincter. At this time the crypts form. The ciliary processes at first reach much farther over the iris than they do in the mature eye. Later the form of the ciliary body alters so as to suggest a backward displacement of the ciliary processes (Fig. 21).

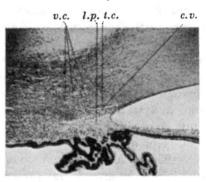

Fig. 21. The angle at the beginning of the seventh month (34·5 cm.). The uveal meshwork is well developed. Schlemm's canal (*c.v.*) lies behind the angle. (Seefelder and Wolfrum.)

At the beginning of the seventh month the anterior chamber is still very shallow. Seefelder found its depth centrally to be less than half the thickness of the adjacent cornea. It was about one-third deeper peripherally. The sclero-corneal meshwork is at its fullest development, which of course is a very different state from that of the fully grown eye. The tissue at this early stage contains more nuclei and large numerous open spaces connect the sclero-corneal and the uveal meshwork. The trabeculae of the latter are thicker than in the sixth month, and the

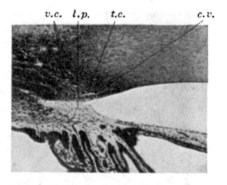

Fig. 22. The angle at the end of the seventh month (38·0 cm.). Atrophy of the meshwork has commenced and the canal is farther forwards. (Seefelder and Wolfrum.)

numerous many-branched cells stain deep red with van Giesen's stain but differ from the sclero-corneal meshwork by not staining with Weigert's "Elastinfärbung". The anterior third of the sclero-corneal meshwork opens directly into the angle, but the posterior two-thirds are still hemmed in by the uveal meshwork. Nearly all of the sclero-corneal meshwork arises from the scleral spur, which forms a slight projection. The majority of the meridional muscle fibres arise from the scleral spur, but they are still relatively far from the angle.

By the end of the seventh month more spaces have appeared in the deep part of the uveal meshwork that lies between the sclera and the ciliary processes. The passages between the two meshworks appear farther forwards. The immature circular portion and the meridional

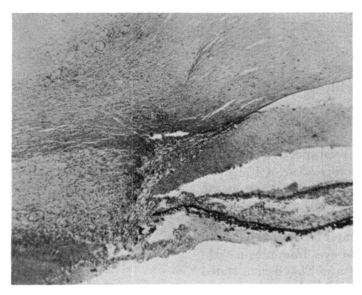

Fig. 23. Seven months' foetus. × 55. Pathological specimen. The angle is full of haemorrhage which has spread into the spaces of the meshwork towards Schlemm's canal. The meshwork is profuse.

portion of the ciliary muscle are closer together and more compact. At this stage the pupillary membrane is still well preserved though the atrophic process, which has already begun in the posterior and the lateral portions of the tunica vasculosa lentis, will soon affect the central portion, which from the beginning is thinnest. These facts are of interest in their relation to the origin of the congenital corneal opacities and synechiae to be considered later (Fig. 22).

During the eighth month, as a result of atrophy of mesoblastic tissue, the spaces in the uveal meshwork become larger and more numerous. In various places this meshwork may be found wedged in between the two parts of the ciliary muscle. This state resembles that seen in lower animals, in some of which, indeed, the appearance has suggested an exchange of fluid between Fontana's spaces and the capillaries on the inner surface of the ciliary body (Hotta, 1906).

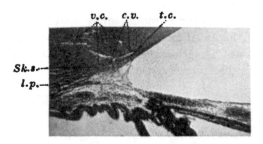

Fig. 24. The angle at the eighth month (40·0 cm.) showing further atrophy of the meshwork. (Seefelder and Wolfrum.)

The pupillary crypts of the iris form after the disappearance of the pupillary membrane, which begins in the eighth month. The ciliary crypts open after the completion of the regression of the uveal framework in the ninth month (Figs. 24, 25).

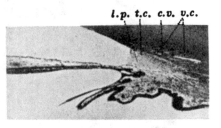

Fig. 25. The angle at the ninth month (45·0 cm.). The canal is still behind the angle and the meshwork is profuse. (Seefelder and Wolfrum.)

Seefelder was struck by the differences between two normal pairs of eyes from nine-month-old foetuses. They demonstrated the individual variation that may occur in development. In one pair the uveal meshwork was fully developed, filling the entire angle. The anterior chamber was shallower than in his eight-month foetus. In the other pair there were only slight remains of the uveal meshwork and the scleral spur almost reached the angle. The lumina of Schlemm's canal were level

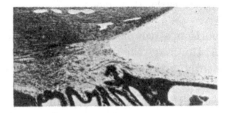

Fig. 26. The angle at birth. (Seefelder and Wolfrum.)

with the angle and the pupillary membrane had completely vanished.

Just before birth Schlemm's canal and the scleral spur lie well in front of the angle and the major circle of the iris is level with it.

These apparent changes in position are due to mesodermal atrophy (Fig. 26).

At birth the ciliary processes are still in contact with the iris and the stroma of the ciliary body is very cellular. In the rabbit and kindred animals the ciliary processes arise from the iris. The presence of ciliary processes on the posterior surface of the iris is normal until after birth in the human eye, and throughout life in certain animals.

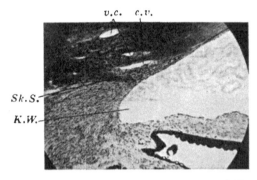

Fig. 27. The angle of a four-months-old child. (Seefelder, 1906.)

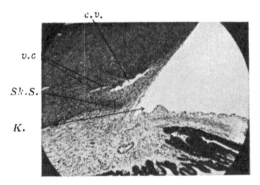

Fig. 28. The angle of a normal adult. (Seefelder.)

In man, however, as Reese (1935) has pointed out, such a finding is not uncommon in the adult eye. They have been found in many hydrophthalmic eyes. The significance of the presence of all the processes on the iris becomes great if an operation such as a trephine is performed.

At birth the angle is usually narrow. It becomes rounded later with the development of the ciliary muscle. This muscle is still flat rather than wedge-like as in the adult.

After birth as the human ciliary processes are displaced backwards, the angle of the anterior chamber deepens and reaches its full development during the first three years of life (Figs. 27, 28).

"The uveal trabeculae fill the angle of the anterior chamber at birth, and the region only widens out between the years of two and four, during which time the ciliary processes and the anterior margin of the retina are relatively moved backwards" (Duke-Elder, 1932).

THE STRUCTURE OF THESE TISSUES

The angle of the anterior chamber. In considering the angle of the anterior chamber the first point to realise is that this angle is

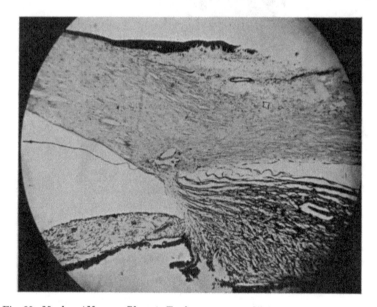

Fig. 29. Monkey (*Macacus Rhesus*). To show an unusual appearance of Schlemm's canal, and the attachment of muscle fibres to trabeculae and meshwork.

not formed by the junction of the iris and the cornea. The iris does not arise from the corneo-scleral junction but from the middle of the anterior surface of the ciliary body. Therefore a portion of this surface usually takes part in the formation of the angle. The outer wall is formed by corneo-scleral meshwork, as it covers the tip of the scleral spur, the anterior half of Schlemm's canal and the margin of the cornea. The amount of scleral overlap varies, but is about 2·0 mm.

above, 1·5 mm. below, and 1·0 mm. at each side. The uveal meshwork may cover over the otherwise exposed portion of the ciliary body.

In a consideration of congenital glaucoma it is necessary to consider in detail various structures, such as the scleral spur, Schlemm's canal and its vascular connections and the meshwork of the angle.

Unfortunately much of our information is inexact and some quite incorrect. Some of the inaccuracies and contradictions are due to imperfect histological methods and hasty conclusions. Let us take, for example, the appearance of Schlemm's canal. Apart from the

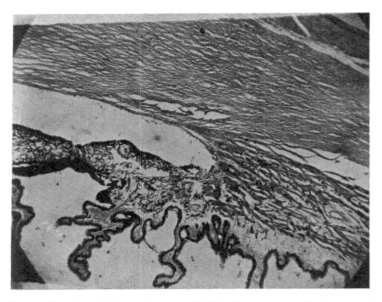

Fig. 30. Eye of aged Orang-Outang. × 35. To show apparent displacement of ciliary processes and the elongation of Schlemm's canal from oblique sectioning.

fact that its shape and size may vary according to the use of atropine or eserine prior to enucleation, its apparent dimensions will vary with the thickness of the section, the distance of any particular section from the antero-posterior axis of the globe and the degree of obliquity of the section to the axis of the canal (Fig. 30).

The scleral furrow and the scleral roll or spur (Fig. 31). One is more familiar with the obvious overlapping of the corneal margin by scleral tissue than with the equally important furrow or groove that lies beneath it. This furrow lies between the anterior limit of the inner surface of the sclera and the deep forward projection known as the scleral roll or spur. Into this spur the ciliary muscle is said to be inserted. The old name of the scleral spur was the annular ligament. This name and that used by Henderson, viz. the scleral ring, are of

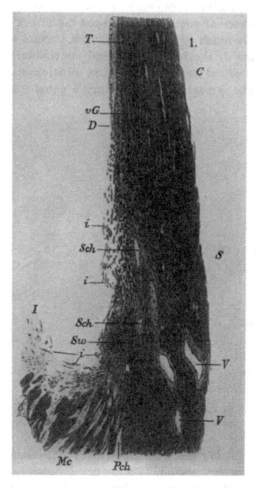

Fig. 31. The scleral furrow with its environment, meridional section. ×96. *C*, cornea; *D*, border of Descemet's membrane; *vG*, the anterior border ring; *T*, deep root of the scleral framework; *i*, uveal framework; *Sch*, lumina of Schlemm's canal; *V*, efferent veins of these canals; *Sw*, scleral roll; *Pch*, beginning of the perichoroidal space; *Mc*, musculus ciliaris; *I*, iris root. (After Salzmann.)

value, for they help to keep in one's mind the annular form of the structure and not simply its appearance in the usual antero-posterior sections of microscopic work. The circular fibres are clearly visible in tangential and transverse sections. It is regrettable that in these days of haste the old teased and surface preparations are neglected. They are of particular value in studying the structures round the angle and the meshwork (Fig. 32).

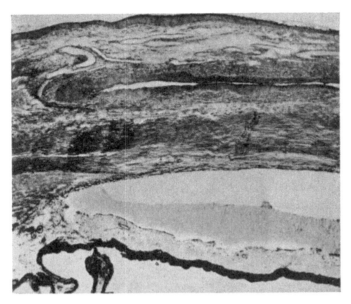

Fig. 32. Man. ×30. Peripheral section through the filtration angle of the human eye to show the equatorial direction of the sclero-corneal trabeculae. These fibres lie between the anterior chamber which contains exudate and an elongated section through Schlemm's canal which is full of blood corpuscles. The eye was slightly inflamed.

The spur will be shown to have the following functions:

1. One point of insertion for the meridional fibres of the ciliary muscle.

2. A strong circular band that tends to maintain the patency of Schlemm's canal and resist the distension of the globe.

3. A valve for varying the capacity of Schlemm's canal.

There is no certainty yet, however, as to the exact nature of the part played by the spur and the trabeculae in aiding the outflow of fluid from the anterior chamber.

The scleral spur points forwards and inwards, which is in the opposite direction to what we would expect if its sole function is to act as a fixed point for the meridional fibres of the ciliary muscle. Tscherning, it must be noted, stated that these fibres are more fixed posteriorly than at the spur. Thomson demonstrated, by differential staining, (1) that fibres of the ciliary muscle do not pass beyond the tip of the spur, and (2) that some of the fibres of the meshwork of the angle "sweep backwards past the projecting summit of the scleral spur and become continuous with the tissue of the iris lying internal to the meridional fibres of the ciliary muscle and establishing a connection with the area occupied by the circular fibres of that muscle". Thomson emphasised the point that, as the contractile fibres of the ciliary muscle lie behind the spur and the elastic fibres in the trabeculae in front of it, its setting and attachments will aid its mobility. He

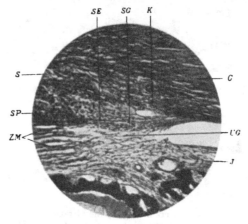

Fig. 33. Angle of 32·0 cm. foetus showing strand of muscle (*SE*) running well beyond the spur towards the angle. (Fischer.)

demonstrated this further under a dissecting microscope, by applying gentle traction to the iris and watching the canal open and close. Thomson's description of the pump-like mechanism of the scleral spur has been supported by Fortin's work. The latter examined specimens that were fixed immediately after death and found varying states of Schlemm's canal and the spaces in the corneo-scleral trabeculae. If the eye when under the influence of eserine were rapidly fixed "the pull of the ciliary muscle on the scleral spur and the widening of the spaces between the trabeculae is very obvious" (Duke-Elder, 1934).

Even though a wider insertion may be demonstrated the influence on the canal of Schlemm and the importance of the spur are little altered. In many sections one finds some muscle fibres torn from the spur and yet others apparently attached to sclero-corneal trabeculae or even strands of uveal meshwork. In subchoroidal haemorrhages and those that lead to expulsion of the contents of the globe we get a further demonstration of the tenacity with which the meridional muscle fibres adhere to the tip of the spur and the adjacent trabeculae. See unpublished specimen V and myopic eye (Figs. 7, 2).

In a 24·0 cm. embryo Fischer (1933) found that some of the meridional fibres were inserted into the spur, and that others ran past it to the scleral and uveal meshwork. This appearance was more definite in his older specimens, e.g. 32·0 or 37·5 cm. (see Fig. 33). He concluded that (1) the innermost meridional fibres pass by the spur to be inserted into the scleral and uveal meshwork, that (2) the intermediate bundles of fibres are attached near the point to the spur, and that (3) relatively few superficial fibres pass between the posterior fibres of the scleral spur and those of the foetal band—Virchow's "Skleralwulst-Formation".

The destination of the sclero-corneal trabeculae will be discussed shortly. It may be stated here that a very considerable number run past the spur and appear to have free connection with the ciliary muscle. The number will be greater if the spur is narrow and straight and does not project centrally from the scleral surface. They may form the majority of Fischer's Type I (see below). There is roughly a corresponding type of sclero-corneal trabeculae for each type of scleral spur.

Virchow considered that the scleral spur was a characteristic of primates. It was better defined in apes than in man and the "Skleralwulst-Formation" remained differentiated from it in them. Because he could find neither the spur nor the canal of Schlemm in hoofed animals and those of prey, he held that the two structures were related. The presence of meshwork in these suggested its independence. Our findings however (q.v.) differed from the above.

Too much importance cannot be attached to the series of equatorial connective tissue bundles lying in this zone. They constitute the scleral spur, the bundles that were the foetal band and now form part of the sclera and those that lie at the base of and even all round Schlemm's canal and between its vascular connections. In front of the canal a series of bundles is frequently found. They constitute an anterior scleral spur. Henderson (1921) found trabeculae rising from a similar clearly defined anterior spur in the Rhesus monkey. The equatorial bundles that form the spur are narrower and closely packed towards the sclero-corneal trabeculae. This renders the line of division indefinite. On the outer side, however, the bundles are loosely arranged and the trabeculae can be seen coursing between them.

The structure of the spur is constant. It contains many elastic fibres. By birth it differs from the "scleral foetal band", for the latter has come to resemble the sclera. The bundles of the band are less strictly equatorial, thicker and more closely packed than those of the spur.

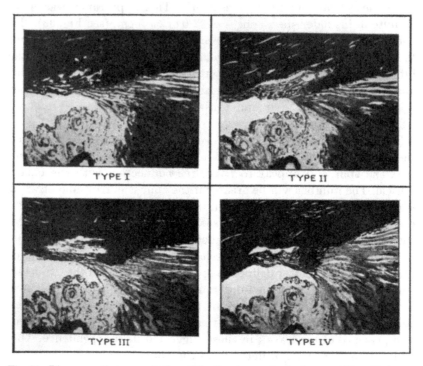

Fig. 34. Diagrammatic representation of the four types of scleral spur. (After Fischer.)

After a critical survey of twenty-eight normal eyes, of which sixteen were sectioned serially, Fischer (1933) described four types of scleral spur (see Fig. 34). They were:

(a) Type I. The spur is short and blunt and runs either straight to the front or curves slightly inwards.

(b) Type II. The spur is longer and thinner and runs forwards farther into the trabeculae.

(c) Type III is arched from the sclera towards the inner part of the eye and is hook-shaped as it curves outwards towards its pointed extremity. It projects beyond the posterior end of the scleral channel in a manner that is intermediate between Types I and II.

(*d*) Type IV is curved like Type III but is coarser. It forms a definite inward projection from the scleral surface. Types I and III are most common. The same type is present in both of each pair of eyes, and Fischer found little variation in different sections of the same eye. In some eyes the spur appeared to be thicker nasally than on the temporal side. Transitional forms are not infrequent.

From this it will be readily understood that there are varying types of Schlemm's canal. The influence of the scleral spur on the canal itself is obscured by its branching nature. It will be found that the relationship of the spur and Schlemm's canal is further demonstrated by the findings in congenital glaucoma. These also show a relative independence of the sclero-corneal trabeculae and a relationship of the latter to the ciliary muscle.

It is of interest to realise that the spur tends to atrophy in glaucoma. Even in absolute glaucoma it may still be visible in some sections though absent in the majority. Fischer found that it and Schlemm's canal varied together in such cases. He failed to find any relationship between the type of spur present and the incidence of glaucoma. It is possible, however, that a well-developed spur and trabeculae may assist to maintain the patency of the canal. The ability of the spur to resist distension is seen in specimens of partial corneal and intercalary staphyloma. It may also determine the shape of the eye in hydrophthalmia. See Figs. 102, 103, unpublished specimen V.

The canal of Schlemm. Close to the bottom of the scleral furrow lies Schlemm's canal, which usually consists of two or more lumina which coalesce and re-divide irregularly. "The canal is surrounded on the outside and behind by the sclera; immediately behind it and to some extent overlapping it internally is the scleral spur; while its inner wall is supported by the trabecular tissue of the angle of the anterior chamber." Its outer wall therefore is rigid and its inner wall consists of highly elastic tissue. "It communicates by many minute branches with an intricate venous plexus situated in the surrounding scleral tissue, derived from the anterior ciliary veins. The connecting channels running between the canal and the intrascleral venous plexus are very minute, have an oblique course, are flattened, and have somewhat valvular openings making retrograde flow difficult" (Duke-Elder, 1932). The very thin endothelial lining of this canal is its only wall (Thomson and others) and it is continued into the small venous channels leading to the anterior ciliary veins. The canal is shut off from the spaces in the meshwork and only solutions or the finest suspensions can pass into the canal.

Trabeculae act as sand does which inhibits "the passage of bacteria and inanimate particles many times smaller than the pores between the granules, the process depending on an adhesion of the particles to the grains of sand" (Wegefarth). This and the closing of the angle when the iris touches the cornea as soon as the aqueous escapes may explain the absence of blood cells in the anterior chamber after puncture.

It is difficult to understand the significance of the red-blood corpuscles that some authors (Thomson, Sondermann, and others) have found within the canal. Sondermann (1933) found that blood corpuscles introduced into the anterior chamber passed into the inner canaliculi, Schlemm's canal, and the outer canaliculi and also into the iris and the ciliary body. Thomson (1911) studied a case of retinal haemorrhage and found corpuscles not only in the recesses of the trabeculae and Schlemm's canal but also in the crypts at the ciliary attachment of the iris and in the spaces between the bundles of the ciliary muscle.

The afferent arteriolar supply to Schlemm's canal. The old controversy that centred on the question of whether there were open connections or not between Schlemm's canal and the anterior chamber was settled for many years by the work of Leber and Schwalbe. It was re-opened recently by Sondermann's (1930–31) and Theobald's (1934) researches. These authors believed that open communications existed and that Schlemm's canal was a venous sinus. Sondermann described "inner canals" in contrast with the "outer canals" that were discovered long ago. These inner canals are always found in the posterior half of the canal but the outer ones with rare exceptions open into the anterior half. The inner canals are narrower than the outer ones (0·005–0·025 mm. as compared with 0·02–0·04 mm.) and appear to be more numerous. These "canals are often in open communication with the spaces in the pectinate ligament. Schlemm's canal, the inner and outer canals and the spaces in the pectinate ligament are very narrow in the newborn, but increase considerably in diameter during the first years of life." Since then, however, Friedenwald (1936) has firmly expressed his opinions that both these views are incorrect. He adopted Maggiore's technique (1917) for injecting opaque material into an artery and found that even if the intra-ocular pressure was lowered by paracentesis no sign of this material was found in the anterior chamber. This agreed with Maggiore's experience and certainly suggests the absence of direct communication. Friedenwald considered that Sondermann's inner canals were blind pockets extending into the spaces of the sclero-corneal trabeculae but separated from the anterior chamber by a continuous endothelial wall. Apart from such histological findings the presence of open communications would theoretically be a great hindrance to the maintenance of normal intra-ocular pressure. In his serial sections Friedenwald found afferent arterioles opening into Schlemm's canal. His conception therefore is of a continuous flow of plasma from these arterioles into the canal and of its dilution within this canal with water osmotically attracted from the anterior chamber. An alteration in the volume or the quality of the plasma may produce serious intra-ocular complications.

Friedenwald's microphotographs show that a branch to the intra-scleral plexus is given off by only some of the arterioles which come from the ciliary arteries and enter the inner surface of the sclera at from 0·5 to 1·0 mm. behind the scleral spur. These arterioles, accompanied by small nerves, pass anteriorly to the canal and some of them give off a branch which runs the following characteristic course—it turns in a retrograde direction at an acute angle and runs directly into the canal. As a rule such a branch has no muscular coat. It may be accompanied by a twig of the nerve that runs close to the arteriole. The afferent arterioles are less numerous than the efferent venules, and the connecting arteriolar branches are minute (5 to 10 microns). Friedenwald assumes that the plasma that flows continuously from these branches into the canal attracts osmotically water from the anterior chamber. Any process that might lessen the flow of plasma would reduce the rate of absorption of aqueous and so tend to raise intra-ocular tension. The conception is that the canal lies between the artery and vein as a specialised form of capillary sustaining a slight but steady circulation of blood or plasma, rather than a blind out-pouching of the episcleral veins as has hitherto been assumed. In a globe with early uncomplicated chronic simple glaucoma he found sclerosis of the afferent arterioles, and this he considered might be one means by which the hypertension of chronic simple glaucoma is produced. It is work of great interest and may throw light on the pathogenesis of congenital glaucoma. The state of the minute nerve fibres when neurofibromatosis is present might be a study productive of gain.

There is considerable evidence to support the view that various unrelated mechanisms are employed for the reabsorption of the different components of the intra-ocular fluid. Colloids appear to be removed by active phagocytosis in the endothelium of the iris. Proteolytic enzymes in the aqueous and the surrounding tissues aid in the removal of the proteins. Crystalloid exchange takes place between the blood vessels of the iris and the anterior chamber by diffusion, and to a lesser degree they escape with the reabsorbed water through Schlemm's canal. The main escape for water is by means of this canal and possibly also by the vessels of the iris (Friedenwald, 1936).

The meshwork of the angle. "The pectinate ligament." Considerable confusion exists in the literature because of the use of the term "pectinate ligament". This was first used by Hueck in 1839 because of the resemblance of the tissue in the filtration angle of ungulates to a comb (pecten). As in the mature human eye, and probably at any foetal stage, this resemblance is not present, it appears wise to discontinue the use of this term. This is particularly desirable, because in the literature "ligamentum pectinatum iridis" frequently refers to the whole of the tissue in the angle, and since Seefelder's recommendation other writers have restricted its application to the inner portion only of this tissue. If the term "ligament" is applicable at all to any part of this tissue it is the sclero-corneal portion, for it may function as one insertion for the longitudinal fibres of the ciliary muscle. This part, however, is neither pectinate, nor does it resemble in structure or function the true mammalian pectinate ligament. Further, it is not a ligament of the iris.

Surely it is preferable to refer to the outer portion, which is the persistent part in man, as the scleral or sclero-corneal meshwork, and to the inner portion, which largely atrophies in man, as the uveal meshwork. A further advantage of the latter term is to emphasise its relationship with the remainder of the uveal tract.

The sclero-corneal meshwork lies on the inner side of Schlemm's canal and fills up the remainder of the scleral furrow. It is a delicate ring of tissue that is roughly triangular in section. Its apex is in the deeper layers of the cornea, where it arises from the circularly arranged bundle of connective tissue and elastic fibres—the anterior border ring of Schwalbe. The base abuts against the scleral spur and the anterior surface of the ciliary body. Most of this tissue is attached to the spur and the remainder blends with the ciliary body. The outer side is continuous with the corneo-sclera and forms the inner boundary of Schlemm's canal, and the inner side bounds the angle of the anterior chamber (Duke-Elder, 1932). In addition to the sclero-corneal meshwork, there are a few delicate elements lying on its inner surface, the uveal meshwork which, in foetal life, until the sixth month somewhat resembles the pectinate ligament found in herbivora. Most of this disappears and can scarcely be said to exist in the adult. In monkey's eyes Heine (1899) has demonstrated a collapse of the meshes of the "pectinate ligament" with atropine and an opening out with eserine.

If one detaches the ciliary body from the sclera, the meshwork and the peripheral portions of Descemet's membrane remain attached to the anterior end of the ciliary body like a whitish seam, 1·0 mm. in width. If one separates the iris from the ciliary body, the delicate uveal meshwork adheres to the iris, and the more extensive scleral portion and the adjacent border of Descemet's membrane remain attached to the ciliary body. In a meridional section the uveal meshwork scarcely exists; a surface preparation is necessary for its study.

The trabeculae of the scleral meshwork are delicate flat bands consisting of collagenous fibres surrounded by a thick covering of elastic fibres, which is covered by a fine homogeneous layer continuous with and having the same staining reaction as Descemet's membrane. Most superficially there is an endothelial layer continuous with the corneal endothelium and the endothelial vestiges of the iris. Anteriorly the meshwork is about three or four elements thick, and posteriorly much thicker. The outer trabeculae penetrate between the loosely arranged bundles of the spur and are soon lost to sight. The termination of the central trabeculae is less certain, being obscured by the tightly packed bundles of the adjacent portion of the spur. The inner trabeculae run past the spur to the anterior extremity of the meridional portion of the ciliary muscle (Figs. 31, 29).

The termination of Descemet's membrane. This membrane thins out peripherally but does not end, for it is continued over the trabeculae of the meshwork as a very thin layer. (*Note.* Eisler (1930) does not agree with this view.) In teased preparations one can see the transition of the most posterior lamellae of the cornea into the meshwork. "The fibre mass of the particular corneal lamella divides up into narrower bundles", which contain a glass membrane and an endothelial covering and form trabeculae. This may be looked upon as a deep or meridional root of the meshwork. A superficial or circular root exists in the form of the anterior border ring. This is a flat bundle of connective tissue, supported by elastic fibres, which varies in position, thickness and breadth in different portions of the same eye. Immediately posterior to it one encounters the most anterior spaces that open into the anterior chamber. It lies on or even in the substance of the peripheral portion of Descemet's membrane (Salzmann).

Collins, Parsons, Thomson, Schäfer and others considered that Descemet's membrane does not end abruptly at some little distance from the angle of the chamber. They demonstrated its division into a leash of fibres which, after joining others coming from the deeper corneal lamellae, forms the pectinate ligament. Elliot (1922) agreed with this finding. In the examination of a large series of trephined discs it was not possible to demonstrate an abrupt ending of Descemet's membrane. The spaces therefore lie partly in the meshes of the broken-up membrane of Descemet and partly in those of the deepest strata of the substantia propria of the cornea (Elliot).

Thomson Henderson was supported by Buchanan (1913) in the view that Descemet's membrane ended abruptly on the inner side of the ligament and that the two structures are unrelated. Their ideas will be described shortly. Salzmann emphasised the marked reduction in width of Descemet's membrane but considered that its ending is only apparent and that it really continues on as a delicate layer over the iris.

The trabeculae branch freely and so increase in number from before backwards, and near the scleral roll there may be fifteen to twenty overlying each other. The spaces between superimposed lamellae do not overlie each other (Salzmann).

Though the corneal endothelium is continued over the trabeculae and covers all the spaces of the meshwork it is not united in any way with that of Schlemm's canal.

Posteriorly the main mass of the meshwork goes over into the scleral roll, which Schwalbe described as the posterior border ring of the meshwork. The roll shows individual variations and anteriorly and inwards shows no sharp limits. It consists of a large number of connective tissue bundles of varying width which pursue a circular course and resemble scleral fibre bundles. A limited number of trabeculae course past the inner border of the roll and are lost in the intermuscular connective tissue of the ciliary body.

The uveal meshwork, or the so-called pectinate ligament, is a vestigial remnant of delicate round trabeculae having a structure similar to that of the scleral meshwork except that the elastic fibres are absent.

The uveal meshwork arises mainly from the inner surface of the scleral meshwork and also from the margin of Descemet's membrane. Its trabeculae, which are rounded and not flattened like those of the scleral meshwork, run over the anterior surface of the ciliary body to the root of the iris. They form a very loose reticulum of wide polygonal meshes. The main histological difference between the two forms of trabeculae is the absence of elastic fibres in the uveal form. At the root of the iris this endothelium is continuous with that of the iris, the glass membrane vanishes and the central collagenous fibres merge into the connective tissue stroma of the iris.

Iris processes. "In places, the regularity of the angle may be broken by the downward continuation of the so-called iris processes, which are cord-like structures projecting from the anterior surface of the iris at the ciliary border. They consist of the same elements as iris tissue and are pigmented and thicker than the trabeculae of the angle" (Salzmann).

Barkan (1936), as a result of his gonioscopic studies, considered that the iris processes, which cross the angle in varying numbers, constitute the main part of the uveal meshwork. When they are highly developed they may form a dense mesh resembling the pectinate ligament in animals. They probably are aberrant remnants of the foetal structure corresponding to this ligament. They arise from the iris root and are inserted into the wall of the angle as far forwards as the anterior border ring of Schwalbe. A microphotograph of an iris process illustrates Barkan's paper. A similar one is seen in Seefelder's paper of 1906. Troncoso and Givner (1936) also described these (Figs. 12, 48).

The anterior attachment of the ciliary muscle. De Villiers (1933) raised the question whether Descemet's membrane should not be regarded as an anterior tendon of the ciliary muscle. In such a form it would be another example of the remarkable modifications of ocular tissue for the purposes of vision. He considered that the anterior attachment of the ciliary muscle is not to the scleral spur any more than its posterior attachment is to the choroid. The scleral spur has sufficient connection with the fibres of the anterior attachment to enable it to dilate and collapse Schlemm's canal as the ciliary muscle contracts and relaxes.

Henderson (1908 and 1921) considered that the inner corneal lamellae, after forming the meshwork which he called the cribriform ligament, terminate as the ligament of origin of the ciliary muscle. None of the fibres bends round into the iris root, as they may appear to do in oblique sections. "The connective-tissue stroma of the iris root is attached to the circular bundles of the ligament at a point just posterior to the scleral ring." This ligament, according to Henderson, is part of the sclera and is therefore composed of circular and longitudinal fibres. One of the characteristics of the sclero-corneal coat is the presence of many circular fibres, of which a prominent collection lying just posterior to the canal of Schlemm has been called the "scleral ring". The longitudinal fibres of the ligament terminate in two divisions—a small superficial portion which blends with the sclera and a larger deep portion that acts as the ligament of origin for the longitudinal and the radiating fibres of the ciliary muscle. At the same time the deep portion acts as a check ligament for the circular fibres. The ring is traversed by fibres which give attachment to the longitudinal bundles of the ciliary muscle and acts as an anchor for the ligament when the muscle is in action. He found it present only in the human eye. It is possibly a ligament for the ciliary muscle and a meshwork through the spaces of which aqueous may pass into Schlemm's canal, and also according to Henderson into the supra-choroidal space. He considered that the experimental injections of Indian ink as well as histological studies prove that the connection with the latter space is not merely a potential one. He held that the corneal endothelium is directly continuous with that of the supra-choroidea and does not spread over the anterior surface of the iris, as is usually stated. He thought that the cribriform ligament was formed as a homogeneous tissue, similar to Descemet's membrane, by the endothelium which lines the alveoli of the pectinate ligament.

Smith (1936) held the view that the action of the band of ciliary muscle on the scleral spur was more like that of a sluice than a pump, as Thomson suggested. He considered that the pressure in the collecting venules of the canal of Schlemm was most probably in the neighbourhood of 5·0 mm. of mercury instead of 22·0 mm. as has been assumed. When the muscular band pulls back the scleral spur fluid rushes through the spaces of Fontana, then the muscle relaxes and the elastic ligament adjusts the scleral spur as a valve. He considered that this view is confirmed by the regular opening and closing of the valve as shown in Rycroft's kymographic tracings of the intra-ocular pressure in an exsanguinated cat. The opening and shutting was not a pressure reflex and occurred four times a minute and once to every twenty cardiac beats. The cause of this rhythmic beat is unknown.

THE COMPARATIVE ANATOMY
OF INVOLVED TISSUES

This study of the structures in the ciliary region and angle of the anterior chamber is an attempt to learn something of the evolutionary history of the drainage mechanism in the human eye, and to see what are its defects compared with other mammals.

In regard to the evolution of these structures the following questions arise:

1. Do the structures at the angle in man belong to his ancestral inheritance or are they the results of adaptation to the circumstances of his setting? "An animal, regarded from the point of view of structure, is a complex of the basal plans of heritage and the adaptations of habitus" (Wood Jones, 1929).

2. Is the state of the angle as we know it in the adult human eye a recent attainment? If so we may expect developmental defects and variations. Its phylogenetic youth will make for structural instability.

3. Are we to expect that each of the stages in the development of any one structure in human embryology will have its counterpart in one of the profuse variations found in lower animals? Do all the developmental defects found in human pathology have a corresponding feature in the normal anatomy of lower animals?

An affirmative answer to these last questions would imply too implicit a belief in the recapitulation law of Meckel and Serres, for we do not know the genealogical tree of man. We need not expect to find, for example, counterparts for the foetal state of the human angle of filtration in the horse or the lion. We may regard the extensive meshwork in the horse as an extreme development to meet some special need. Not only are the majority of lower animals related to men merely by means of a very remote common ancestor, but many of them show varying degrees of specialisation of tissue that suit their own environment and make them quite unlike man or any other primate.

Even over-specialisation is possible. This has probably produced not only the snout of platypus and the tree-clinging habits of the koala, but also the eye of *Tarsius*, and so, by a restriction of plasticity, further adaptation to a changing environment has become unlikely. They may therefore join those that, for a similar reason, are represented only in "the record of the rocks". Transgression of

the law of successful minimal adaptive specialisation leads to phylogenetic senility (Wood Jones).

An anatomical study of the eyes of mammals of widely different
genera shows that the following interdependent structures are

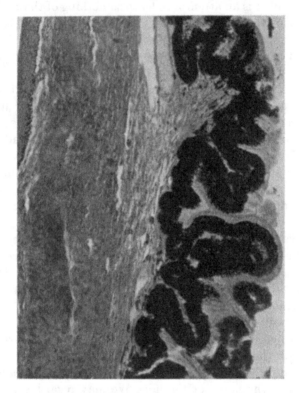

Fig. 35. Ornithorhynchus. × 200. Two lumina resembling a posteriorly situated canal of
Schlemm, are separated from the angle by tissue that is less dense than the sclera,
though scarcely trabecular. Observe the extensive ciliary processes, scanty muscle
fibres and an iris vessel in a characteristic situation.

remarkably constant in their presence and remarkably variable in
their relative degree of development. These structures are:

1. The iris.

2. The ciliary body, in which connective tissue and vessels and
the inmost layer of epithelium are continuous with the same tissues
in the iris. The outer part of the ciliary body consists of longitudinal
fibres of connective tissue and muscle. Circular and radial muscle
fibres may also be present.

3. Ciliary processes, from the inner surface of the ciliary body and sometimes from the iris, supporting the suspensory ligament of the lens.

4. The insertion of the ciliary body into the scleral spur and into the cornea by means of the sclero-corneal trabeculae.

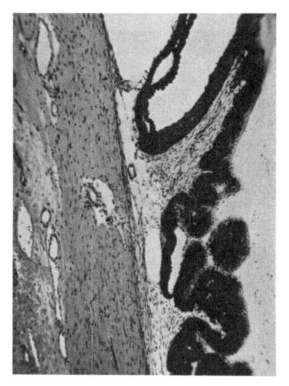

Fig. 36. Echidna. × 100. The anterior part of the very primitive ciliary body is shown. No ciliary muscle is visible and the iris consists almost entirely of vessels and pigment. Schlemm's canal is not present, but the aqueous probably escapes into the vessels in the iris or into others behind the angle, which are continuous with those that perforate the sclera.

5. Sclero-corneal trabeculae—interlacing elastic fibres arising from the posterior deep layers of the cornea and running back to merge with the longitudinal fibres of the ciliary body at the cilio-scleral junction.

6. Uveal tissue of the angle, connecting the root of the iris to Descemet's membrane and the inner fibres of the sclero-corneal trabeculae.

7. The spaces and channels among these tissues by which aqueous fluid may escape from the anterior chamber into the blood stream.

To show at once the similarity and diversity of these structures in different eyes let us investigate a few examples (see Figs. 29, 30, 35 to 46).

The most primitive mammals of which the angle of the anterior chamber has been examined are the Platypus (*Ornithorhynchus*) (see Fig. 35) and the Spiny Ant-eater (*Echidna*) (Fig. 36). As in the Platy-

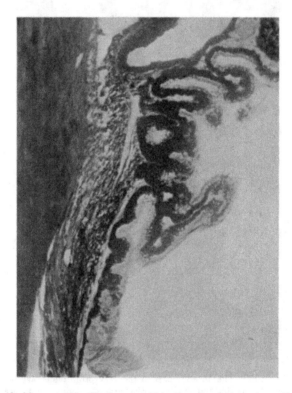

Fig. 37. Pseudochirus. × 100. The lumen within the scleral tissue is a ciliary capillary. There is no definite canal of Schlemm. The cilio-scleral sinus is of moderate size and is bridged by stout iris pillars.

pus, the ciliary body of the Echidna is flat, consisting of a long series of convolutions almost as far back as the tip of the scleral cartilage. Within the scanty fibrous tissue between the pigment layer and the sclera no muscle tissue has been found. This, however, does not mean that none exists, for to be adequate little involuntary tissue is required and such may be difficult to recognise in loose areolar tissue. Branches of anterior ciliary vessels which penetrate the sclera behind the level of the iris root, divide and one series of the division runs to form a freely branching plexus on the surface of the iris. There is little iris stroma, these vessels lying exposed on a double row of pigment cells. The only other structure visible is a prominent fibrous ring—the sphincter—in which no typically staining muscle tissue has been

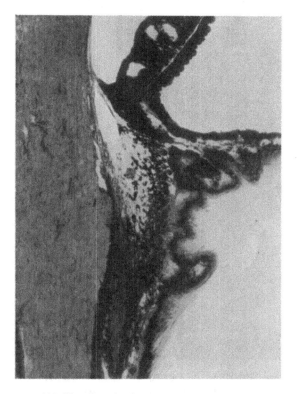

Fig. 38. Dasyurus. × 100. The cilio-scleral sinus is separated from the anterior chamber by a dense iris process and from the primitive canal of Schlemm by loose pigmented tissue. Profuse meshwork.

found. No canal of Schlemm has been found, though close to the lumen of the vessel that, in most sections, lies at the angle, there is a channel which could drain the angle. This opening is much farther forwards than in animals such as the horse and dog. A small cilioscleral sinus is present and a little meshwork lies in front of and behind the vessel at the angle. These animals rely much more on other senses than on vision. The eyes of the next group are in a much more advanced stage of development.

Eyes of the following marsupials were examined: the native cat (*Dasyurus viverinus*), the Ringtailed Phalanger (*Pseudochirus*), the Longtailed Phalanger (*Trichosurus*), the Wombat (*Phascolomys* and the Grey Kangaroo (*Macropus giganteus*).

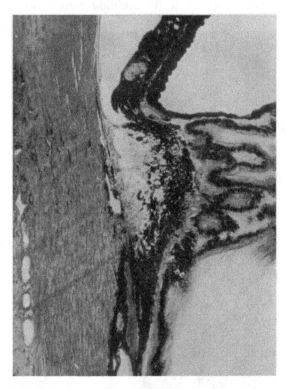

Fig. 39. Dasyurus. ×100. Another section for contrast. Observe the definite scleral promontory, the strand of ciliary muscle and the loose tissue separating cilio-scleral sinus from the primitive canal of Schlemm and the anterior chamber.

In these one found many differences from the state just described and many variations in the different species. In most sections the *Pseudochirus* revealed a very primitive state and the *Dasyurus* a more advanced one (see Figs. 37, 38, 39). The latter will be described here. The iris and the ciliary region are richly pigmented in these animals. The development of muscle tissue is much more advanced than in Echidna. The ciliary processes occupy less of the ciliary area than in monotremes, but protrude farther into the interior of the eye. Beneath the more posterior processes lies a well-defined band of muscle tissue which appears to be inserted into a very marked scleral prominence. Immediately in front of this, in most sections, several flat lumina are found. They are bounded externally by sclera, and on their inner aspect is a strand of pigmented tissue which stretches between the scleral promontory and the margin of the cornea. This tissue is less

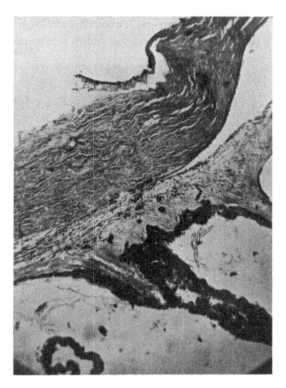

Fig. 40. Rabbit. ×65. The deep and narrow angle is shown with Descemet's membrane extending to its apex. Greater magnification revealed two endothelium-lined lumina, one of which lies in the corneal tissues just anterior to the end of Descemet's membrane. A small cilio-scleral sinus is present.

dense than sclera, but is not as open as true meshwork. It represents the sclero-corneal trabeculae and is probably permeable to the intra-ocular fluid. Between this strand and the more anterior ciliary processes is a triangular space occupied by a meshwork. The extent of this cilio-scleral space or sinus varies in different sections. In many sections dense iris processes were found, which separated the sinus from the angle. The scleral promontory is well marked in the Wallaby (*Thylogale*) and almost like a spur. It is composed of equatorially directed fibres. A singularly long and slender strand of muscle runs from the level of the ora serrata to this "spur".

Turning to the rabbit (see Figs. 40, 41), we again find ciliary processes on both iris and ciliary body, but their development is not so great compared with other structures. The ciliary muscle is poorly developed but longitudinal muscle fibres can be seen, inserted over a fairly wide area in the sclera. The sclero-corneal trabeculae are long, and covered by Descemet's membrane almost to the point where they pass into

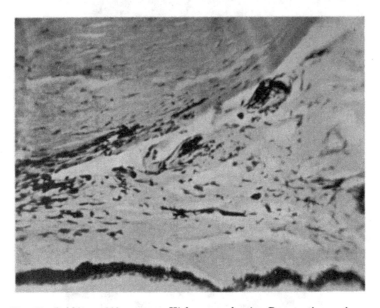

Fig. 41. Rabbit. × 180, approx. High power showing Descemet's membrane extending beyond the first iris process, and curled processes.

the ciliary body. Between them and the sclera, to which they are for the most part closely applied, is a plexus of channels, which is separated only by the sparse fibres of the sclero-corneal trabeculae from the deep cilio-scleral sinus. This is a narrow prolongation of the angle of the anterior chamber, bridged by processes which pass from the iris to Descemet's membrane. These processes are of a hyaline substance which stains similarly to Descemet's membrane, they are clothed with endothelium. They pass into Descemet's membrane near the sclero-corneal junction, and through the spaces among them the aqueous may permeate to the depths of the cilio-scleral sinus.

In the sheep (Fig. 42) the sclera is slightly prominent in the region of the comparatively narrow ciliary muscle insertion, from which well-developed sclero-corneal trabeculae run forward. Between the latter and the sclera exterior to them are large spaces forming a plexus, which resembles Schlemm's canal in the human eye, except that Schlemm's canal lies in man in front of the apex of the angle, and this plexus lies behind. Few veins are visible in this part of the sclera, but

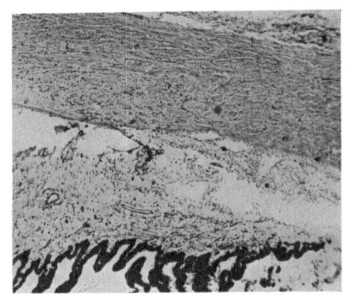

Fig. 42. Sheep. × 68. The ciliary muscle is poorly developed and has a wide insertion. There is a slight scleral prominence. The trabeculae are well defined, forming an open mesh. Iris pillars arise opposite the ciliary processes and are attached to the end of Descemet's membrane. The cilio-scleral sinus extends back to the level of the well-developed canal of Schlemm. The apex of the sinus is full of open mesh.

occasionally a small one is found in communication with these lumina of Schlemm's canal. The cilio-scleral sinus extends backwards almost to the level of the plexus and is bridged anteriorly as in the rabbit by hyaline processes, and posteriorly by more delicate tissue whose meshes become more dense till the spaces of the sinus, known also as spaces of Fontana, disappear among them. The iris is thick, shows a sphincter and dilatator, and carries some of the ciliary processes. Opposite the most anterior of these the hyaline processes or pillars arise, to be inserted into the end of Descemet's membrane. These, when seen at the boundary of the anterior chamber on macroscopic dissection, give the appearance of a comb—hence the term "pectinate ligament".

The angle in the eye of the goat, the cow and the horse (see Fig. 43) largely resembles that of the sheep. The cilio-scleral sinus extends beyond the hyaline pillars which run to the margin of Descemet's membrane. The ciliary muscle is inserted mainly into the scleral promontory which lies behind a well-marked canal of Schlemm. The

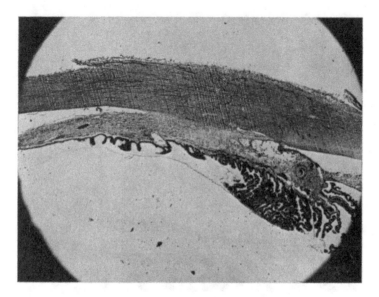

Fig. 43. Cow. ×12. Showing moderate development of the longitudinal fibres of the ciliary muscle with a wide scleral attachment. The muscle is posterior to a thickening of the sclera. The tissue lying between this and the well-marked cilio-scleral sinus is open in texture and resembles the iris. A well-defined canal of Schlemm is visible. A pillar of hyaline material runs from near the end of Descemet's membrane to the iris. This lies opposite the most anterior of the ciliary processes.

remaining muscle fibres end in the meshwork that is attached to the periphery of the cornea near the apex of the sinus. In the horse much of the deep uveal meshwork is replaced by pillars of hyaline material with a collagenous core.

In the pig (see Fig. 44) Descemet's membrane and the hyaline pillars are much thinner. The sinus is very deep and the sparse ciliary muscle lying behind it is inserted as in the other herbivora. Schlemm's canal is represented by a series of channels that are smaller than those in the sheep.

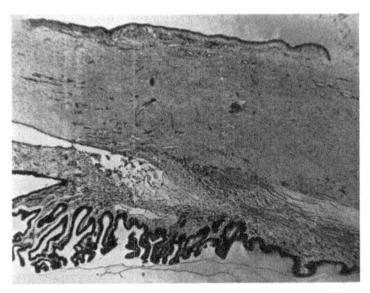

Fig. 44. Pig. × 30. The inner part of the ciliary muscle is more developed than in the sheep, though hardly wedge-shaped (see the dog). There is a slight scleral spur, but a wide area of insertion of ciliary muscle. The sclero-corneal trabeculae are extensive but ill-defined. Superficial to them are several small lumina but no well-defined canal of Schlemm. The cilio-scleral sinus is deep and contains much meshwork.

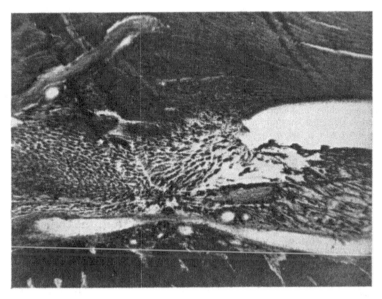

Fig. 45. Hippopotamus. × 140. The ciliary muscle is poorly developed, and owing to oblique sectioning the insertion is indefinite. For the same reason the sclero-corneal trabeculae are cut across and appear to radiate from the cornea close to Descemet's membrane. The shallow cilio-scleral sinus is bridged by iris processes. There are well-marked lumina between the trabeculae and sclera. A ciliary nerve and vein are also seen.

In the dog (see Fig. 46) while the hyaline tissues are as in the pig, the muscle tissues of the iris and of the ciliary body are more highly developed and more pigmented than in herbivora. Some fibres of the ciliary muscle run towards the base of the iris, others end in the mesh-work, and the remainder are attached to the poorly marked scleral promontory. The first group of fibres can be traced to a point well in

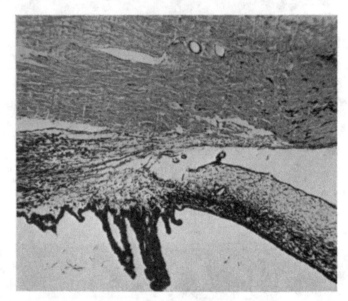

Fig. 46. Dog. ×65. Showing forward position and narrowing of anterior attachment of ciliary muscle to the sclera. The scleral spur is well marked. The ciliary muscle is not spindle-shaped as in ungulates but is wedge-shaped with the wide end forwards. A deep cilio-scleral sinus is present. The most anterior iris pillars are attached to the end of Descemet's membrane. The sclero-corneal trabeculae are well marked and form an inner wall to the canal of Schlemm. The superficial vessels are part of the circle of Hovius.

front of the bottom of the deep cilio-scleral sinus. Between the sclero-corneal trabeculae and sclera is a large plexus freely communicating with numerous superficial scleral veins (the circle of Hovius). Well-developed corneo-scleral trabeculae originate from the cornea just in front of the end of Descemet's membrane, which is sometimes level with the anterior lumen of Schlemm's canal.

In the monkey (see Fig. 29) (*Macacus Rhesus*) the muscle is more strongly developed with inner circular and radial fibres as well as numerous longitudinal ones. The scleral spur and sclero-corneal trabeculae are well defined and between them and the sclera lies a large Schlemm's canal. Only the most anterior ciliary processes reach the level of this canal, which lies well behind the end of Descemet's membrane, and the iris pillars appear as occasional fine processes inserted in the sclero-corneal trabeculae. In the *Macacus Rhesus*, the Grey-cheeked Mangaby and some other monkeys, a corneal spur projects backwards over the front portion of Schlemm's canal. This spur is most marked in Jentinck's cercopithique (Henderson, 1921). The fibres of the "cribriform ligament" radiate back-

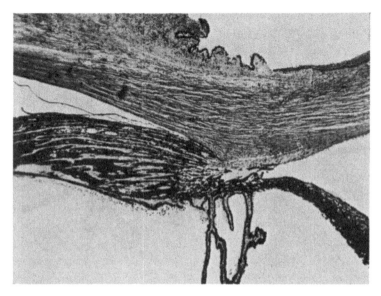

Fig. 47. Tarsius. ×50. The insertion of the powerful ciliary muscle into the prominent scleral spur is shown. No canal of Schlemm has been found. The spur is traversed by a fine radial vessel.

wards from the corneal spur. The angle of the human eye (see Fig. 48) resembles that of the monkey, except that the muscle is still better developed and the iris pillars more rare.

These descriptions, it is hoped, will be sufficient to give a general idea of what may be found in mammalian eyes. Eyes from a number of other genera were examined, but nothing remarkable was noticed in them. Just as the ciliary body, etc. was very much the same in all Ungulata, the region of the angle in other Carnivora (*e.g.* cat, lion) was found closely to resemble that of the dog.

This brings us to an interesting point in connection with the marsupials. A glance at the microphotographs shows that the carnivorous *Dasyurus* has the narrow ciliary muscle insertion in a well-defined scleral prominence, the well-formed sclero-corneal trabeculae and canal of Schlemm, and the wide cilio-scleral sinus bridged by few iris pillars, that are found in the true mammalian carnivores, whereas the herbivorous phalanger has a ciliary muscle extending behind the ora serrata, and a wide flattish scleral insertion, poorly defined trabeculae, a few irregular lumina in place of Schlemm's canal, and a narrow sinus bridged by well-defined iris pillars.

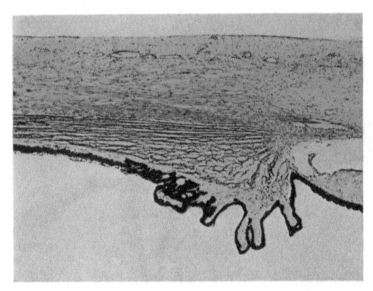

Fig. 48. Man. × 35. The ciliary muscle is highly developed and wedge-shaped and shows radial and circular as well as horizontal fibres. The former help to form the square end of the wedge. The sclero-corneal trabeculae form a well-marked band joining the scleral spur. There is a large canal of Schlemm. The iris process in this section indicates the relationship of the angle of the anterior chamber in man to the cilio-scleral sinus of lower mammals.

Dasyurus and the domestic cat provide an example of convergent evolution under a similar mode of life. The structures we have discussed are so similar in the two animals that we might suppose them to be of related genera, but possibly the cat is more closely related to the cow than to *Dasyurus*.

We must remember that this has so far been a purely comparative, not an evolutionary, study. As we have no record of man's remote ancestors we cannot hope to trace his detailed ocular development. But the points of resemblance in all the eyes studied lead us to suppose that far back in evolutionary history we should find a fairly flat ciliary body with a wide insertion in the sclera, a canal of Schlemm or its homologue, and a uveal meshwork blocking the angle of the anterior chamber at the end of Descemet's membrane, but containing a system of spaces, the cilio-scleral sinus, by which aqueous fluid permeates to the region of Schlemm's canal. The eye of *Dasyurus* probably bears most resemblance to this type.

We may discuss the later developments under the following headings:

1. The consolidation, growth and forward spread of the ciliary muscle.
   The development of the scleral spur.
2. The modification of the drainage of the angle.
   The emergence of Schlemm's canal.
3. The modification of the cilio-scleral sinus and the meshwork of the angle.

Amongst recent works that of Troncoso and Castroviejo (1936) on the comparative anatomy of the angle of the anterior chamber is of interest. They examined with the slit-lamp a large series of mammals' eyes, both living and dead, and compared their findings with the results of dissection under a microscope and with gonioscopic appearances. Such methods are a valuable aid to the study of the normal state of this region.

The consolidation, growth and forward spread of the ciliary muscle. This is associated with the need for accommodation. We find a flat muscle lying far back in animals whose eyes are of little importance in the search for food. In the phalangers which are nocturnal almost half of the ciliary muscle lies behind the ora serrata. In Carnivora, who require some power of accommodation for seizing their prey, the muscle is thicker, swelling out from its scleral insertion so as to fill some of the space otherwise occupied by the cilio-scleral sinus. In Primates alone, circular and radial muscle fibres are present, and the bulk of the whole muscle is very much greater and lies anteriorly.

Scleral spur. In most marsupials and in rodents and ungulates there is a slight scleral prominence at the site of the wide ciliary muscle insertion. This prominence is more marked in carnivorous marsupials and mammals, and in some sections of the dog's filtration angle it closely resembles the scleral spur that projects over the posterior half of Schlemm's canal in man. Thus the more developed the ciliary muscle is, the narrower is its area of insertion and the more prominent the sclera at this point. In certain mammals the main part of the ciliary muscle is situated posteriorly and only an apparently detached slip of tissue approaches the end of Descemet's membrane. In the evolutionary history of man we may assume that as sight became of increasing importance, along with the attainment of binocular vision, an ever greater power of accommodation was required, so that the ciliary muscle thickened and developed till it filled most of the space in this region. Its scleral insertion became stronger and denser, but at the same time narrower, to give the muscle greater play. The ciliary muscle is attached to the outer coats in two places, at its scleral insertion and by the sclero-corneal trabeculae. In man the maximum of free play for the muscle has been attained by the projection of the spur into the trabecular region so that the muscle is attached only at a single point, somewhat farther forward than in ancestors in whom the spur had not developed. The muscle is fixed, as it were, not directly to the sclera proper, but to a point on an arc whose two ends are fixed. This arrangement is of importance as regards the "pump-like action" of ciliary contraction, discussed elsewhere, but the dense spur and trabeculae of man probably form a less permeable wall than do the more open trabeculae which act as the only barrier between Schlemm's canal and the cilio-scleral sinus of most mammals. The iris crypts found in higher mammals only may be a supplementary exit for aqueous.

The emergence of Schlemm's canal. If we define it as one or more endothelial-lined lumina separated from the angle of the anterior chamber only by trabeculae and loose meshwork, a canal of Schlemm is to be found in all mammals we have examined except monotremes, but if it is essential for the posterior half of the canal to be separated from the anterior chamber by a scleral spur a canal of Schlemm is present in Primates only.

Within the sclera in certain mammals there is a venous plexus known as Schlemm's venous plexus. As it has been mistaken for Schlemm's canal it is wise to call it the intra-scleral venous plexus. Its vessels are most marked in Carnivora. They can be studied with the slit-lamp in the dog and the cat but are less developed in Herbivora. Nuel and Benoit (1900) suggested that Schlemm's canal develops from certain branches of this plexus.

In addition, one frequently finds several lumina apparently separated from the spaces of the cilio-scleral sinus by strands of meshwork.

The distance of these lumina from the end of Descemet's membrane appears to vary with the state of development of the iris pillars. These lumina are probably so closely related to Schlemm's canal that nothing is gained by calling them by any other name.

In the dog Wegefarth (1914–15) observed tufts of mesothelial cells which projected from the pectinate ligament into small openings in the middle third of the inner scleral surface between the ciliary body and Descemet's membrane. He called them "pectinate villi" because he considered they bore a structural and functional resemblance to the arachnoid villi of the brain. He was not able to find more than six such openings or stomata in the circumference of the angle. "Drainage, therefore, in the eye of the dog cannot be considered as a process taking place throughout the entire circumference of the angle, but is limited in its extent to these irregularly placed stomata in the wall of the sclera." Wegefarth thought that drainage took place through these tufts rather than round them. He described a similar state in the eyes of the rabbit and the cat. Even in the monkey (*Macacus Rhesus*) he observed: "suggestions of cell growths from the body of the trabecula into the lumen of the canal".

It is possible that such stomata lead into spaces which branch and that the branches unite and so complete the circular sinus known in primates as Schlemm's canal. In many human foetal eyes the lumina of this canal are found in only some of the sections. Wegefarth considered that the masses of cells, pigmented and unpigmented, found by Seefelder in certain hydrophthalmic eyes, were scattered villus-like projections that were inadequate for the task of absorbing the aqueous. Seefelder, on the other hand, considered them to be obstructions to the escape of fluid.

Our observations differed from those of Wegefarth.

We found in all the mammalian eyes examined a plexus which seems to correspond to the canal of Schlemm, lying anterior to the main insertion of the ciliary muscle, and between the corneo-scleral trabeculae and the sclera. There is by no means always a true canal in this area, but there are always a number of channels, frequently anastomosing, and with numerous communications with vessels in the sclera exterior to them.

Studying serial sections of any eye one finds that while these channels may be few and small in one section, they will probably enlarge or unite a few sections later. There is often a characteristic difference between the nasal and the temporal portions. Even where the channels are fewest, they are more numerous in this particular area than anywhere in the neighbouring tissues, and in most mammalian eyes one may find a few sections at least showing a canal as distinct as that of Schlemm in a human eye. But the canal is more definite where there is a well-developed scleral prominence, and most definite in the human eye where the scleral ring, or spur, reaches its maximum development, and the canal lies in the groove between this ring and the rest of the sclera. It seems that where the attachment of the uvea to the outer coats is clearly defined and concentrated in a small space, the neighbouring canals also are clearly defined and are concentrated into one or two large lumina.

It should be pointed out that we do not know for certain that these small channels or vessels actually resemble Schlemm's canal in containing aqueous fluid only. Blood corpuscles were not found in them, but neither were they in the neighbouring scleral arteries, nor in most veins. It is mainly because they are separated from the anterior chamber by meshwork only that these channels appear analogous to Schlemm's canal.

Their position relative to the angle of the anterior chamber, on the other hand, varies greatly, or appears to do so, if one considers that the angle is situated at the point where the iris pillars or pectinate ligament arise. But if one compares the farthest points to which the aqueous fluid has free access, that is to say, the bottom of the cilio-scleral sinus, we find the conditions more nearly similar. The deepest part of the sinus is on a level with the middle of the Schlemm-like plexus in the sheep and cow, and extends slightly beyond it in the dog and in man.

In the *Macacus Rhesus* the cilio-scleral sinus has almost gone and Schlemm's canal sometimes appears as two narrow parallel slits. The lumen can be opened by pulling inwards the root of the iris, but it does not widen when the fibres of the ciliary muscle are drawn down with forceps. This suggests that contraction of the pupil as well as of the ciliary muscle may widen the lumen of Schlemm's canal.

It is probable that as the iris grows more muscular it becomes less vascular and the ciliary processes become more profuse and more vascular (compare Echidna and dog).

The cilio-scleral sinus. In most mammals there is the cilio-scleral sinus which lies between the sclera and the ciliary body and is not a canal. In the rabbit at times interlacing fibres separate the large spaces in this sinus. Similar spaces found by Fontana in the cow are known as "Fontana's spaces". The slit-lamp shows that the sinus in Ungulata is filled with spongy tissue. This sinus being a prolongation of the anterior chamber is filled with aqueous. The exact function of the spongy tissue is obscure. It does not contain vessels, but it may, by capillary attraction, soak up aqueous and so aid the circulation of fluid from the anterior chamber into the sinus, which, in large eyes containing a great amount of aqueous, may be a difficult process. In the cat and the dog the cavity of the sinus is filled with fine thread-like fibres which may play some part in absorption. It is more probable, however, that Henderson was correct when he assumed that these fibres play some rôle in accommodation, and from their position it is still more probable that their function is to give adequate support to the iris and large lens.

Maggiore and others incorrectly described the upper space of this sinus as a canal. The angle of this sinus does not develop into the angle proper of the anterior chamber. As a result, however, of the enormous development of the ciliary muscle in monkeys and man, and the movement forward of the insertion of the ciliary body to the scleral spur, the greater part of the sinus is replaced by muscle. In man, only the most anterior part of the sinus remains, and it is opened so that it becomes the angle of the anterior chamber. In a few human eyes one finds occasional fine strands of uveal framework bridging the extremity of the angle (see Figs. 12, 48).

Henderson considered that even in man the aqueous may come into direct contact with ciliary tissue by passing between the heads of origin of the ciliary muscle, into the suprachoroidal space as well as into the loose stroma of the ciliary body generally. If this view is correct, there is some slight resemblance to the deeper parts of the primitive cilio-scleral sinus.

The uveal meshwork. We have seen that in most mammals the cilio-scleral sinus is filled with this meshwork. It reaches its state of highest development in the "iris pillars" or "pectinate ligament" of ungulates. Since the deepest part of the angle of the anterior chamber in man represents the remains of the sinus, the meshwork which fills the angle in the foetal human eye is therefore comparable with the "pectinate ligament" of a cow. It should not, however, be called by the same name, for its structure is dense and indefinite, and it is unwanted in the adult eyes, whereas the true pectinate ligament has a well-developed structure peculiarly its own and is presumably of functional importance, perhaps as indirect support, through the iris and ciliary processes, of the large heavy lens.

In lower mammals the meshwork suspends the root of the iris and connects the detached portion of the ciliary body to the corneo-scleral wall. The sinus has almost vanished in monkeys, but a small space exists between the iris root and the anterior, concave border of the ciliary body. The iris is still suspended from the cornea by the uveal meshwork which, conversely, prevents the iris from coming in contact with the cornea. In the chimpanzee the root of the iris is attached to the anterior border of the ciliary body by a narrow strip of tissue. Treacher Collins has pointed out that the reduction in size of the cornea as compared with that of the globe seems to be associated with a prolongation outwards of the angle of the anterior chamber and a simplification of the structure of the meshwork.

In monkeys and especially the chimpanzee the innermost trabeculae are more widely separated, bend down sooner to be attached to the root of the iris and have larger spaces between them than in the human eye.

In man, although the rudimentary fibres of the uveal meshwork are still inserted into the last roll and the upper part of the iris root, they do not suspend this membrane, which has become firmly attached to the ciliary body and no longer needs support. Below the last roll, between the iris root and the scleral wall, there is a small depression. This is the only vestige of the cilio-scleral sinus. In the recess, the anterior border of the ciliary body is directly exposed to the anterior chamber, being covered only by the fibres of the uveal meshwork.

The researches of Troncoso and Castroviejo (1936) have shown that the fibres of the uveal meshwork in man, though much less developed than in monkeys and Carnivora, are much more numerous than they appeared to those observers whose investigations were purely histo-logical.

Conclusions

In attaining the unequalled range of accommodation of the human eye, the primitive features have undergone profound modifications, all tending to give greater power and free play to the ciliary muscle. This muscle, its scleral insertion and Schlemm's canal have moved forwards towards the true angle of the anterior chamber. The canal of Schlemm is still in much the same position relative to the cilio-scleral sinus as in other mammals, but in man the sinus is generally so empty of uveal tissue that it appears like part of the angle. The disappearance of this meshwork gives the ciliary muscle maximum freedom, but may be a real loss to the eye, if we are right in supposing that a true pectinate ligament aids the circulation of aqueous by capillary attraction, and by preventing the iris root from coming in contact with the cornea.

The modifications found in the human eye are so considerable, and being associated with accommodation and binocular vision, must be so recent phylogenetically, that it is not surprising they should be somewhat unstable. Any slight extraneous or hereditary influence might cause one or more of the structures concerned to develop abnormally. Man's ciliary region exhibits a fine balance between the claims of accommodation and of drainage, and the proper functioning of each part is so dependent on the integrity of the others that the slightest abnormality may have far-reaching effects.

REFERENCES

The Development of the Involved Tissues

1899 COLLINS, E. T. Utrecht Congress. Abst. *Zeitschr. f. Augenheilk.* 2. Beilageheft.
1904 PARSONS, J. H. *Pathology of the Eye*, 1, pt. 1. London: Hodder and Stoughton.
1906 HOTTA, G. *Arch. f. Ophthal.* 62, 250.
1906 SEEFELDER, R. *Arch. f. Ophthal.* 63, 481.
1906 SEEFELDER and WOLFRUM. *Arch. f. Ophthal.* 63, 440.
1917 SPECIALE-CIRINCIONE. *Ann. Ottal. e clin. Ocul.* 40. Quoted by *Kurzes Handb. der Ophthal.* 1, 503. Berlin: J. Springer, 1930.
1923 KREKLER, F. *Arch. f. Augenheilk.* 93, 144.
1925 CUCCHIA, A. *Soc. Ital. di Oftal.* 336. Abst. *Ophthal. Lit.* 1927, p. 79.
1926 KAYSER, B. *Arch. f. Ophthal.* 116.
1930–31 SONDERMANN, R. *Arch. f. Ophthal.* 124, 151; 126, 341.
1932 DUKE-ELDER, W. S. *Text Book of Ophthal.* 1, 369. London: Kimpton.
1933 FISCHER, F. *Arch. f. Ophthal.* 131, 326.
1935 REESE, A. B. *Amer. Jl. Ophthal.* 18, 6.

The Anatomy of Involved Tissues

1899 HEINE. *Arch. f. Ophthal.* 40, 1.
1899 COLLINS, E. T. Utrecht Congress. Abst. *Zeitschr. f. Augenheilk.* 2. Beilageheft.
1904 PARSONS, J. H. *Pathology of the Eye*, 1, pt. 1, 285.
1906 SEEFELDER, R. *Arch. f. Ophthal.* 63, 205.
1908 HENDERSON, T. *Trans. Ophthal. Soc. U.K.* 28, 47.
1911 THOMSON, A. *The Ophthalmoscope*, 9, 472.
1912 SALZMANN, M. *Anatomy and Hist. of the Human Eyeball*, p. 233.

1913 BUCHANAN, L. *Brit. Med. Jl.* Aug. p. 399.

1917 MAGGIORE. *Ann. di Ottal. e clin. Ocul.* **40,**,317.

1921 HENDERSON, T. *Trans. Ophthal. Soc. U.K.* **41**, 465.

1922 ELLIOT, R. H. *A Treatise on Glaucoma*, p. 621. London: Frowde and Hodder and Stoughton.

1923 KREKLER, F. *Arch. f. Augenheilk.* **93**, 144.

1925 CUCCHIA, A. *Soc. Ital. di Oftal.* p. 336. Abst. *Ophthal. Lit.* 1927.

1926 KAYSER, B. *Arch. f. Augenheilk.* **116**.

1929 SONDERMANN, R. *XIII Concilium Ophth. Amsterdam*, **1**, 249. F. van Rossen.

1930 EISLER, P. *Kurzes Handb. der Ophthal.* **1**, 102.

1930 SEEFELDER, R. *Kurzes Handb. der Ophthal.* **1**, 503.

1930 SONDERMANN, R. *Arch. f. Ophthal.* **124**, 151. Quoted by Fischer, 1933.

1931 SONDERMANN, R. *Arch. f. Ophthal.* **126**, 341. Quoted by Fischer, 1933.

1932 DUKE-ELDER, W. S. *Textbook of Ophthal.* **1**, 77. London: Kimpton.

1933 DE VILLIERS, H. *Brit. Jl. Ophthal.* **17**, 675.

1933 FISCHER, F. *Arch. f. Ophthal.* **131**, 318.

1933 SONDERMANN, R. *R. Acta Ophthal.* **11**, 3, 28.

1934 DUKE-ELDER, SIR STEWART. *Recent Advances in Ophthal.* p. 127. London: Churchill.

1934 THEOBALD, G. D. *Trans. Amer. Ophthal. Soc.* **32**, 593.

1936 FRIEDENWALD, J. S. *Arch. of Ophthal.* **16**, 65 and 8.

1936 BARKAN, O. *Arch. of Ophthal.* **15**, 103.

1936 SMITH, H. *Arch. of Ophthal.* **15**, 42.

1936 TRONCOSO and GIVNER. *Amer. Jl. Ophthal.* **19**, 549.

COMPARATIVE ANATOMY

1900 NUEL and BENOIT. *Arch. d'Ophtal.* **20**, 183.

1914–15 WEGEFARTH, P. *Jl. Med. Research*, **26**, 127.

1921 HENDERSON, T. *Trans. Ophthal. Soc. U.K.* **41**, 465.

1929 WOOD JONES, F. *Man's Place among the Mammals*, p. 36. London: Arnold.

1936 TRONCOSO and CASTROVIEJO. *Amer. Jl. Ophthal.* **19**, 371, 481, 583.

CHAPTER IV

THE PATHOLOGY OF CONGENITAL GLAUCOMA

The information for this chapter has been gleaned from previous writings and particularly the reports of specimens in the literature. The series of Seefelder, Takashima, Magitot and Lagrange have been most instructive. In addition five specimens have been described by the author for the first time. They are referred to in the following manner: unpublished specimen I, which may have been an example of infantile staphyloma; unpublished specimens II and V supplied by Dr W. A. Fairclough of Auckland—the former was described microscopically by Dr Eisdell Moore; unpublished specimens III and IV supplied by Mr Humphrey Neame, London; and unpublished specimen VI supplied by Dr E. O. Marks of Brisbane. Dr J. M. Wheeler of New York very kindly sent the author slides of his specimen with neurofibromatosis described in the *Transactions of the American Ophthalmological Society*, **34**, 151 (1936) (Figs. 88 to 94).

INTERFERENCE WITH FUNCTION

The child with hydrophthalmia when first brought to the doctor presents a characteristic picture. The enlarged and hazy cornea is usually obvious. As a rule the head is held down because of photophobia and therefore examination may be difficult. On closer inspection the widening and flattening of the sclero-corneal angle, the bluish sclera and the deep anterior chamber are noticed. Frequently a tremulousness of the iris and a yellowish pupillary reflex are observed in the late stages. The tension is usually raised, and the optic disc may be cupped. Some difficulty in fixation and later partial or complete blindness completes the clinical picture of advanced bilateral hydrophthalmia.

Refraction. Myopia is the most common refractive condition found. It is usually present in only a moderate degree, viz. from 1–7 dioptres, and is not as marked as the increased length of the eye would suggest. The relationship between the length of axis and the degree of ametropia which is nearly constant in myopia, does not hold in hydrophthalmia.

Parsons (1920) gave three reasons why the hydrophthalmic eye is not nearly so myopic as its axial elongation would suggest. They were:

(1) The flattening of the cornea. Its radius of curvature approximates that of the sclerotic and is not uncommonly 11·0 mm. instead of 7·8 mm.

(2) The flattening of the lens, due to the stretching of the suspensory ligament. "There are no accurate measurements of the lens on record, but we shall not be far wrong in taking the average thickness to be

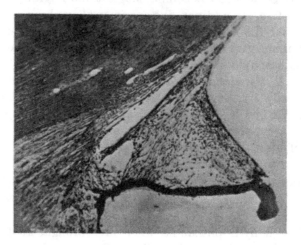

Fig. 49. Case of aniridia, showing mesodermal tissue separating the well-developed canal of Schlemm from the anterior chamber. (Seefelder, 1908.)

reduced from 4·0 mm. to 3·0 mm. and the radii of curvature of the anterior and posterior surfaces to be increased from 9·51 mm. and 5·87 mm. to 11·0 mm. and 7·0 mm. respectively."

(3) The displacement backwards of the lens. "In most cases there is a slight real displacement backwards of the suspensory ligament relative to its normal attachment to the ciliary body. This is due to the enlargement of the globe and the expansion of the scleral ring." In addition, there is an enormous displacement relative to the anterior surface of the cornea. The normal distance from the anterior surface of the cornea to the anterior surface of the lens is 3·78 mm. In congenital glaucoma it is approximately 7·3 mm.

Seefelder and Hess considered that the effect of the altered curvature of the cornea was much greater than that due to any displacement of the lens, though Gros believed this to be great. Seefelder found hypermetropia of 2 to 4 D. in four cases, slight or moderate myopia in twenty and myopia of − 12 to − 20 D. in six eyes of his series of thirty. In two of Seefelder's four cases with hypermetropia of 2 to 4 D., hydrophthalmia had been arrested rapidly by therapeutic measures. In another the disease was supposed to have appeared at the age of sixteen years! He observed an emmetropic eye which became myopic in the space of three years, while its fellow, which was not hydrophthalmic, remained emmetropic. In the course of seven years he noticed mixed astigmatism become myopic. In another patient

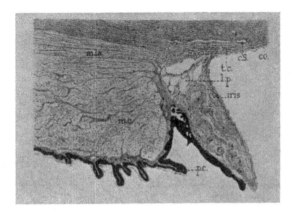

Fig. 50. Specimen of partial aniridia, showing persistent uveal meshwork (*l.p.*) and spaces of Fontana. The canal of Schlemm is undergoing anastomosis with an anterior ciliary vein. (van Duyse, 1907.)

(case 2) the left eye, in which hydrophthalmia was arrested at an early stage, remained emmetropic, while the right eye, in which hypertension persisted, developed a cupped disc and myopia. Gallenga's findings were exceptional, for nine of his ten cases were hypermetropic. Dettmering in a series of fifty-five eyes found twenty to be myopic and in six the myopia was over − 10 D. In three of his cases fundus changes resembling those of myopia were present and in seven a temporal conus. In ten of twenty-two cases reported by Seefelder a conus was present.

Seefelder found no evidence of inheritance to explain the frequency of myopia in hydrophthalmic eyes. With only one exception did an examination of parents, brothers and sisters reveal the presence of myopia.

The fact that myopia is commonly found in association with juvenile glaucoma may mean simply that both are due to a common cause. A study of hydrophthalmia suggests, however, that in some cases of myopia a rise of tension has produced a definite stretching of the coats of the globe. See "Differential Diagnosis".

Astigmatism is usually present, but it varies greatly in degree and type. Seefelder found it to be against the rule in eighteen of twenty eyes. Parsons and Elliot, however, stated that astigmatism was

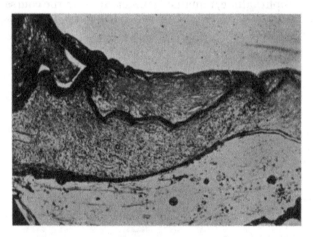

Fig. 51. A layer of newly-formed hyaline material covered by endothelial cells extends over the iris. Connective tissue fills the angle and numerous cells are seen in the iris. Aged twenty years. (Jaensch, Specimen VIII, 1927.)

usually according to the rule. de Grosz and de Gama Pinto shared this view. The divergence in these views is probably due to the variation in the type of refraction with the stage of the hydrophthalmia of the majority of cases in the series. If, for example, most of the cases are early and tension is high and corneal distension not marked, the astigmatism will tend to be against the rule, as it is in adult glaucoma and when the sclera and cornea are hardened by age. If, however, advanced and degenerate cases are in the majority the influence of the lids on the enlarged and plastic cornea will be great and the vertical meridian will be less hypermetropic than the horizontal, as is normal in youth and the rule in megalocornea and keratoconus. In these advanced cases of hydrophthalmia ocular tension may be low, the cornea very distended and the influence of lid-pressure at a maximum. An alteration in the position of the lens may sometimes be a factor in producing a refractive change. In the questionnaire in only six cases was the type of astigmatism stated. It was oblique in one and against the rule in five. All these were advanced cases, the ages varying from eight to seventeen years.

Parsons (1920) calculated the cardinal points of a hydrophthalmic eye of average size. He found that not only would such an eye have to be 31·0 mm. long to be emmetropic, but that an aphakic eye with normal corneal curvature must also be 31·0 mm. long if parallel incident

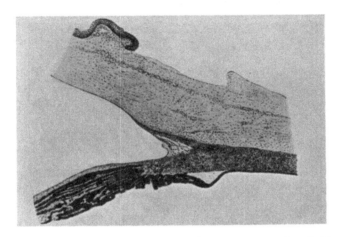

Fig. 52. Filtration angle in hydrophthalmia, containing persistent meshwork. The canal of Schlemm and the scleral spur are absent. The ciliary processes are drawn forwards and adhere to the atrophic iris. Age five months. (Spielberg, 1911.)

rays are to be focused upon the retina without correction. For this to occur this eye must have myopia of 24 D. prior to removal of the lens.

The cardinal points of the hydrophthalmic eye, measured from the apex of the cornea, were found to be:

1st focal point	= − 16·8689 mm.	(− 12·8095 mm.)
2nd focal point	= + 31·1215 mm.	(+ 22·2119 mm.)
1st principal point	= + 3·3714 mm.	(+ 1·9578 mm.)
2nd principal point	= + 3·8669 mm.	(+ 2·3276 mm.)
1st nodal point	= + 10·3857 mm.	(+ 7·0748 mm.)
2nd nodal point	= + 10·8812 mm.	(+ 7·0748 mm.)

The distance between the principal points = the distance between the nodal points = 0·4955 mm. (0·3698 mm.). The normal measurements are within brackets.

Vision. There is no division of opinion regarding the severity of the visual loss, and its progressive nature in spite of treatment. Seefelder, for example, found that 81 % of his series of sixty eyes were quite or almost blind. Ten of the forty-six patients were in blind asylums. In only fifteen was the corrected vision as good as 6/60.

The field loss resembles that in adult glaucoma; the lower and inner quadrants being most affected. Seefelder considered that the colour sense was usually well retained even when the form sense was very defective. In two long-standing cases he found reduced light sense.

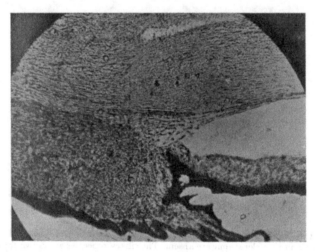

Fig. 53. Hydrophthalmic eye at ten months. Schlemm's canal is represented by a narrow slit lying behind its normal site. It is closed by thickened meshwork. Schlemm's canal was absent in some sections through the upper half of this specimen. (Jaensch, specimen I, 1927.)

Many of the patients are so young that it is difficult to estimate the visual loss. In these and in older patients the colour of the disc and the size of the retinal vessels are probably better criteria than the depth of the cup. The visual loss is due to the atrophy of nerve fibres rather than to the recession of the lamina cribrosa. The occasional association of either a deep cup with a normal field and central vision or the presence of atrophy and marked visual loss with a normal cup must be remembered (Fuchs). The suggestion that deep cups are of necessity due to cavernous atrophy (Schnabel) and not the direct result of hypertension is disproved by the reduction in the depth of the cup when tension returns to normal after miotic or operative therapy.

In addition to optic atrophy reduced vision may be due to one or more of the following disorders: (1) various forms of corneal opacification, (2) cataract, (3) vitreous opacities, (4) retinal detachment, (5) refractive changes, (6) an associated anomaly.

Intra-ocular pressure. The ocular tension in congenital glaucoma is not uncommonly within normal limits. Eventually, however, one will find it raised unless the patient in question presents an example of the abortive form. Later still the tension may be found to fall when a retinal detachment or other form of degeneration occurs. A sudden fall in tension may accompany the formation of a retinal tear and detachment. The fall was so marked and the collapse of the globe so complete in a case reported by Hühn (1929) that the presence of a spontaneous scleral rupture was suggested. The right cornea became depressed and the globe shrank to one-tenth the size of its fellow which it had equalled three days previously.

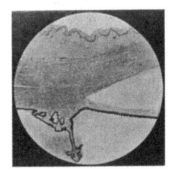

Fig. 54. Signs of inflammation. Schlemm's canal is represented by round and connective tissue cells. There are probably signs of aplasia. The outer trabeculae are dense and the ciliary muscle foetal. Aged two and a half years. (Reis, specimen I. 1905.)

The tension is frequently about 50 mm. Hg, but Gilbert (1912) has reported a reading of 100 mm.

There is a daily variation similar to that which occurs in primary glaucoma. As a rule the pressure tends to be higher in the morning than in the evening and to rise again in the early hours of the morning.

Tonometry is almost exclusively of value as a comparative estimation for an individual patient rather than a means of ascertaining the absolute tension at one time. The following are causes of individual variations: the altered shape of the cornea, the lessened resistance of this tissue and of the sclera, and the effect of a general anaesthetic which is essential in young children. We do not know what is a normal reading for a distended hydrophthalmic eye.

The oedema of the cornea and its consequent cloudiness is often a valuable guide to hypertension. Jaensch, however, stated that tension could be raised for some time before the steaminess became visible.

ALTERATIONS IN STRUCTURE

The orbit and the globe. An increase in the size of the orbit may be observed clinically and seen by X-rays. Wessely (1920) held the view that this is probably not simply a widening due to pressure from a distended globe but rather a correlated growth, independent of pressure.

When one remembers how enormously the globes may distend with congenital glaucoma it is not to be wondered that at times one finds

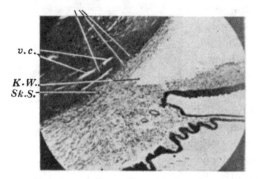

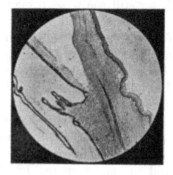

Fig. 55. The angle (*K.W.*) is open. Observe the foetal position of Schlemm's canal, the poorly developed spur, and the compact outer trabeculae. Aged ten months. (Seefelder, specimen I, 1906.)

Fig. 56. The inner lamellae of the meshwork are dense. The canal of Schlemm is almost absent. There are no signs of inflammation. Aged five and a half years. (Reis, specimen II, 1905.)

an enlarged orbit. Coronat and Aurand (1912) recorded a globe that measured 44·0 mm. by 30·0 mm. The measurements of Lagrange's third and sixth specimens were: antero-posterior axis 44·0 mm. in each and equatorial diameter 25·0 and 27·0 mm. respectively. Cross (1896) examined a globe that was 40·0 × 27·0 mm. In one series the average antero-posterior diameter was 32·0 mm., the maximum being 38·8 (normal 24·3) and the average vertical diameter was 26·0 and the maximum was 28·6 (normal 23·6). The eye of the newborn is 16·0 mm. long and by the age of eight years the average length is 24·0 mm.

The ocular distension leads to an increase in all dimensions. The following figures are the averages of seventeen specimens:

Antero-posterior axis: 29·8 mm. (normal 24·15).
Horizontal diameter: 27·3 mm. (,,   24·13).
Vertical diameter: 26·0 mm. (,,   23·48).

The increase in the antero-posterior axis is apparently greatest.

The ratios of the diameters of the cornea to those of the globe show an increase with one exception:

The horizontal diameter of cornea: sagittal diameter of globe is 1·6 : 3 (normal 1·4 : 3).

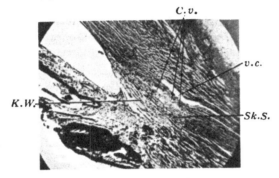

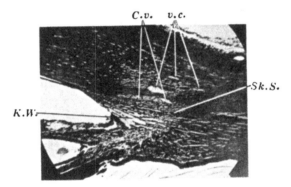

Figs. 57 and 58. Persistent uveal meshwork with torn trabeculae. The angle (*K.W.*) is full of persistent meshwork. Observe the foetal position of the well-developed Schlemm's canal (*C.v.*) and scleral spur (*Sk.S.*). The iris and ciliary body are also foetal. "Remains of an almost vanished irido-cyclitis." Aged seven days. (Seefelder, specimen II, 1906.)

The horizontal diameter of cornea: horizontal diameter of globe is 1·7 : 3 (normal 1·4 : 3).

The vertical diameter of cornea: vertical diameter of globe is 1·3 : 3 (normal 1·36 : 3).

According to Thomson the cornea of a full-time foetus occupies approximately one-fifth of the circumference of the globe. In the adult we may take the corneal arc as being 11·6 mm. and the circumference of the globe as 74·91 mm., that is $\dfrac{0·77}{5}$ or $\dfrac{4·6}{30}$. In the unpublished specimens the following measurements were made:

In   I the cornea occupied $\dfrac{9}{30}$ of the globe.   Cornea = 24·5 mm.
                                                              Circumf. = 82·5 mm.

II   ,,   ,, $\dfrac{4·5}{30}$,,   ,,   Cornea = 10·0 mm.
                                                    Circumf. = 71·5 mm.

III   ,,   ,, $\dfrac{4·8}{30}$,,   ,,   Cornea = 13·5 mm.
                                                    Circumf. = 85·0 mm.

IV   ,,   ,, $\dfrac{9}{30}$,,   ,,   Cornea = 26·5 mm.
                                                    Circumf. = 92·5 mm.

V   ,,   ,, $\dfrac{8}{30}$,,   ,,   Cornea = 19·0 mm.
                                                    Circumf. = 74·0 mm.

VI   ,,   ,, $\dfrac{7}{30}$,,   ,,   Cornea = 18·0 mm.
                                                    Circumf. = 85·0 mm.

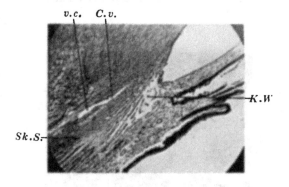

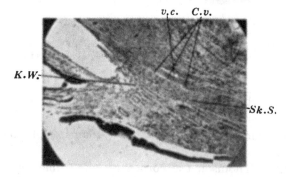

Figs. 59 and 60. The angle of the left eye of specimen II. In addition to other changes an iris process is present. Aged seven days. (Seefelder, specimen III, 1906.)

"The diameter of the cornea at birth is three-fifths of the antero-posterior axis" (Wolff), that is 10·0 mm. to 12·5–15·8 mm. In the adult the proportion is approximately $\frac{4\cdot8}{10}$, that is 11·6 mm. to 24·15 mm. (outer ocular axis). In our specimens the following proportions were found. In the unpublished specimens we found:

In I the relation of the corneal arc to the antero-posterior axis was as				$\frac{7\cdot5}{10}$.	Cornea = 24·5 mm. A.P. Axis = 32·0 mm.	
II	..	,,	,,	$\frac{4}{10}$.	Cornea = 10·0 mm. A.P. Axis = 25·0 mm.	
III	.:	..	..	$\frac{4\cdot4}{10}$.	Cornea = 13·5 mm. A.P. Axis = 29·0 mm.	
IV	:.	..	..	$\frac{7\cdot6}{10}$.	Cornea = 26·5 mm. A.P. Axis = 34·0 mm.	
V	,.	..	..	$\frac{5}{10}$.	Cornea = 19·0 mm. A.P. Axis = 37·0 mm.	
VI	.,	.:	,,	$\frac{5}{10}$.	Cornea = 18·0 mm. A.P. Axis = 35·0 mm.	

It is seen that the increase in the corneal diameter was much greater than was the increase of either the circumference or the antero-posterior axis in all the specimens, except I which had an extensive peripheral synechia, and II which was affected by neuro-fibromatosis. The latter was the earlier specimen, being from a patient five weeks old (see Figs. 3. to 8).

The following are the ocular dimensions of an animal that exhibits the form of megalocornea that is so common in the animal world.

	YOUNG TARSIUS	ADULT TARSIUS
Sagittal diameter	18·0 mm.	20·0 mm.
Vertical diameter	18·0 mm.	19·0 mm.
Horizontal diameter	18·0 mm.	19·0 mm.
Circumference	48·0 mm.	55·0 mm.
Corneal arc (not base or diameter)	16·0 mm.	19·0 mm.

It is seen that the cornea in each specimen occupied almost exactly one-third of the circumference of the globe (one-seventh in man approximately). It is of great interest to observe that in each specimen the corneal arc was almost as great as the sagittal diameter of the globe (three-fifths in man approximately).

NOTE. The use of the term "corneal diameter" is misleading, for it may refer to either the arc or the base of the cornea. In future greater accuracy would be obtained by specifying which is meant.

The size of the angle and the degree of distension. If we exclude specimens showing extensive peripheral synechiae it is of interest to notice the evolution of the eye with developing glaucoma. At first the angle is acute, later it becomes a right angle, and as the stretching continues it becomes obtuse. Its apex even may be torn so that the ciliary muscle is split. In Seefelder's case IV (Figs. 64, 65) many areas were found in which the inner trabeculae of the persistent meshwork were torn from the outer ones, and several areas in which the separated trabeculae appeared to be rolled up as a ball behind the root of the iris. It appears that if distension ceases a proliferation of the new tissue may appear, as in Reis, case IV (Figs. 61, 62).

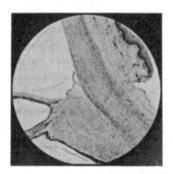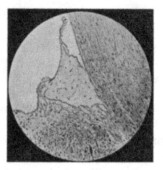

Figs. 61 and 62. The angle is torn open. There are dense trabeculae and persistent uveal meshwork. The new tissue is composed chiefly of fine elastic fibres and its staining qualities suggest that it has developed from the meshwork. The canal of Schlemm is absent and there are no inflammatory signs. Aged four years. (Reis, specimen VI, 1905.)

Most of the acute-angled cases are early cases, the majority being under the age of one year (see Figs. 55, 57 to 60). The following specimens illustrate the various degrees of distension:

(i) Acute angle and slight distension.
Early specimens: Seefelder I, II, III, Meller, Kalt, Mayou.
Older specimens: Lagrange, I, VI, VIII, X, Reis II.

(ii) Wide open angle but not torn.
Early specimens: Würdemann, Spielberg.
Later specimens: Reis V, Lagrange II, III, V, Magitot IV, unpublished specimen IV (Figs. 71, 99).

(iii) Obtuse and torn angle.
(a) Gap filled with new tissue: Reis IV.
(b) Gap unfilled: Reis VII, Seefelder IV, V (Figs. 61, 62, 64, 65, 66).

It is more difficult to find a relationship between the degree of distension and the size of the angle if we consider the specimens with peripheral synechiae. The chief point of interest is that these adhesions are not found in early specimens. Probably they arise as a rule when the iris fails to separate from the cornea. It is difficult to imagine how an extensive adhesion could arise in other cases once distension is at all marked. It is very difficult to account for the varying degrees of distensibility of the globe. A marked difference is found in the

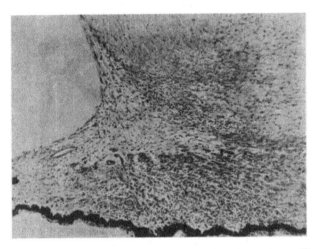

Fig. 63. The angle is open. Schlemm's canal and spur are almost absent. There is more meshwork than is normal at that age (eight weeks). (Stimmel and Rotter, specimen I, 1912.)

sclero-corneal ring, and also the thickness of the cornea if we compare unpublished specimens III, IV, V. The age of onset is probably an important factor in explaining this feature (Figs. 95, 98, 102).

We will study the alterations in those structures that as a rule are affected secondarily before those that show the primary lesions.

The Sclera. As the globe elongates it assumes an oval shape. It tends to fill the orbit and become immobilised. At times the proptosis is quite marked. The sclera, particularly near the limbus, develops a bluish-white appearance due to its thinness and that of the overlying conjunctiva. In the later stages dark areas may appear showing marked ectasia. As a result of exposure and possibly ulceration, the conjunctival vessels may become engorged. A similar appearance of congestion may arise when there is a sharp rise of intra-ocular pressure. A very distended globe was dislocated after a blow against a chair. It was replaced and sutured in position but later it became atrophic (Ball, 1922).

The resistance to distension is least at and immediately behind the sclero-corneal junction. The stretching of this part is one of the most striking features of hydrophthalmia. This leads to a displacement of the cornea forwards and an increase in the basal

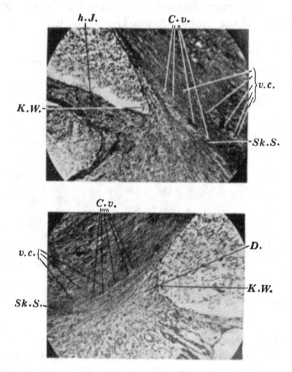

Figs. 64 and 65. The angle is open. The canal of Schlemm is so poorly developed that the spur is in a foetal position. There are profuse sclero-corneal trabeculae and uveal meshwork, the latter is torn (D). There is also a secondary iridocyclitis. Aged eight years. (Seefelder, specimen IV, 1906.)

circumference of the cornea, so that the corneal surface is flattened. While the thinning at the limbus may be great, *e.g.* to 0·21 mm. (Reis), true staphylomata are rarely found.

Lagrange in his study of six specimens found marked reduction of the thickness of the corneo-sclera in two cases (I and VI) and little alteration from normal in three. Chronic hyperplasia with hypertrophy as a secondary change was found in his case II. This result in such an advanced case is easily understood when one recalls the exposed position and the recurrent attacks of ulceration that may have affected such an eye.

Opinions are divided regarding the thickness of the posterior portion of the sclera. Some have considered their findings to be within physiological limits, and Gallenga, Schnabel and others found the thickness of the whole sclera reduced. The following tables show that the posterior sclera is thickened in the early and mild specimens.

As a rule, according to Takashima (1913), the posterior portion of the sclera is not reduced in thickness. Amongst twenty-seven specimens, from the literature and from Takashima's series, nineteen showed normal or even greater thickness at the posterior pole while in five the walls were very thin, being reduced to 0·35 or even 0·18 mm. The three remaining ones showed practically normal thickness. He considered that those that were stretched in the posterior segment were examples of hydrophthalmia complicated by myopia.

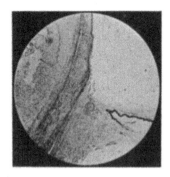

Fig. 66. The angle is torn open so that it extends into the ciliary muscle. There is evidence of the formation of new tissue as in Reis, specimen IV. There are traces of Schlemm's canal and of old inflammation. Aged sixteen years. (Reis, specimen VII, 1905.)

The wide variation of the normal sclera has not been recognised by all writers. Yet it is of great interest, for, in the past, a gigantism (Marschke) and a compensatory hypertrophy (Reis) have been thought to occur.

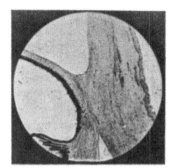
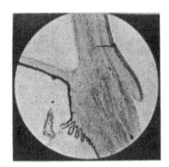

Figs. 67 and 68. The connection of the iris to the cornea is indirect, by means of fibrous tissue containing very few nuclei. The latter stains brightly with van Gieson and so is unlike sclera and also differs from the iris as the latter contains abundant connective tissue. This new tissue is a proliferation from the endothelium of the angle. Is this primary or due to inflammation? There is no canal of Schlemm. Aged fifteen and twenty-one years respectively. (Reis, specimens III and V, 1905.)

AH   8

If we study the eyes that have been removed in early life we find that the sclera tends to be thicker than normal even though as in one of these (Reis IV) the globe may be very distended. Takashima (1913) collected a series of eyes that had been carefully measured.

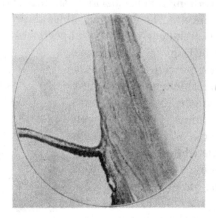

Fig. 69. Neurofibroma of the choroid. Aged sixteen
years. (Treacher Collins and Batten, 1905.)

Five of these had been removed before the age of two years. The findings are in the following table:

Case	Axis	Post. pole	Equator		Ora serrata			Age
			Temp.	Nasal	Temp.	Aver.	Nasal	
	mm.	mm.	mm.	mm.	mm.	mm.	mm.	
Reis IV	30·5	0·85	0·68	0·36	0·68	0·54	0·38	4 weeks
Rabinowitsch	27·0	0·84	0·468	0·48	0·34	0·49	0·64	23 months
Seefelder I	23·0	1·00	—	—	—	0·25	—	9 months
,, II	23·0	0·52	—	—	—	0·3	—	7 days
,, III	23·0	0·64	—	—	—	0·32	—	7 days
Average	25·3	0·77	0·574	0·42	0·36			—
Normal	24·3	0·64–0·12 (2)	0·46–0·06 (3)		0·48–0·71 (2)			

(1) = Average of measurements of temporal and nasal ora serrata.
(2) = Heine and Marschke. Alcohol and formalin hardening.
(3) = Salzmann.

If we consider only the mildest cases we find also that the sclera is thicker than normal, except near the limbus. The cases of Dürr and Schlegtendal are exceptional in that they all showed an unusual degree of thinning. Their Case V will be excluded because little information was supplied and its antero-posterior axis was only 22·0 mm. We will also exclude the very youthful cases in the previous table.

ANTERO-POSTERIOR AXIS OF BETWEEN 25·0–29·0 MM. (INCLUSIVE)

Case	Axis	Post. pole	Equator		Ora serrata		Age (years)
			Temp.	Nasal	Temp.	Nasal	
	mm.	mm.	mm.	mm.	mm.	mm.	
Reis I	29·0	0·93	0·38	0·51	0·34 (0·34)	0·34	2½
Seefelder IV	29·0	0·90	—	—	0·37	—	8
Dürr and Schlegtendal III	28·0	0·35	—	—	0·50	—	12
Takashima III	28·0	0·67	0·56	0·58	0·58 (0·52)	0·46	14
,, IV	28·0	0·88	0·75	0·70	0·45 (0·54)	0·62	11½
Seefelder VII	27·0–28·0	0·975	—	—	0·32	—	—
Raab	25·4	1·20	0·50	0·40	0·30	—	10
Dürr and Schlegtendal II	25·0	0·30	—	—	0·35	—	19
Average of eight cases	27·5	0·78	0·55	0·55	0·405	—	—
Average if D. and S. II cases are excluded	27·8	0·926	0·55	0·55	0·40	—	—
Normal	24·3	0·64–0·12	0·46–0·60		0·48–0·71		

It is of interest to compare Seefelder's mild and advanced specimens.

ANTERO-POSTERIOR AXIS OF UNDER 25 MM.

Case	Axis	Post. pole	Ora serrata	Age
	mm.	mm.	mm.	
Seefelder I	23·0	1·00	0·25	9 months
,, II	23·0	0·52	0·32	7 days
,, III	23·0	0·64	0·32	7 days
Average	23·0	0·72	0·29	—

ANTERO-POSTERIOR AXIS OF AT LEAST 34 MM.

Case	Axis	Post. pole	Ora serrata		Age (years)
			Temp.	Nasal	
	mm.	mm.	mm.	mm.	
Seefelder V	36·9	0·18	0·15	0·30	8
,, VI	34·0	0·315	0·15		8½
Average	35·5	0·24	0·19		—

In the following table are summarised the measurements of eyes removed later in life, between eight and fourteen years of age inclusive.

Case	Axis	Post. pole	Equator		Ora serrata			Age (years)
			Temp.	Nasal	Temp.	Aver.	Nasal	
	mm.	mm.	mm.	mm.	mm.	mm.	mm.	
Seefelder V	36·9	0·18	—	—	0·15	0·22	0·30	$8\frac{1}{12}$
,, VI	34·0	0·315	—	—	0·15		—	$8\frac{5}{12}$
Takashima I	33·0	0·56	0·49	0·50	0·48	0·45	0·42	10
Reis III	32·0	0·59	0·42	0·32	0·36	0·37	0·39	13
,, VI	31·0	0·85	0·68	0·48	0·69	0·62	0·55	14
Takashima II	30·0	0·70	0·38	0·54	0·30	0·24	0·18	$9\frac{7}{12}$
,, V	—	0·74	0·48	0·70	0·45	0·37	0·30	9
Seefelder IV	29·0	0·90	—	—	—	0·37	—	8
Dürr and Schlegtendal III	28·0	0·35	—	—	—	0·50	—	12
Takashima III	28·0	0·67	0·56	0·58	0·58	0·52	0·46	14
,, IV	28·0	0·88	0·75	0·70	0·45	0·53	0·62	$11\frac{7}{12}$
Raab	25·4	1·20	0·50	0·40		0·30	—	10
Average	30·5	0·63	0·53	0·53	39		—	$10\frac{7}{12}$

There is therefore evidence of great thinning of the sclera in all except those eyes that show a mild degree of hydrophthalmia and those that were studied in very early life. These exhibited adequate evidence to confirm the theory of compensatory hypertrophy.

Some authors claimed that the thinning is always limited to the anterior portions of the globe and that the remainder is thickened.

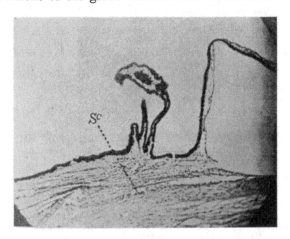

Fig. 70. Congenital glaucoma showing incomplete separation of the iris from the cornea, a posteriorly situated canal of Schlemm (Sc), and atrophy of the iris and ciliary body. Aged ten days. (Clapp, 1924.)

The tables already referred to disprove this statement, as also does the most extreme case in Takashima's list, which is case II of Reis. The axis was 39·0 mm., the posterior pole 0·24 mm. thick, the equator, temporal 0·18 and nasal 0·28 mm., the ora, temporal 0·34 mm. and nasal 0·25 mm.

The scleral thickness is more influenced by the degree of distension than the age of the specimen. This is shown by the following tables of average figures:

Age	No. of specimens	Limbus	At or near ora serrata	At macula
		mm.	mm.	mm.
Under 3 years	4	0·46	0·30	0·77
4–10 years	7	0·34	0·30	0·51
Over 10 years	7	0·35	0·41	0·79
Antero-posterior axis				
Under 31·0 mm.	6	0·40	0·32	0·76
31·0 and over	8	0·37	0·335	0·58
Normal	—	0·60	0·30	1·00

As age advances the sclera near the limbus becomes thinner, but elsewhere no change is observed. As the antero-posterior axis increases, however, both the limbus and the posterior sclera appear to become thinner.

From a study of fourteen specimens it appears that the nasal sclera in the neighbourhood of the ora serrata is more affected by the distension than the temporal sclera. It was thinner than the temporal sclera in ten of these. In the neighbourhood of the equator little inequality was observed. The alteration at the limbus corresponds with another evidence of stretching, viz. the displacement backwards of the insertions of the four rectus muscles. Thirteen specimens studied by Reis, Seefelder and Cross were considered and the following alterations in the distance between the limbus and the insertions were found:

Superior rectus: 11·0 mm. from limbus, that is, an increase of 3·3 mm.
Internal   „   9·3 mm.   „   „   „   3·8 mm.
Inferior   „   10·6 mm.   „   „   „   4·1 mm.
External   „   10·0 mm.   „   „   „   3·1 mm.

These variations may at times influence the choice of site for operation. In some cases the displacement of the superior rectus was over 2·0 mm. greater than that of the inferior rectus.

The following is a summary of measurements made by Reis, Seefelder and Takashima. It shows the marked variations in thickness of the sclera.

	7 dys.	7 dys.	9 mos.	2½ yrs.	4	*5½	8	*8	*8¼	9½ yrs.
	mm.	mm.	mm.	mm.	mm.	mm.	mm.	mm.	mm.	mm.
At limbus	0·39	0·4C	0·50	0·55	0·36	0·30	0·57	0·30	0·27	0·40
At ora serrata or behind muscle insertion	*0·30	*0·32	*0·24	0·36	0·32	0·29	*0·37	*0·12	*0·15	0·52
At macular region	0·52	0·64	1·00	0·93	0·59	0·24	0·90	0·18	0·31	0·67

	9⅔ yrs.	*14	11 yrs.	14 yrs.	*15	*16	18	*21	Normal
	mm.	mm.	mm.	mm.	mm.	mm.	mm.	mm.	mm.
At limbus	0·17	0·50	0·26	0·12	0·40	0·46	0·23	0·48	0·60
At ora serrata or behind muscle insertion	0·42	0·60	0·58	0·24	0·32	0·36	0·45	0·34	0·30
At macular region	0·70	0·85	0·88	0·70	0·59	1·02	0·60	0·89	1·00

The majority of these figures are from the series of Seefelder and Takashima. The most distended globes, that is 31·0 mm. and over, are marked *.

Lagrange considered that as the sclera stretched it hypertrophied. Reis found thinning of most cases, especially in the anterior and the equatorial regions. Stimmel and Rotter (1912) thought that such a change was preceded by corneal thinning.

The development of an anterior staphyloma may lead to a greater enlargement of the eye. As the sclera in such an area may become as thin as paper, spontaneous rupture is apt to occur. Axenfeld (1905), Zentmayer (1914) and Höeg (1911) have each reported such an occurrence.

An instance of an extensive spontaneous subconjunctival rupture with recovery at the age of five years was reported by Blair (1910). The application of a pressure bandage may be of value.

The origin of the halo and the conus that are found in congenital glaucoma is obscure. A conus may be found in eyes with comparatively thick sclera, e.g. Seefelder case VII, antero-posterior axis 27·0–28·0 mm.; scleral thickness at posterior pole 0·975 mm., at ora 0·32 mm., and Reis case VI, antero-posterior axis 31·0 mm.; scleral thickness at posterior pole 0·85 mm., at ora, temporal 0·69, nasal 0·55 mm. A halo was present in two of Takashima's cases: case III, antero-posterior axis 28·0 mm.; scleral thickness, posterior pole

0·67 mm., ora, temporal 0·58, nasal 0·46 mm.; case IV, antero-posterior axis 28·0 mm.; scleral thickness, posterior pole 0·88 mm., ora, temporal 0·45, nasal 0·62 mm.

Myopia with staphylomata has not been found in cases of blue sclera, which suggests that a thin sclera as a result of its richness in elastic fibres may support normal intra-ocular tension (Oppenheim, 1920). One exception, however, a case of keratoconus, has been described by Behr (1913). The scleral thinning, with normal dimensions of the eye, is a deficiency not of the elastic fibres but of the collagenous ones (Borel, 1925).

A consideration of the cause of "blue sclerotics" raises an interesting point. If the colour in this condition is due to scleral thinning as so many observers hold, it is strange that one does not find hydrophthalmia or more frequent signs of axial myopia in these cases. Rangarchari (1936) recently described a boy who presented the association of blue sclerotics with unilateral hydrophthalmia. It has been suggested that the transparency is due to the absence of lime salts in the connective tissue elements of the sclera. A hypofunction of the parathyroid has been blamed for this condition and for the reduced serum calcium and high urinary calcium content. Friedberg (1934), however, failed to find an altered serum calcium and in this was supported by Rados and Rosenberg (1936). Though Patterson found the sclera in one of Bronson's cases (1917) to be of normal thickness, yet Buchanan (1923) found it reduced to one-third and the cornea to three-fifths normal. In another case he also found the sclera reduced in thickness. Casanovas (1934) recently confirmed these observations. Findings made with the slit-lamp, however, cast some doubt on these views (Wirth and Vogt, 1936).

It is known that the sclera may become as transparent as the cornea if its water content is altered more than 20 % from normal, viz. 65·5 % (Fischer, 1928–31).

The cornea. The alterations may be summarised as follows:

(a) Increase in size.

(b) Thinning of the cornea.

(c) Changes of curvature.

(d) Opacities of the cornea.

    (1) Superficial opacities.

    (2) The steaminess of the cornea from oedema.

    (3) Ruptures in Descemet's membrane.

    (4) Congenital opacities.

(a) *Increase in size.*

Little difficulty is experienced in deciding that the cornea is abnormal in extent, particularly if the hydrophthalmia is unilateral. Greater difficulty will be met when one attempts to measure its diameter, for, as a rule, there is so much stretching of the sclerocorneal junction that the limbus is difficult to locate. Axenfeld held that the first stage of hydrophthalmia was an increase in the size of the cornea—a megalocornea which was followed by megalophthalmia. This view was supported by Stimmel and Rotter's observation in an early case, six weeks, that only the cornea was increased in size.

The normal corneal diameter in infants is between 8·0 and 10·0 mm. The period of greatest growth is during the first year, when the measurement may be 11·4 mm. (Kaiser). Parsons referred to a series of twenty hydrophthalmic globes of which the minimum horizontal diameter was 12·0 mm., the maximum 23·5 mm. and the mean was 16·0 mm. Of nine specimens removed at not later than $2\frac{1}{2}$ years, the average diameter was 12·7 mm. Of thirty-one specimens of a greater age than this the average was 15·7 mm. In each series the larger of the two diameters was considered.

Of 140 eyes in the questionnaire (including Zeeman's series) reference was made to the size of the cornea in 110. Of these

> 3 were described as normal;
> 56 were described as being large or having a diameter between 12·0 and 13·75 mm.;
> 43 were described as very large or having a diameter between 14·0 and 15·75 mm.;
> 8 were described as having a diameter of 16·0 mm. or more.

(b) *Thinning of the cornea.*

A flattening of the cornea is apt to develop as a result of stretching of the base-circle (Parsons, 1904). It appears as if the cornea has been displaced forwards by a giving way of the weak sclero-corneal junction (Elliot). As one would expect, the sensation of the cornea tends to become diminished. Derby considered that the loss of sensation varied directly with the degree of hypertension. The cornea may be clear or dull and its state may vary from time to time with sudden variations in ocular tension. Elliot stated that the centre is usually of normal thickness.

Series	Centre of cornea	Difference from normal	Peripheral	Difference from normal
12 cases from the literature	0·67 mm.	− 0·23 mm.	0·47 mm. (8 cases)	− 0·63 mm.
15 cases (Reis, Seefelder and Takashima)	0·54 mm.	− 0·36 mm.	0·53 mm.	− 0·57 mm.

In the first series the minimum peripheral thickness was 0·2 mm. and in the second the central measurements varied from 1·1 to 0·17 mm. and the peripheral from 1·0 to 0·21 mm.

It is of interest to compare the corneal thickness of unpublished specimens III and IV (Figs. 95, 98).

The thickness of the cornea in the fifteen specimens measured by Reis, Seefelder and Takashima was as follows:

	S. II	S. III	S. I	R. I	R. IV	R. II	S. IV	T. III
Centre	1·10	0·84	0·17	0·80	0·78	0·42	0·42	0·29
Peripheral	0·94	1·00	0·50	0·80	0·68	0·37	0·43	0·41
Age	7 days	7 days	9 mos.	2½ yrs.	4 yrs.	5½ yrs.	8 yrs.	9½ yrs.

	T. V	T. IV	R. VI	T. II	R. III	R. VII	T. I
Centre	0·45	0·73	0·80 0·21	0·58	0·50	0·72 0·25	0·52
Peripheral	0·45	0·53	0·51	0·40	0·50	0·38	0·39
Age	9⅔ yrs.	11 yrs.	14 yrs.	14 yrs.	15 yrs.	16 yrs.	18 yrs.

This summary shows that in eight of these fifteen cases the thickness was greater towards the centre—the reverse of the normal state. The thickness at the centre was actually greater than normal in two cases. They were the two earliest specimens, viz. 7 days, Seefelder II and III. It was least in the next earliest specimen, Seefelder I. Numerous ruptures in Descemet's membrane were present in this specimen and in the earliest specimens too. In Clapp's early specimen (1924) the centre was thinner than the periphery.

It is difficult to know how frequently spontaneous perforation of the cornea appears. As a rule trauma, slight though it be, plays an important part. Such cases must be distinguished from those with developmental corneal defects that can be attributed only to intra-uterine perforation as in Mayou's case (1910).

(c) *Changes of curvature.* Already considered under Refraction and Megalocornea.

(d) *Opacities of the cornea.*

(1) Superficial opacities. In quite early cases one may find swelling of the epithelium and minor abrasions and scars. There is a tendency to superficial vascularisation and various degenerative changes in long-standing cases. Ulceration is apt to develop and to be recurrent. Diminished sensitivity and exposure play parts in its production. Degenerative changes, such as pannus and opaque areas, develop late. Such changes may lead to an actual thickening of the cornea. Therefore in the old cases which have been exposed to repeated abrasions, one need not be surprised if one finds the thickness of the cornea increased.

(2) The steaminess of the cornea from oedema. The form of corneal oedema similar to that which occurs with sudden hypertension in adult glaucoma is relatively common. This form disappears with operation, a common finding in hydrophthalmia. Stimmel and Rotter observed dense corneal cloudiness and inflammatory symptoms to disappear and only tears to persist after operation. Seefelder and others mention such cloudiness clearing in a few days or even hours.

(3) Ruptures in Descemet's membrane (see Figs. 77, 78, 79). The "Bändertrübung" of Haab are of great interest and merit attention. Apart from the diagnostic value of such tears, in excluding megalocornea, they are an important indication of the influence of hypertension on the cornea in early life. They are present in about 75 % of cases (Seefelder). Stähli (1915) examined forty cases from Haab's clinic and found them in 75 %. This form of opacity, unlike the steaminess already referred to, does not disappear quickly after operation.

Erdman's experimental work throws light on their origin. He put electrolytic iron into the anterior chamber of two rabbits and watched the development of ruptures in the greatly enlarged corneae. The rupture led to a transient swelling and cloudiness of the parenchyma.

Haab (1899) wrote: "At first there is only the characteristic dulness of the corneal surface upon which diffuse opacity of the stroma soon intervenes. Shortly afterwards the cornea begins to expand and with this there appears a patchy opacity in which on close examination curious band-like stripes are visible." In reflected light they are glass-like and in direct illumination they are grey and show a double contour. They resemble a thread of Canada balsam on a glass slide (Haab). Stähli considered that they are a cause of reduced vision in more than one-third of all cases. Such tears may produce an appearance very like that of interstitial keratitis.

The ruptures permit imbibition of fluid and consequent cloudiness of the cornea. This occurs in the interval prior to the closing of the rupture by proliferating endothelium.

The secondary changes that occur along the tears make them easier to see. Stähli (1918) held that the tissue newly laid down by the endothelium may contract and so produce secondary tears. Such an exacerbation is rarely described, though it is also found in keratoconus, the ruptures becoming visible when the opacification clears.

Grahamer (1884) appears to have been the first to associate ruptures in Descemet's membrane and hydrophthalmia. Arnold (1891) recognised them clinically, but Haab (1899) was the first to realise their clinical significance. In nine cases examined microscopically Seefelder found them to be a constant feature, and Coats (1907) found them in at least twelve of thirteen specimens. Of forty cases examined clinically tears were found in twenty-nine and were absent in seven. In four the cornea was too opaque for tears to be seen.

Gallemaerts (1925) studied, with the slit-lamp, these tears in ten cases of hydrophthalmia. He described varying forms from the simple splits to most complicated attempts at healing. Landolt (1910) and Coats usually found evidence of repair, new endothelium being present on both surfaces of the torn Descemet's membrane. Detachments of this membrane were also found and the newly-formed cleft was lined with endothelium and filled with loose fibrous tissue. In one eye of a patient aged forty-eight years, half of Descemet's membrane was detached. There is a tendency for each endothelial layer to lay down a new membrane similar in structure to that of Descemet. As a result of such reparative processes there may be, as Coats pointed out, three membranes of Descemet, viz. the original one, and one on each side of it. The inelasticity of the so-called elastic membrane is shown by its tendency to rupture, and that of the margins of the tears to curl up. "A rare form of rupture is that in which overlapping instead of spreading apart of the edges occurs. This is probably due to a relaxation of the heightened intra-ocular tension after the occurrence of the rupture" (Coats). The endothelial cells may form masses of connective tissue, the secondary shrinkage of which produces alterations in the appearance of the tear and its surroundings (Stähli). Coats and Rumschewitsch (1909) have described excrescences on the posterior corneal surface with extensive tears. Elschnig thought that tears could not always be distinguished from the congenital defects described by Peters (see below) that sometimes produce a secondary hydrophthalmia.

As a rule the ruptures are situated centrally. When they are numerous they may also be found peripherally and then they are usually concentric with the limbus.

Most tears run in a horizontal direction, a fact probably related to the flattening or the greatly increased radius of curvature of the vertical meridian of the cornea. Axenfeld was the first to point out that the tears ran in the same direction to the ones found in Bowman's membrane in senility. Vogt (1921) attributed the horizontal ruptures of Bowman's membrane in senility and those in keratoconus to flattening of the corneal curvature. In senility the cornea tends to flatten in the vertical meridian, and in keratoconus the cornea flattens between the conus and the limbus. In the former state the ruptures are in the horizontal meridian, and in the latter they are more or less concentric with the apex of the conus and in sites where the surface has flattened. Elschnig wrote: "In old corneae the cornea flattens out in the vertical meridian and this leads to the cracking and rupture affecting the horizontal meridian: in keratoconus the cornea flattens between the keratoconus and the limbus, and as a matter of fact the rupture in the membrane runs concentrically to the apex of the conus, generally in places of similar or nearly similar flattening."

In hydrophthalmia both the forces of stretching and flattening may be agents in producing tears. In the future special attention should be paid to the relationship between the direction of the ruptures and the alteration in corneal curvature in the different meridians.

As a rule, as Seefelder showed, the vertical meridian of the stretched cornea is less curved than the horizontal. The effect of a flattening force is seen also in birth tears in Descemet's membrane, which were first observed by von Hippel in 1893.

The age of onset of the tears. The tears and the corneal thinning are apt to vary directly with the distension of the globe. Takashima reported three globes with tears, and the corneal thickness was from 0·3 to 0·55 mm., the base of the corneae from 14·0 to 17·0 mm. and the ocular axes from 28·0 to 33·0 mm. This marked thinning and ocular distension can be contrasted with the state of a fourth globe examined by him. The cornea was 0·68 mm. thick, the ocular axis was 27·0 mm. and no tears were present. Reis's and Seefelder's measurements led to no definite conclusions.

Thiele and Elschnig (1924) considered that ruptures as a rule arise early, frequently being present at or before birth. Meisner and Meller have reported the histological examination of such ruptures in the newborn and Stimmel and Rotter and Seefelder in very small children. In a very early case reported by Stimmel and Rotter the cornea only was enlarged and then slightly so; nevertheless, a rupture in Descemet's membrane was found.

Ruptures may, however, be found with very slight distension. Whether this means that a sudden rise in tension is more apt to produce tears or that in the youngest children the membrane is more easily torn (Seefelder) is uncertain. Elliot considered that it was the suddenness with which the agent making for distension was applied that had prevented the development of tears in experiments on animals. Römer and others have reported considerably enlarged corneae with tears. Elschnig held the view that tears developed before, at, or soon after birth. The sudden development of such tears, followed by imbibition, would be recognised if occurring later in life. Possibly, however, later in life the tears appear so gradually that the compensatory endothelial proliferation keeps step with it and prevents imbibition such as appears to occur when the tears of early life become wider in later life with further ocular distension. Elschnig reported a case, however, showing extensive rupture and opacification very early in life. He considered that as a rule this picture has gone before the child comes under observation.

Takashima, Reis and Seefelder considered that recent tears are rarely found. In the cases of Takashima that did not show ruptures in Descemet's membrane, gaps were found in Bowman's membrane which corresponded with the so-called tears of this membrane referred to by Reis, Seefelder and Rabinowitsch. "We cannot, however, say that these changes are directly due to mechanical stretching of the cornea; much more probably they are due to a parenchymatous inflammation" (Takashima). This author admitted, however, that he found no vesicle formation, as in keratitis bullosa, and no new vessels. There was a more or less marked interstitial inflammation, which was particularly noticeable towards the outer surface. Tears in Bowman's membrane are rarely found (Seefelder, Stähli, Jaensch). They may have been present in specimens III and IV of the last named.

Stähli after his study of this subject concluded: "Concerning the conditions of development, that is, time, etc., we unfortunately have hardly any exact knowledge." Frequently in the literature there is no reference to the presence of tears till late in the histories, but probably careful examination in infancy would have revealed them. Elschnig, Axenfeld and others emphasise the value of narcosis, rectal and otherwise, for this investigation.

Guist (1920) reported a thirteen-year-old boy with bilateral hydrophthalmia. Towards each limbus was a pair of concentric refractile lines with double contours. After a haemorrhage into the anterior chamber they resembled red stripes. Crvaric (1934) observed Krukenberg spindles near an embryotoxon in a twenty-nine-year-old patient with a moderate degree of hydrophthalmia.

Congenital pupillary synechiae and corneal defects—"ulcus corneae internum". Central corneal defects and adherent strands of tissue running to the iris have been found in hydrophthalmic eyes. The state is identical with the "ulcus corneae internum" of v. Hippel. The following early examples were found: (1) Cosmetattos: both eyes were examined after death, from pneumonia, at the age of seven days. All communication between the anterior and the posterior chamber was blocked by adhesions stretching from the iris and pupillary membrane to the cornea and the lens. The canal of Schlemm was present and empty. The iris tissue was dense and poorly differentiated. (2) Mayou described a specimen removed at seven weeks. Corneal defects and an adherent iris and an anterior polar cataract were present. (3) v. Hippel (4 weeks). (4) Jones (4 months). (5) Meisner I (1 year), Meisner II (1½ years), Meisner III (2 years).

Of the later specimens (1) Schlaefke's was of particular interest. Neither the canal of Schlemm nor lens was present, though the latter was probably represented by a faintly staining mass in the cornea. A pupillary anterior synechia was present and a defect in Descemet's membrane. (2) Christel's specimen was probably of a related condition. In it the epithelial cells of the posterior part of the lens were still visible and posterior pupillary synechiae were present. (3) It is conceivable also that Juler's specimen with "intra-uterine corneal perforation" was an extreme result of such a state. Possibly there had been a defective cornea into which aqueous could soak and facilitate distension and even rupture before birth. The following were probably examples of a similar state. (4) In Seefelder's specimen, for example, there was an extensive defect in the centre of the cornea and an anterior polar cataract. In addition, remains of a severe iridocyclitis were present and complete peripheral synechiae. (5) The cornea of Lagrange's specimen IX was staphylomatous, and completely adherent to the iris. This may be an example of a more advanced state of the condition under consideration. Böhm's specimens I, II, III may also belong to this group.

Meisner (1923) reported three eyes with hydrophthalmia and corneal opacities. In the first the cornea was in contact with the iris, which consisted almost entirely of epithelial layers. In the centre of the cornea was a broad space which extended almost through the cornea. It was lined with iris epithelium. In the second eye the posterior corneal wall was covered with the iris, which consisted almost entirely of epithelial layers. No anterior chamber was present in this or the preceding case. The third eye showed central defects in Descemet's membrane and the endothelium and anterior synechiae. The meso-dermal part of the ciliary body and iris was replaced by connective tissue. Clinically a diagnosis of iridocyclitis had been made, but histologically a malformation without signs of inflammation was found. Such a finding demonstrates how unreliable our interpreta-tions of clinical appearances in hydrophthalmia may be.

Other examples of central corneal opacity and hydrophthalmia were described by Reis (1905), Stimmel and Rotter (III), Mohr (III), Wirths (1918), v. Hippel (III, 1918), Clausen (1922) and others.

The uveal tract. The changes throughout the uveal tract may be considered as developmental, inflammatory or atrophic. It is often difficult, however, to classify them with confidence. The separation of aplasia from the results of atrophy is not always simple. So little is known of foetal inflammation that its tracks are hard to follow. The response of the almost avascular foetal tissues to infection and the influence of the disappearance of the transient vascular systems are obscure.

The iris. In the early stages the iris appears to be normal, but it soon becomes dull with an indistinct pattern. As a rule the pupil is round and active. Later it tends to dilate and become sluggish in its movements and its responses to drugs. Occasionally a hyper-trophic condition of the sphincter has been found. It was present in eight cases described by Fuchs and in Meller's early specimen. Signs of iris atrophy are common in the later stages, and as a rule only in these stages are evidences of inflammation found. The plane of the iris tends to be flat or even concave. The sinking back of the lens and the stretching of the iris contribute to this state. These influences also explain the frequent presence of iridodonesis.

(a) Developmental changes. Meller (1916) believed that the origin of congenital glaucoma was closely associated with iridic disturbances. He found a high degree of "atrophy" or aplasia with complete absence of crypts and of musculature. Compare Fig. 86. As his specimen was only eight days old there had been little time for atrophy to occur.

Colobomata are quite commonly found but corectopia is less frequent. Many pathologists have considered that there is some developmental connection between coloboma of the iris, polycoria, and persistent pupillary membrane. Though Deutschmann and van Duyse stated that they were due to intra-uterine inflammation, Ida Mann thought that though this may occur, the facts in support of the theory were very few. She upheld the contention of Awguschewitsch and Haab that persistence of the fibro-vascular sheath of the lens was the cause of many cases of congenital coloboma. Mann (1924) held the view previously suggested by Collins, that failure to disappear of one of the anterior set of branches from the circulus iridis major would cause a coloboma of only the stroma, but "if all the vessels persisted the iris would be short and thick—a condition of aniridia". In aniridia she described a forked process of mesoderm in the region of the short thick iris. One limb joined Descemet's membrane while the other passed backwards to the region of the lens and the ciliary membrane. This condition so resembles that in the 26·0 mm. human embryo that Mann wrote: "Aniridia is really a persistence of the embryonic condition of the latter part of the second month, before the iris has developed, and its cause is probably failure of the vessels at the margin of the cup to disappear at the proper time."

Collins thought that there were two ways in which congenital colobomata might be produced. They might follow (1) an adhesion of the pupillary membrane to the lens capsule which would check the inward growth of the iris, or (2) delayed separation of the lens from the back of the cornea. In the last-named group a small stump of iris always persisted.

Aniridia. Remky (1933) observed an instance of postnatal emergence of the iris of each eye in a patient with hydrophthalmia. At the age of two weeks aniridia was diagnosed, but at the age of six months a dark band of iris was detected. As posterior embryotoxon and peripheral anterior synechiae were present the author suggested that the adhesions that held the iris in the angle had separated, permitting its escape except at the site of the two synechiae. The grey annular opacities lying deep in the periphery of the cornea resembled those described by Axenfeld (1920), Guist (1920) and others. They were probably tears in Descemet's membrane, and may be due to the traction of the synechiae.

Collins (1891) was amongst the first to recognise the tendency for eyes with aniridia to develop primary or secondary glaucoma in later life. Parsons considered that the association with congenital glaucoma was not very common and that the apparent depth of the anterior chamber when aniridia was present had led to an incorrect diagnosis of hydrophthalmia. Thiele held that the form of hydrophthalmia associated with aniridia was probably secondary as, in such eyes, hypertension is apt to follow injury. In aniridia there is nearly always a stump of iris present which is not infrequently found adherent to the sclera in the angle. As a rule there is a faulty development of the meshwork in the angle. Filtration carries on until some upset makes this insufficient and then hypertension ensues. (Figs. 49, 50).

The peripheral stump of iris may seriously interfere with the result of an operation. Penman (1930) trephined both eyes and obtained a great improvement in one with a normal iris, but no benefit occurred in the other eye, which had almost complete aniridia; but Hudson (1921) trephined a seven-week-old child with this association and reported immediate corneal clearing. Both eyes in case II in Dettmering's series presented this association. They were trephined but both became blind. Würdemann's patient (1927) had bilateral hydrophthalmia and aniridia.

Seefelder (1909) collected the following nine cases of congenital glaucoma with aniridia: Brünhuber (1877), Cabannes (1895), Pflüger (1888), Venneman (1902), Lembeck (1890), Reck, Holzel, Dzondi and Lusardi. Case XVI in Seefelder's series had juvenile glaucoma and aniridia. Duggan and Nanavati (1927) found one child with hydrophthalmia amongst a family of four with aniridia. Denis (1926) reported a patient with bilateral hydrophthalmia, aniridia and cataract. Jaensch (1927) reported one example (case XIX) of this association. Weekers (1921) reported a man, with bilateral glaucoma, aniridia and congenital cataract, whose eight-year-old child had bilateral hydrophthalmia, aniridia and cataract.

Amongst those who have reported aniridia with adult glaucoma are the following: Klein, A. v. Graefe (two cases), de Benedetti, Samelson, Laskiewicz-Friedensfeld, Lembeck, Uhthoff and Axenfeld, Bergmeister (two cases), Pagenstecher (1903), H. Juler, Hirschberg, Goldzieher, Chowdbrury (1933), Krauss (1923), Somogyi (1922), Gloor (1922), Clausen (1921). Clausen's family had bilateral complete aniridia, cataract, glaucoma and nystagmus. The father and seven of the eight children had complete aniridia.

(b) Inflammatory changes. In the series of nineteen early specimens, signs of iritis were found in only four. The iris was described as atrophic in three and as dense and poorly differentiated in two. Its anterior surface was smooth in three, and the stroma rich in nuclei in two. The iris root was displaced forwards in one (Seefelder II), and aniridia was present in one specimen. Of the early specimens, Cross's with obvious iridocyclitis and iris bombé was the only one to show pupillary synechiae.

(c) Degenerative changes. The iris degenerates and is represented very often as a thin membrane with connective tissue on its anterior surface. This may tend to fill up the angle at the periphery, and by contraction produce ectropion uveae (see illustration of unpublished specimen III, Fig. 95). Takashima described scarring at the root of the iris as a result of inflammation. Jaensch described a striking abundance of mast cells in the anterior uveal tract and the episclera.

From a study of eighty-five specimens of two and a half years and over, we find that the iris

> was apparently normal in 9;
> showed no signs of inflammation in 16;
> was rudimentary in 4;
> showed dense stroma in 10;
> showed signs of old iritis in 22;
> showed ectropion pupillae in 12;
> was cystoid in 2;
> showed hyaline tissue on the anterior surface in 3;
> showed hyaline tissue on the posterior surface in 1;
> was atrophic in 36;
> was not mentioned in 3.

It is difficult to say whether a reference to dense stroma or a highly nuclear structure means a rudimentary state or post-inflammatory changes. The degenerative changes were found most frequently in the older and most advanced specimens; the changes then resembled those of absolute glaucoma.

Hyaline tissue may be found running round the angle on to the iris surface, or extending deeply into the ciliary body, or as a mass in the angle (Fig. 51). It is probable "that both epithelial and endothelial cells in the anterior part of the eye can produce hyaline material under stress of inflammation" (Mann, 1933). It stains deeply with orcein acid. Such material is found also in association with adult glaucoma and chronic iridocyclitis. Herbert found it continuing on from the trabeculae into the sclerotic and the ciliary muscle. When it is found in specimens of congenital glaucoma it is probably only as a secondary change. It may extend as a delicate layer over the surface of the iris. The anterior chamber may become a closed space surrounded by a single layer of endothelium and a sheath of hyaline material of varying thickness. The latter may even spread on to the surface of the iris (Wiener, 1903; Halben, 1903; Licsko, 1923; Jaensch, 1927; Böhm and others). The presence of such tissue in the angle must seriously interfere with the escape of aqueous (Wagenmann, 1892; Collins, 1927; Friedenwald, 1930). Such a state is shown in the illustrations of Wheeler's specimen (Figs. 93, 94). Collins (1900) found a hyaline membrane beneath the endothelial cells of the iris in an eye, with hydrophthalmia, removed from a seven-year-old girl. He regarded this as a congenital defect. "There was an adhesion of the iris to the back of the cornea a little above its centre." The endothelium of the iris and of the cornea were in continuity along this synechia. Collins found no sign of uveal pigment in a hydrophthalmic eye of a boy aged fourteen years. "The posterior limiting membrane, instead of splitting up into a number of fibres at the angle of the anterior chamber, continued round it and extended for a short distance along the anterior surface of the iris as a hyaline structure lined by endothelial cells which terminated rather abruptly. Externally to the angle of the chamber in this eye there was a broad adhesion of the root of the iris to the sclerotic, to which the ciliary muscle was attached, but neither fibres of the ligamentum pectinatum nor a canal of Schlemm could be detected." Mann suggested that if the tissue that forms the pupillary membrane and the anterior layer of the iris stroma remains too long in contact with the periphery of the cornea, the formation of hyaline material may result. Probably the hyaline tissue of the meshwork is produced by the endothelial cells, lining the spaces of Fontana. On staining it behaves as Descemet's membrane does. The continuity of Descemet's membrane with hyaline tissue in the vicinity of the angle is referred to in the section on Comparative Anatomy.

Zeeman (1919) reported two sisters who showed signs of iris atrophy. He regarded the changes as secondary and not causative as Meller had suggested. Particularly in bleached specimens Jaensch was able to find large crypts full of chromatophores of pigment. In the less atrophic specimens he decided that both the iris and the canal of Schlemm function as channels of outlet, though in an inadequate manner.

The ciliary body. The following is a summary of the state of the ciliary muscle and processes in the early and late specimens under investigation.

	2½ YEARS AND UNDER	3 YEARS AND OVER
CILIARY MUSCLE		
Normal and well formed	3 of 19 specimens	15 of 58 specimens
Poor development of circular fibres of foetal type	12 or 63 %	10 or 17 %
Inflammation	3 or 16 %	6 or 12 %
Atrophy	4 or 21 %	19 or 33 %
Large and vascular	0	2
Displaced forwards	3	3
CILIARY PROCESSES		
Normal	5	18
Foetal	4	1
Old inflammation	1	2
Sclerosed	—	2
Atrophy	2	16
Stretched	—	9
Adhesions	0	5
Cystic degeneration	1	2
Pigmented	0	4

The chief points of interest are the following:

(1) The tendency for a foetal type of ciliary muscle and processes to remain. This is most evident amongst early specimens. The circular muscle fibres were commonly poorly developed. The circular portion may lie in front of the insertion of the horizontal fibres of the muscle. This constitutes a foetal type (Seefelder) and was present in 63 % of early specimens and 70·21 % of all published cases (Stimmel and Rotter, 1912). It must be realised that not all the lack of development is prenatal. In many specimens a proportion of it results from disuse, as in myopia.

(2) The relative infrequency of signs of inflammation, though atrophic changes are common in older specimens.

(3) The unexpectedly frequent finding of normal ciliary muscle and processes.

The ciliary and vorticose veins. The anterior ciliary veins received little attention from most observers, so little can be learned from the following summary:

	2½ YEARS AND UNDER	3 YEARS AND UNDER
No mention	11 of 19 specimens	31 of 58 specimens
Normal	3	9
Full and numerous	2	9
Small and few	1	2
Signs of inflammation	1	3

The posterior ciliary veins and the vorticose veins were rarely referred to. Fuchs, Jaensch and others found them to be normal.

Magitot, however, emphasised the importance of endo- and periphlebitis as a primary cause of congenital glaucoma. In his specimens I and II the anterior emissary, vorticose and posterior ciliary veins were obstructed, though the anterior ciliary veins were distended. Schlemm's canal was blocked and surrounded by round cells and pigment. In his specimen III the anterior ciliary veins were distended but showed signs of endophlebitis. The posterior ciliary veins and one vorticose vein were blocked. The canal of Schlemm was open.

The globes described by Magitot were early specimens, viz. ten and fourteen months with the corneal measurements of 19·0, 17·0, 19·0 mm. respectively. It is remarkable that his cases should be so similar and yet almost unique in the literature. Magitot believed it was because other observers did not look carefully for such changes. This, however, did not apply to Seefelder.

Dürr and Schlegtendal's specimen I also showed blocked anterior ciliary veins, but it was old and one cannot be certain of the initial lesions.

In Seefelder's case VIII Schlemm's canal was almost absent. There was an old thrombosis of the central retinal vein and a fresh thrombosis of a lower vorticose vein. The latter changes and the haemorrhages in the retina and the choroid were probably the result of an iridectomy six days prior to death. The angle apparently contained persistent meshwork. The ciliary muscle was foetal in type and the iris atrophic or poorly developed. A thrombosis of the central retinal veins was present also in Seefelder's cases V and VII—both relatively old cases.

If Kalt had not examined the optic nerve carefully in his early specimen he would have classed it as an example of pure developmental defect. The meshwork was a dense layer resembling sclera, with endothelial cells on its surface. It blocked communication between an open angle and a narrowed but otherwise normal canal of Schlemm. Iris crypts were present. There were obliterating changes in the central artery and vein which may have produced hypertension, as a central retinal thrombosis may in later life. No signs of inflammation were present, nor any haemorrhages in the retina. As the artery as well as the vein was occluded, and as this association does not usually produce hypertension, these vascular changes may have been secondary. The anterior segment of the other eye showed similar changes, but it was not possible to judge the state of its central vessels.

Kalt's old specimen showed general atrophy of the uveal tract and marked reduction in the calibre of the vessels. The vorticose veins were surrounded by fibrous tissue but no obstruction was found in Fontana's spaces. A chronic iridochoroiditis, so Kalt considered, had produced a progressive obliteration of the vessels that had led to hypersecretion and ocular hypertension. In Zentmayer's first specimen obliterating endophlebitis of the scleral emissaries, near the angle, and of some of the anterior ciliary veins was found.

Spontaneous intra-ocular haemorrhages may occur in congenital glaucoma. Goldzieher held the view that they were due to tearing of a long posterior ciliary artery, as a result of the stretching of the coats of the eye. The manner in which the blood, in unpublished specimen V, has spread around the globe beneath the choroid, and has dissected the ciliary muscle from the sclera as far as the spur, certainly suggests a very free haemorrhage. A further source of extensive haemorrhage may be the wide vessels with thin walls which have been found in the anterior part of the ciliary body by Leber and Bentzen, Reis (specimen IV) and Dürr and Schlegtendal (specimen IV) and others.

The choroid. Goldzieher emphasised the frequent occurrence of choroidal lesions. He formulated the theory that congenital glaucoma was due to choroidal inflammation, which produced vascular sclerosis and serious interference with the drainage of the choroid. The investigation of early specimens disproved this theory, for, in these, such changes were very rarely found. In ten of a series of eleven eyes no considerable change was found in the choroid (Seefelder). This was not because of failure to search for this tissue, for Seefelder was greatly interested in Goldzieher's theory and studied in detail (1) the state of the choroid, (2) the relationship between the vorticose veins and the line of insertion of the oblique muscles and (3) the state of the veins themselves. His findings are markedly in contrast, firstly, with those of Dürr and Schlegtendal, who emphasised the importance of compression of the vorticose veins by the adjacent oblique muscles and, secondly, with the views of Magitot regarding the primary part played by endo- and periphlebitis. Regarding the former theory, Seefelder wrote: "How much more easily would lasting congestion and hypertension from such compression be obviated by means of the numerous anastomoses with the sister veins—their normal state being assumed? In both eyes where a vortex vein appeared in a microscopical preparation no pathological changes in them were found."

Reis considered that changes in the choroid were frequent though not constant. The majority of observers now hold that the choroidal changes are almost entirely atrophic and resemble those found in myopia. Crescents on the temporal side of the disc have been described by several observers.

Numerous early observers, including Haab, May, Dürr and Schlegtendal, and Cross, found recent or old uveal inflammation which they believed had appeared in foetal life. Takashima was unable to find any signs of recent inflammation. He found the choroid thin and deficient in vessels. Atrophic changes were present also in the ciliary body, and in one case the ciliary body was represented by a mass of pigment. He concluded that the atrophy of the uveal tract was undoubted, but that there was insufficient evidence to show whether it was the result of inflammation or due to stretching. The choroidal atrophy is certainly not necessarily the result of inflammation and may be the results of stretching, as the changes in myopia so frequently are.

One's estimate of the importance of the choroid as a factor in producing glaucoma has waned considerably. At one time it was considered to be the site of the main primary lesions, but now the changes in this tissue are held to be atrophic and secondary in all but very few instances.

	$2\frac{1}{2}$ YEARS AND UNDER	3 YEARS AND OVER
Choroid normal	16 of 19 specimens	10 of 58 specimens
Signs of inflammation	2 or 11 %	17 or 30 %
Engorged and haemorrhagic	3	1
Atrophic	1	28
Conus myopicus	—	2
Neurofibromatosis	3	5
Angioma	—	3

The following points are of interest:

1. The high percentage of early specimens with a normal choroid.

2. The infrequency of signs of inflammation in early specimens and its increase in late specimens. The choroid may be included when the anterior uveal tract is infected, as apparently occurs infrequently in early life. Much more frequently is it involved in a secondary inflammatory process of later life. As a rule the anterior part of the uveal tract shows more signs of inflammation than the choroid.

3. The high percentage of atrophy in the later specimens and its rareness in the early stages.

4. The relatively frequent occurrence of neurofibromatosis in the choroid. See below.

The lens. "The lens is the only ocular structure which is not distended by the increase of intra-ocular pressure" (Elliot). It is usually transparent, but in the later stages, and particularly when it becomes subluxated, opacities are apt to appear.

Alteration in shape. Flattening of the lens and consequent bowing of its fibres may occur as a result of traction from the overstretched suspensory ligament. Wessely showed that the zonular fibres may reach the astonishing length of 20·0 mm.

The sagittal diameters of two lenses measured by Collins were 3·5 and 4·0 mm. and the equatorial diameters were 9·0 and 10·0 mm. The measurements of the lenses (after section) in the three cases reported by Cross were: equatorial diameter, 6·0, 7·0, 8·0 mm.; sagittal diameter, 2·5, 4·0, 5·0 mm. The third lens was approximately normal in size. The mean equatorial diameter of five lenses was 6·8 mm. (Gros).

The normal measurements at the age of one year are approximately 2·5 and 7·5 mm. and in the adult 4·5 and 9·0 mm.

The average measurements of eight lenses collected from the writings of Reis and Seefelder were: equatorial diameter, 8·28 mm.; sagittal diameter, 4·0 mm. Little can be learned from these figures. If we attempt to compare the various lenses with the normal dimensions at the age of each specimen we learn more.

The normal measurements adopted were:

Age	Equatorial Diameter	Sagittal Diameter	
	mm.	mm.	
9 months' foetus	5·75	4·3	
1–2 years	7·87	2·57	
2–3 years	8·2	2·72	Dub (1891)
5–6 years	8·4	3·2	
12 years	8·8	3·6	

In six of eight lenses the ratio between the equatorial and the sagittal diameters became less than normal, that is, the lens became less flat. The only flattening effects were in the earliest specimen (9/12 old) and in the most distended one, which was grossly affected. Its sagittal diameter was 39·0 mm. at the early age of 5½ years and Reis considered that formalin had possibly upset its dimensions.

It appears, therefore, that in older specimens the lens is not flatter as is usually stated but rounder. This may be the condition when the suspensory ligament, as a result of overstretching, loses its influence on the lens.

The only lens with a marked increase in the equatorial diameter was the earliest specimen (8·5 × 4·0 mm.). Possibly the flattening shown by it is the initial alteration that takes place in the shape of the lens.

Seefelder found a lens coloboma in three of his cases, viz. cases XIX, XXIII, XXXV. In the third case both eyes were affected. Probably this defect is frequently missed, because so many eyes are examined without a mydriatic.

Alteration in position. The distension of the anterior ocular coats leads to a posterior displacement of the lens which is increased by the slight posterior displacement of the origin of the suspensory ligament (Parsons). The stretching of this ligament permits iridodonesis and possibly dislocation of the lens.

Belskiy (1934) considered that the lenses were small in his case, in which they periodically became displaced into the anterior chamber. Dislocation of each lens was recognised by Edgar Brown (questionnaire case) eighteen months before much increase in the size of the globe was observed. It is probable that such dislocation and possibly associated defects at the angle constitute predisposing causes for congenital glaucoma. In five of Wright's series bilateral iridodonesis was present. In three other cases a dehiscence of the zonule was thought to be present because of the presence of fluid vitreous in the anterior chamber or the ease with which the lens became dislocated after operation.

Aplasia of the lens. In Schlaefke's case no lens was present. Possibly it was represented by the faintly staining amorphous mass in the cornea. In Christel's case the immaturity of the lens was shown by the presence of posterior epithelial cells.

One form of maldevelopment that may produce hydrophthalmia is that in which a rudimentary lens is found enclosed by a persistent fibro-vascular sheath. Hypertension would result from the definite connection between the iris and the sheath. Marshall (1924) described an eye in which such a state was found. The distended cornea and the small pupil were displaced into the superior nasal quadrant as a result of the presence of an intercalary staphyloma. Collins considered that the iris had failed to separate completely from the back of the cornea. Such cases are similar to those described by Collins and Mayou as congenital staphylomata of congenital origin. See under Cornea.

One of the characteristic features of an advanced hydrophthalmic eye is the tremendous increase in the circumlental space. This forms a striking contrast to the condition in a glaucomatous eye.

Priestley Smith's statement is worthy of recall: "The salient fact is that while the lens grows larger as life advances, the globe does not, so that the older the eye becomes, the more likely it is to suffer from the disproportion in question: and the smaller it is, the earlier in life is the disproportion likely to arise."

Though a relatively large lens has been held responsible for many cases of senile glaucoma, yet a similar state seems to play little part in congenital glaucoma.

Isolated cases have been reported in which a large lens has been associated with juvenile glaucoma, *e.g.* Kunz (1931), Urbanek (1930). The tendency in these cases to a paradoxical rise in tension and miosis after the instillation of pilocarpine is probably further evidence of the interference by the unduly large lens, with fluid circulation between the anterior and posterior chambers.

In Kunz's case each lens was pushed forwards and the measurements were:

Thickness of lens	R. 5·43 mm.	L. 5·34 mm.
	(Normal 3·4–3·9 mm.)	
Radius of curvature of anterior surface	10·69 mm.	10·06 mm.
	(Normal 7·8–9·0 mm. Knapp)	
Radius of curvature of posterior surface	7·47 mm.	7·89 mm.
	(Normal 5·3–6·9 mm. Knapp)	

Eighteen dioptres of myopia were present in the right eye and fifteen in the left. This was probably not axial in nature though the fundus showed signs of stretching.

The relationship of glaucoma and myopia is difficult to understand. It has long been recognised that as a rule few changes are found in the fundus when these two conditions are associated. It is probable also that the age incidence is definitely lower in these cases.

Gnad found five cases of glaucoma amongst fifteen patients with globophakia. Kunz considered that the two reports of the association of a large lens and juvenile glaucoma in Löhlein's collection (1913) probably related to the same case. Fleischer (1916), Urbanek (1930) and Gilbert reported similar cases. Dalén's case (1903) was similar to those of Priestley Smith in that microphthalmia was present.

The retina and the optic nerve. The changes found in the retina are of relatively little importance. They include (1) disappearance of the cells, particularly of the ganglion type, (2) the formation of connective tissue on the inner surface, (3) retinal detachment and (4) sclerosis of the vessel walls. As is usual, infiltration of the central vessels is found in specimens complicated by iridocyclitis.

Parsons stated that the reduction in the calibre of the arteries and in their pulsation was less frequently observed than in adult glaucoma. The fundus becomes pale and albinotic, as in myopia, as a result of increasing pigment atrophy.

Even when the cornea is definitely enlarged the disc may be normal in appearance. If the disease is arrested spontaneously or as a result of treatment no cup may appear. In the advanced stages, however, the disc becomes cupped and later atrophic. Complete optic atrophy may make the cupping unusually deep. Owing to the presence of connective tissue at the point where the vessels enter it is rare to find lacuna-formation. ·

A filling-in of the cup from neuroglial proliferation does not often occur. Jaensch found it in his specimen I as a result of an operation reducing the tension and in specimen V as a sequel to inflammation. Takashima reported deep hollow spaces in the cupped discs of some hydrophthalmic eyes. Such a space may be divided by a wall of connective tissue, supporting the vessels, which appears to have maintained a definite resistance to the hypertension. More or less outward curving of the lateral walls of the cup was found in four of his five cases. In the remaining case very shallow cupping was found. This eye presented myopic-like changes round the disc with atrophic retina and choroid, but no true conus was found. It was of interest that in this case the anterior segment had yielded, producing a staphyloma. One may surmise that this saved the optic disc.

In this connection the following history supplied by Gault (1937) is of interest. It concerns a patient who at the age of fifteen months was found to have congenital glaucoma of the left eye. A widespread naevus covered the greater part of the left side of the face and the left half of the upper lip was greatly hypertrophied. At the age of seven years the note was made, "no cupping of the disc". Seven years later marked cupping was present. One may surmise that in early life the cornea and the anterior sclera had responded by stretching and the optic disc did not yield until these tissues had passed out of the stage when distension was possible.

It is likely that the distensibility of the sclera and the choroid around the entrance of the optic nerve can both delay the appearance of the cupping of glaucoma and, when it does appear, influence its shape, so that it may resemble a flat funnel rather than the usual cup with parallel or even concave lateral walls.

It is very difficult to estimate the percentage of patients with cupping and atrophy of the optic disc. It is difficult also to ascertain the average age of onset of these changes. So often in the literature the only reference to the state of the disc is made after the operation. The state of the cornea and the age of the child frequently made earlier examination difficult.

If we analyse Dettmering's eighteen cases with cupping we find that:

1. 9 were not detected until at least seven years of age.
2. 2 showed cupping at 7 months.
3. 1   ,,   ,,   9 months.
4. 1   ,,   ,,   14 months.
5. 1   ,,   ,,   16 months, 2 operations at 14 months, pale by 19 months.
6. 1 was normal at 9 months, cupped by 2 years, operation at 10 months.
7. 2 were normal at $2\frac{1}{2}$, cupped by $6\frac{1}{2}$, operation at $6\frac{1}{2}$ and $2\frac{1}{2}$ years.
8. 1 was normal at 4, cupped by 5 years, operation at 4 years.

The final record of vision for these cases was:

1. V. = 0·2, 0·2, 0·2, 0, 0·3, 0·2, 0·2, C.F., C.F.
2. Early operation, but T. remained +, V. fair.
3. Early operation, and T. = ?, V. = C.F.
4. Late operation, T. = ?, V. = C.F.
5. Early operations, and T. = N., V. = C.F.
6. Early operations, T. +.
7. Late operations, T. +, no useful vision.
8. Late operations, T. +, C.F.

In three cases in this series the cup appeared after operation. The only ones who retained even fair vision developed a cup later, that is, at seven years or over.

In the seven instances of cupping in Fleischer's series the cup was first mentioned

At 7 years or over in 4 cases,	
At $4\frac{1}{2}$ years	in 1 case,
At 1 year	in 1 case,
At 6 months	in 1 case.

SUMMARY

State of optic disc

	Question-naire	Dett.	Wright	Stölt.	Fleisch.	Seef.	Total	Per-centage
No mention or not visible	69	18	20	6	4	32	149	42·5
Normal	29	14	16	5	8	6	78	22·0
Cupped	18	19	14	5	7	22	85	26·0
Cup and atrophy	9	8	—	2	—	8	27	8·0
Atrophy	3	4	—	1	1	2	11	3·0
Total	128	63	50	19	20	70	350	—

Duration of normal disc appearance

It is interesting to note that in many eyes reported in the question-naire no cupping was found even though definite signs of marked hydrophthalmia were present and the age was relatively advanced, for example, ten years.

Normal disc at 21, no treatment. ? spontaneous cure.
,, ,, 13½, no treatment; mild hydrophthalmia. ? spontaneous cure.
,, ,, 11¾, treatment at 11 weeks.
,, ,, 9, sclerotomy at 9 weeks, tension remained + +, excision.
,, ,, 10, treatment at 10 years.
,, ,, 20, trephine at 3½ years.

The anterior chamber. The anterior chamber in hydrophthalmia is very often deep, as it is in secondary glaucoma in adults. It may be very deep, *e.g.* 18·0 (Schmidt-Rimpler, 1908) and 12·8 mm., com-pared with a normal depth of from 3·036 (Plantenga) to 3·637 mm. (Lindstedt). Owing to the shrinkage of the lens the depth may become greater. The depth of the anterior chamber was stated in the reports of nineteen of the fifty-eight old specimens investigated in this study and it varied from 2·0 to 12·8 mm. The average was 5·75 mm.

Of the eyes reported in the questionnaire no mention of the state of the anterior chamber was made in twenty-nine. It was described as

Normal in 9 cases,
Shallow in 2 cases,
Obliterated in 1 case,
Deep in 86, that is in 87 % of those with information on the state of the anterior chamber.

Seefelder considered that a deep anterior chamber was characteristic of those cases of glaucoma that were congenital and primary, and that in the acquired cases a shallow anterior chamber was often found. He added that no hard and fast line could be drawn.

It is of interest to compare the average depth of the anterior chamber in hydrophthalmia with that found in non-glaucomatous eyes.

The variation in depth with different refractive states has been estimated by Lindstedt (1916). In this table the depth of the anterior chamber is in mm. and the age in years.

Age:	0–12	15–30	31–50	51–80	Total
Myop.	3·130 (1)	3·857 (32)	3·846 (5)	3·673 (3)	3·831 (41)
Over –10D.	3·540 (1)	3·970 (1)	—	3·648 (4)	3·683 (6)
Emmetr.	3·683 (9)	3·704 (72)	3·546 (25)	3·213 (8)	3·637 (114)
Hyperm.	3·494 (4)	3·412 (33)	3·114 (36)	3·283 (20)	3·272 (93)
Total	3·585 (15)	3·675 (138)	3·340 (66)	3·342 (35)	3·537 (254)

THE ANGLE OF THE ANTERIOR CHAMBER

The angle in chronic glaucoma. Herbert (1929) described three out-standing features of many globes with chronic glaucoma. They are: (1) A thick posterior inner wall of the sinus of the anterior chamber, made up mainly of an extension of the ciliary body supporting the iris base, instead of iris alone as in many eyes. (2) A posterior displacement of the open angle of the anterior chamber, by pressure of the aqueous, so that it lies far beyond the level of the scleral furrow and Schlemm's canal. Such a displacement is only found in chronic glaucoma. (3) A failure of the meridional fibres of the ciliary muscle to approach Schlemm's canal and so a defective inward pull of the muscle on the pectinate ligament. The middle and inner divisions of the muscle are neither particularly broad nor closely packed. This last feature is clearly shown in Fig. 9 of Herbert's article. It represents the opposite condition to that which he considered normal, in which the middle and inner fasciculi of a forward-reaching ciliary muscle exerts an opening influence on the spaces of the pectinate ligament. He rarely found a mobile scleral spur, as described by Thomson, which is an essential state if the pump-action is to take place. Herbert concluded that the marked defect in the action of the ciliary muscle on the pectinate ligament and on Schlemm's canal may be the crucial influence determining the onset and development of glaucoma in eyes otherwise predisposed to the disease.

Elliot agreed that a lessened elasticity of the pectinate ligament hampering the scleral spur could be a predisposition to glaucoma and opposed Henderson's view that a sclerosis of the ligament produced mechanical obstruction and so a tendency to glaucoma.

The angle and Schlemm's canal. As in the adult form of glaucoma the angle of the anterior chamber in congenital glaucoma may be open or closed. Reis and Schmidt-Rimpler found an open angle in 50 % and Polya in 47 % of cases. In five of Lagrange's series of ten specimens in different stages the angle was described as open or widely open. The angle was closed in two-thirds of a group of thirty specimens in which the state of the angle was clearly described. Particularly in early cases is the angle apt to be open.

Whether the angle be open or closed some defect is found which interferes with the escape of the intra-ocular fluid. Gros (1897) appears to have been the first to emphasise this point.

Though the angle appears to be open in somewhat less than 50% of hydrophthalmic eyes, yet very often there is obliteration of Schlemm's canal or some adjacent defect which is the result of either chronic inflammation or congenital deformity.

The following are the defects commonly found:

1. Persistent or aberrant meshwork in the angle.
   "Persistent ligamentum pectinatum."
2. Poorly developed or absent Schlemm's canal.
3. Posteriorly placed (foetal) Schlemm's canal.
4. Rudimentary development of scleral spur.
5. Peripheral anterior synechiae.

In the following discussion particular value is attached to the state of the angle in a series of twenty-seven specimens removed and examined during the first $2\frac{1}{2}$ years of life. In addition eighty older specimens and eleven of unknown age are included. Let us consider these defects in order.

(1) *Persistent or aberrant meshwork in the angle.* Of twenty-seven early specimens at least fourteen showed some defect in this tissue. Amongst forty-five specimens of eleven years and older it was possible to recognise such changes in only nineteen. Eleven specimens of unknown age are included and of these nine showed similar changes in the angle. Sometimes the resemblance to the foetal state was not great, because superadded inflammatory changes were present. The early specimens showed a minimum of destruction due to distension and of infiltration from secondary inflammation and repeated injuries.

It is wise to go to the early specimens for information concerning the causes of and the different types of hydrophthalmia and to rely mainly on the older cases when we are studying the progress of this disease. In the following analysis only the early specimens are classified with any degree of certainty. The element of doubt increases as a rule with the age of the specimen.

The persistent tissue was sometimes in the form of an open meshwork resembling a foetal condition and sometimes much denser resembling iris tissue. The latter state is well exemplified in the cases associated with neurofibromatosis.

The sclero-corneal trabeculae and the uveal meshwork may present the following defects:

1. A compact or undifferentiated system of sclero-corneal trabeculae.

Examples. The specimens of Spielberg (5 months), Seefelder I and Jaensch I (10 months), Reis I (2½ years), Reis II (5¼ years), Seefelder V (8 years), Seefelder VI (8¼ years), Stimmel and Rotter II (9 years; the exact state of the meshwork was indefinite, but Schlemm's canal was foetal in type). (Figs. 52 to 56.)

2. A persistent or an aberrant uveal meshwork.

Examples. The specimens of Seefelder II and III (7 days), Meller 8 days), Würdemann (3 months), Wiener (2½ years), Stimmel and Rotter I (8 weeks). Lagrange VI and VIII (6 and 11 years; angle in each as at 5–6 months of foetal life) and possibly X (age unknown), and Reis IV and VII (4 and 16 years; network of new elastic tissue also present), Seefelder IV (8 years), Dürr and Schlegtendal I and III (18 and 12 years), Priestley Smith (21 years), unpublished IV (28 years), and Rumschewitsch (age unknown). (Figs. 57 to 66, 99.)

3. An aberrant development of the uveal meshwork, or the tissue from which it forms, so that a process of iris-like tissue or of endothelial tissue fills the angle.

Examples. Unpublished II (5 weeks), Kalt (6 months), Michelsohn Rabinowitsch (23 months), Wagenmann (2½ years), Snell and Collins (7 years), Reis III (16 years), Collins and Batten (16 years), Reis V (21 years), Schiess-Gemuseus (27 years), Siegrist (age unknown). (Figs. 81, 82, 67, 68, 69.)

4. A failure in differentiation, so that the periphery of the iris appears not to have separated from the cornea. This may be due to a failure of the uveal meshwork to form or it may be a form of iris process and similar to type 3.

Examples. Clapp (10 days), v. Hippel (3 months), Marshall (3 years), Pesme (4½ years), Böhm I (5½ years), Lamb (6 years), and Stimmel and Rotter III (5½ years). (Fig. 70.)

Of the remaining twelve early specimens the uveal meshwork and the spaces of Fontana were not found in four: Meisner's I (1 year), II (1½ years), III (2 years), Jones (4 months), which presented central anterior synechiae. In two other specimens with similar synechiae the meshwork and trabeculae were imperfectly formed: Cosmettatos (7 days), Mayou (7 weeks). Secondary changes were described in v. Hippel's case (4 weeks) and the findings in Manz's specimen (5 months) were indefinite. The meshwork and trabeculae are not described in the four remaining specimens: Juler (10 weeks), Cross (13 months), Magitot I and III (10 and 14 months).

It was impossible to classify with certainty the original state of the angle in the following specimens of 3–10 years of age, as little or none of the meshwork was visible: Cross I (5 years), Böhm VII (6 years), Cross II (7 years), Sachsalber (7 years), Murakami (9 years), unpublished I (10 years), Böhm II (8 years), and III (4 years), Stoewer (9 years), Takashima I (10 years), III (9½ years), Cabannes (6 years), Christel (8 years).

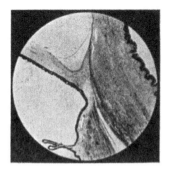

Fig. 71. Direct union of the iris and cornea. The trabeculae are compressed by the iris, the canal of Schlemm is patent, and there is no recent inflammation. Aged fourteen years. (Reis, specimen VI, 1905.)

Few of the specimens examined after eleven years can with certainty be allotted to any of the above groups, though glaucoma, in quite a number, was probably due to a persistence or aberration of tissue in the angle. Ten of these specimens have been included. The analysis of many of these specimens is difficult now because of insufficient data and the varying interpretations due to the different conceptions of the observers concerned.

5. New tissue, either fibrous or endothelial, is found in the angle. The endothelium of the trabeculae and of the meshwork apparently plays some part in the production of this tissue.

All the examples are old specimens, *e.g.* Oguchi (18 years), Böhm IV (22 years), Lagrange II and III (20 and 17 years), Collins (14 years).

In five of his series of eight specimens Fischer (1933) found that the sclero-corneal trabeculae were difficult to recognise, because they were closely packed and tended to blend with each other and even to be replaced by hyaline material. The uveal meshwork was profuse, filling the angle and directly continuous with iris tissue. The scleral spur and the canal of Schlemm in each specimen was poorly developed and in a posterior situation.

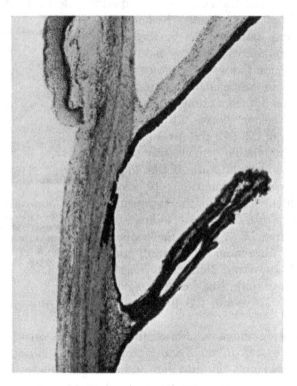

Fig. 72. Congenital glaucoma. ×45. Pigment fills Schlemm's canal. It and the scleral spur lie between the angle and the ciliary body.

In a portion of one specimen in this series the spur was thin and situated well in front of the angle. The canal of Schlemm was almost closed. The trabeculae were homogeneous and partly replaced by hyaline tissue, which extended far back past the spur, to cover the exposed inner surface of the projecting ciliary muscle. Remnants of uveal meshwork filled the angle. Fischer could find neither spur nor canal of Schlemm in two of his specimens.

Cucco (1922) investigated ten specimens removed from patients whose ages ranged from seven to twenty-six years. His conclusions were that, as a rule, the angle was filled with connective tissue and

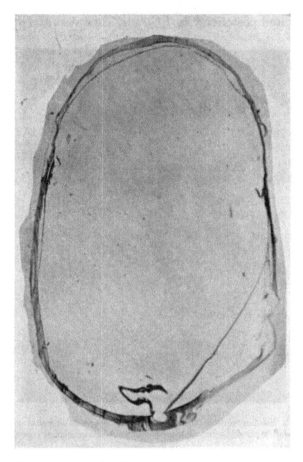

Fig. 73. Unpublished specimen I. × 3. Congenital glaucoma with staphyloma due to corneal perforation. Observe adherent iris, thinning of the periphery of the very distended cornea, atrophic ciliary body. Aged ten years.

persistent remnants of "pectinate ligament", that Schlemm's canal was usually absent, closed or very narrow, and that only a few specimens showed peripheral anterior synechiae.

(2) *Defects of Schlemm's canal.* Defective development of this structure has been described by many authors. Its absence was first emphasised by Seefelder and Reis. Poor development is frequently

associated with a foetal position of this canal, so that it lies behind the angle of the anterior chamber. In a series of forty-four cases in the literature in which reference is made to the state of this canal it was described as absent or obliterated in 79·5 %, as very reduced in 9 %, as situated posteriorly in 7 %, and as present and open in 7 %.

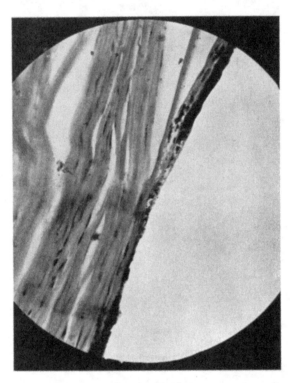

Fig. 74. ×2. Section showing anterior synechia. Descemet's membrane and the anterior layer of the iris disappear where the union is most complete.

Hamburger estimated that the canal was defective in 50 % of cases. Marked variation exists in the reports of different observers. This to a large extent is due to the age of the specimens concerned.

In Seefelder's eight specimens, the majority of which were early, the canal was narrow in all, almost absent in one and posteriorly situated, *i.e.* behind or partially behind the angle, in five.

In Reis's seven specimens, the majority of which were late cases, the canal was absent in two, almost absent in four, one of these from obvious inflammation, and open in one.

In Böhm's seven specimens, the majority of which were late cases, the canal was not found or absent in five. Traces of a posteriorly situated canal were found in one.

In Lagrange's ten specimens, the majority of which were late, absence of the canal was noted in all.

In Magitot's four specimens the canal was absent in two early and one old case, and present in one early case.

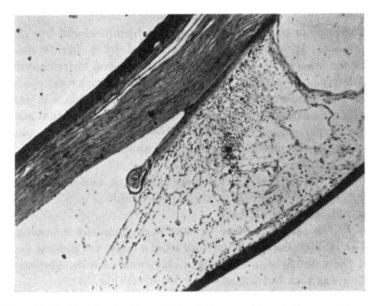

Fig. 75. × 28. Section showing the central anterior synechia and the very thin cornea. Descemet's membrane runs along the iris for some distance and then ends in a curled edge.

In Takashima's five specimens, which were old, the canal had disappeared in two cases. In one it was obliterated by a peripheral synechiae, in two it was narrowed and surrounded by infiltrated sclera. In one of the latter it was situated posteriorly.

In Cross's three specimens, which were old, the canal was absent in one and almost so in two.

In Stimmel and Rotter's two specimens, which were old, the canal was absent in one and almost so in the other.

In five of Fischer's specimens (1933) the canal and the spur were poorly developed and in a posterior position. The canal was almost closed in one and in two neither spur nor canal could be found.

Many other careful observers have reported a complete or partial absence of every trace of Schlemm's canal. These include Lagrange, Reis, Böhm, Römer, Gros, Dürr and Schlegtendal and v. Hippel.

Analysis of specimens showing absence of or a defective canal of Schlemm as the principal lesion

Christel. In this specimen the patency of the meshwork at the angle was possibly demonstrated by the fact that it contained blood from a haemorrhage. The lens was in an immature state.

Schlaefke. Not only was the canal of Schlemm absent but no lens was present. It was probably represented by a faintly staining amorphous mass in the cornea. There was a central anterior synechia with a defect in Descemet's membrane. The meshwork was apparently normal, as it contained blood. One peripheral synechia was present.

Spielberg considered that an absence of Schlemm's canal was the cause of hypertension in his case. He thought that the unusual appearance of the meshwork was due to an anterior displacement of the angle and the ciliary body (Fig. 52).

Seefelder VIII. The development of the iris and ciliary muscles was defective and there was no canal of Schlemm (Fig. 63). There was also an old central thrombosis.

Reis I. The canal appeared to have been closed by inflammation; round-cell infiltration of the iris and ciliary body was present and the site of the canal was marked by a collection of cells. The angle of filtration was torn but the gap was not filled (Fig. 54).

Reis II. A wide open angle with normal meshwork and an almost completely absent Schlemm's canal suggested that the latter defect was primary. No signs of inflammation were present. The angle was acute though great distension was present. The antero-posterior axis was 39.0 mm. and the cornea was 14.5×16.0 mm. at $5\frac{1}{2}$ years (Fig. 56).

Takashima II showed the typical posterior position of scleral spur and Schlemm's canal. The latter was narrow and the surrounding sclera was infiltrated.

Safar's specimens also showed a narrow and posterior canal of Schlemm. Seefelder V and VI showed similar changes. Amongst the others with no sign of a canal were Lagrange I and X, Böhm, Römer, Dürr and Schlegtendal III and IV.

The only series in which the canal was usually present was Seefelder's, which consisted chiefly of early cases.

It appears therefore that as a rule, and particularly in late specimens, the canal of Schlemm is either absent or only traces of it are found. The following analysis of eighty-four specimens demonstrates this fact:

Schlemm's canal	$2\frac{1}{2}$ years and under	3–11 years	Over 11 years
Series	25 specimens	27 specimens	32 specimens
Absent	25 %⎫	54 %⎫	59 %⎫
Almost absent	30 %⎭ 55 %	21 %⎭ 75 %	16 %⎭ 75 %
Small and posterior	25 %⎫	18 %⎫	6 %⎫
Present	20 %⎭ 45 %	7 %⎭ 25 %	19 %⎭ 25 %

It is seen that the canal is present in a considerable number of early cases. In 45 % of specimens not over $2\frac{1}{2}$ years it was either present or small and in a posterior position. In only 25 % of specimens over this age was a similar state observed. This suggests that the canal becomes closed as a secondary process in the late stages.

In only 25 % of the earliest specimens was the canal absent, but no sign of it was found in well over half of those specimens aged over $2\frac{1}{2}$ years.

(3) *Posteriorly placed Schlemm's canal.* Foetal type. A typical example of this was seen in Seefelder's first specimen. There was practically no sign of uveal meshwork and no scleral spur. The sclero-corneal meshwork lying central to the canal of Schlemm was sclerosed. The main defect appeared to be that all the lumina of Schlemm's canal lay behind the angle.

There was a similar displacement in the following specimens: Seefelder's IV, V and VI, Stimmel and Rotter II, Takashima II, Safar, and Reis VII (Figs. 64, 65, 66).

In Seefelder's series the canal was in this position in five specimens. The relative infrequency of this finding in other series may be due either to the greater age of the specimens or the lack of interest of the observer. The foetal position of the canal was observed in 25 % of specimens of $2\frac{1}{2}$ years and under, in 18 % of those between this age and eleven, and in 6 % of those over eleven years.

If Schlemm's canal had been in the normal position to start with it would have been found much farther forward than is normal, as a result of the enormous distension in this region.

(4) *Rudimentary development of scleral spur.* Several observers have described specimens in which the canal is poorly developed and situated as in a sixth- or seventh-month foetus. It is then associated

with a poorly developed and posteriorly situated scleral spur. Estimates regarding the first appearance of Schlemm's canal are very variable, as has been seen. Probably Schlemm's canal is present at the fourth month, but for a long time consists only of a very small lumen. The sclero-corneal meshwork and the scleral spur are very poorly developed at this stage.

(5) *Peripheral anterior synechiae.* It is remarkable that very few of the early specimens showed peripheral synechiae. A small synechia was found in the nasal side of the angle in Rabinowitsch's specimen. This may not have been a true synechia but associated with the neurofibromatosis. Synechiae were present in three other early specimens, none of which was a typical example of congenital glaucoma. In Cross (case M.P.) hypertension was obviously due to iridocyclitis and accompanied by posterior synechiae and an iris bombé. In Cosmettatos's specimen and Meisner's specimen III a central anterior synechia or "ulcus internum" was present. Even if these specimens are included, synechiae were found in only 15 % of twenty-seven specimens not over 2½ years of age.

The presence of anterior synechiae is insufficient evidence to justify the belief in an inflammatory origin for hydrophthalmia.

We find peripheral synechiae much more commonly when we study older

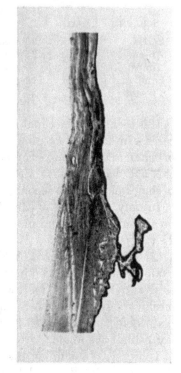

Fig. 76. × 35. Section showing extensive peripheral synechia with atrophy of the ciliary body. Schlemm's canal is closed and filled with pigment (opposite the superficial vessel). Signs of corneal inflammation and remains of iris.

specimens of congenital glaucoma. The following are some of those that showed more or less extensive peripheral synechiae: under eleven years, Böhm I, II, III, Takashima II and V, Dürr and Schlegtendal IV, unpublished specimen I, Marshall. Over eleven years, Reis VI, Takashima IV, Lagrange IV, VII, Jaensch IX, P. Smith, unpublished specimen III, Dunphy, etc. (Figs. 71, 72, 76, 96, 97).

Peripheral synechiae were found in at least thirty-two of eighty specimens over $2\frac{1}{2}$ years, that is in 40 %. This includes three cases associated with facial naevi and one with neurofibromatosis.

The width of the adhesion may be great, as in Dürr and Schlegtendal's fifth specimen (2·0–5·0 mm. in width) and in Lagrange's seventh specimen (3·5 mm.); see his Plate 3, Fig. 1.

A study of the significance of each of these lesions will be found in the chapter on "The Theories of Origin".

SUMMARY

In this survey of the structural alterations found in specimens of congenital glaucoma an endeavour has been made to separate the early lesions that may be primary from older ones that are degenerative or due to a late infection. When this is done the following appear to assume most importance:

1. An absence of Schlemm's canal.

2. A persistence or undue development of meshwork in the angle.

3. A peripheral union of the iris and the cornea that may be due to lack of differentiation, or to post-inflammatory synechiae.

4. Central corneal opacities with adhesions to the iris or the pupillary membrane. Changes in the other tissues appeared to be comparatively late in origin and of secondary importance.

ASSOCIATION OF HYDROPHTHALMIA WITH OTHER ANOMALIES

OCULAR DEFECTS

The association with other ocular anomalies, and still more with malformations elsewhere, gives strong support to the theory that hydrophthalmia is caused by a developmental defect.

Numerous ocular anomalies have been reported in association with congenital glaucoma. They are fully discussed by Reis (1905) and include the following lesions: posterior lenticonus (Pergens), ectopia pupillae and iridemia (Seefelder), corectopia (Kessler, Magerhausen, Warlomont), coloboma of the iris and lens (Gallenga, Penman, 1930, and others), coloboma of lens (St Germain, 1929), absence of ciliary body (Pflüger), incomplete ora serrata, persistent hyaloid artery (Mayou, 1910). Aubaret and Sedan, Meisner and many others have described congenital corneal opacities coinciding with hypertension and hydrophthalmia.

Lacroix (1936) was surprised to find tumour formation in an orbit one month after the removal of an apparently simple hydrophthalmic eye. The patient was aged three years and died three months after the enucleation. Oguchi's specimen (1933) contained a mixed-cell growth—a "haematoma".

The following ocular anomalies are of special interest:

1. *Foetal structure of the ciliary muscle.* One of the characteristic findings in old specimens of hydrophthalmia is a poor development of the ciliary muscle. The circular fibres are frequently absent or poorly developed. This is not unexpected when one remembers the tendency to myopia. In many instances this is a secondary or atrophic state. In others, however, a definite statement that foetal structure was present has been made, *e.g.* Böhm III (1915). In some early specimens, also, persistence of a foetal state has been diagnosed, *e.g.* Seefelder II (and III) and VIII (Figs. 57 to 60, 63). In the last speci-men Stimmel and Rotter described a forward extension of the circular part of the muscle so that it encroached on the anterior insertion of the radial part. They claimed that this was present in almost 75 % of cases of hydrophthalmia. Spielberg referred to a similar state in a young patient aged $5\frac{1}{2}$ months but born fifteen days before term (Fig. 52). The ciliary body appeared to be pushed forwards so that the ciliary processes were flattened and elongated. In addition the sclero-corneal trabecular fibres were foetal in type and they traversed the angle of filtration. The scleral spur was not found. In Dürr and Schlegtendal's fourth specimen the trabeculae had been displaced forwards and diminished in width. The anterior part of the ciliary body had moved backwards and pushed the base of the iris before it. In the other eye of this patient a similar state was found. The iris had been pushed forwards and had taken root from the cornea in its new position. In Lagrange's eighth specimen, in addition to a foetal type of angle with cilio-scleral trabeculae, the iris and the ciliary body appeared to be pushed much farther forwards than was normal.

2. *Defects in the iris.* Meller held that too much attention had been paid to the state of the angle and that even though an abnormality did exist here it should not necessarily be considered the cause of hydrophthalmia. He stated that the angle is normally narrow in the newborn and that it may be largely filled with uveal stroma which retains its foetal character, and that even in normal eyes at birth Schlemm's canal may not be visible in all sections. On the other hand, he wrote: "The crypts in the iris may be absent, and Leber has already

shown that the passage of fluid into them and thence by the veins of the iris and ciliary body to the venae vorticosae is normal."

His specimen from a seven-day-old child was only slightly hydrophthalmic, and though the angle retained its foetal state and the canal of Schlemm was not very clear in all sections and was displaced

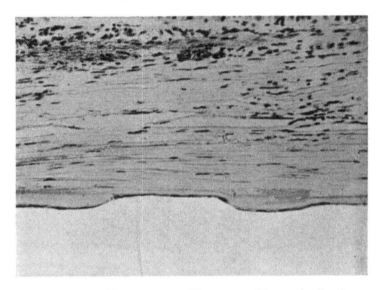

Fig. 77. 1. × 200. Narrow rupture with gap covered by new hyaline tissue.

backwards, yet to him the most important modifications were the following: (1) the iris was very compact and dense, rich in nuclei and devoid of crypts so that its surface was absolutely smooth; (2) the iris was unusually thin, especially towards the periphery; (3) a partial absence of pigmentation of the posterior layer, such as is found in foetal life, was found. Similar though less marked changes were found in the other eye.

Non-ocular anomalies. The following non-ocular anomalies are found: micrognathia and cleft palate (Seefelder), acrocephalia, micrognathia, cleft palate, hyperteliorism, defective joints, etc. (Waardenberg, 1934), Schüller-Christian's disease (Hymes), anencephalia (Meller, Clapp), congenital alopecia (Pincus), epicanthus (Panas and Gros), defective cranial development and supernumerary digits (Himly, Reis), patent foramen ovale and enlarged thymus (Würdemann).

Two other diseases, homolateral neurofibromatosis and naevus flammeus, are of particular interest and they will be considered in detail.

ASSOCIATED HYDROPHTHALMIA

The wisdom of isolating this type of congenital glaucoma may be doubtful for, as the following discussion is developed, a marked resemblance to the main type and further support for the developmental theory of origin will be found.

Congenital glaucoma is associated with two developmental disorders which are characterised by diverse but typical lesions scattered widely within and over the body. These disorders show hereditary and familial tendencies. The description of incomplete forms—*formes frustes*—emphasises these tendencies and explains their oversight in

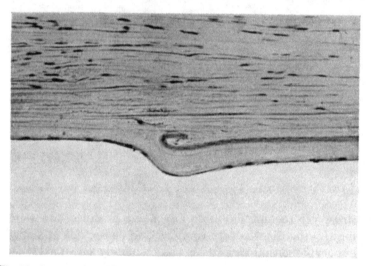

Fig. 78. 2. × 200. Typical curled pigmented line at one edge of the wide rupture.

the past. As some of these forms are found only at autopsy or on microscopical examination the difficulty in recognising the complete form of the disease may be great.

Another point worthy of emphasis is the difficulty experienced here, as elsewhere in pathology, in deciding at what period of life developmental defects cease to arise. Is the body complete at birth and therefore incapable of giving origin to further errors of development? The appearance of certain lesions throughout life suggests that this view is incorrect, and that the process of development continues into the post-natal period, if not throughout life. Many of our boundary lines in pathology are arbitrary and not a few are misleading. Though the dramatic change in sphere at birth is sudden and great yet no revolutionary changes are found in many tissues. Therefore we must not over-emphasise the difference between lesions found at birth and those that are manifest soon afterwards. Capillary and venous angiomata are found at birth and the arterial form is usually only discovered later in life. This, however, does not mean that it develops then and is not a congenital anomaly. A similar attitude of mind is required in considering glaucoma. Not only can

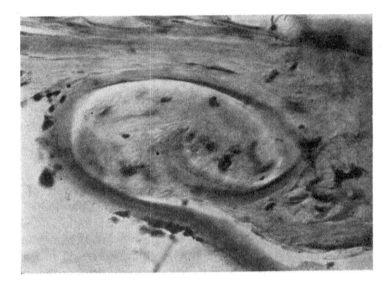

Fig. 79. 3. × 240. More advanced folding of the hyaline tissue.

congenital developmental defects first manifest themselves late in life, but, it appears, anomalies may arise during life that are pure errors in growth or development. This fact makes it essential for us to consider not simply congenital glaucoma as present at birth or soon after as developmental, but also many cases of glaucoma as they appear throughout life. Some predisposing anomaly may be present, particularly when such dysplasic conditions as angiomata or neuro-fibromata are found. See Achermann's family (1929).

The two congenital developmental defects that concern us are:

(1) Generalised neurofibromatosis or von Recklinghausen's disease and especially when the upper part of the face is involved.

(2) Capillary or venous angiomatosis, particularly when it affects
    the areas supplied by the first and second branches of the tri-
    geminal nerve. This necessitates a study of naevi of the face,
    the scalp and the mucous membranes of the head, and of angio-
    matous changes in the uveal tract and the meninges.

In passing it is of interest to note that congenital glaucoma does
not appear to be associated with certain other congenital developmental defects such as tuberose sclerosis (Bourneville's disease),
chronic interstitial neuritis (Critchley, 1932) and retino-cerebellar
haemangiomatosis (Lindau's disease). The ocular lesions in the first
of these diseases will be referred to later.

In all of these disorders hypertrophy, or even a neoplastic overgrowth of one particular tissue, appears to produce the characteristic
clinical picture by which the disease is recognised. For example,
in Lindau's disease certain angioblasts of the retina and cerebellum
become uncontrolled.

GENERALISED NEUROFIBROMATOSIS OR
VON RECKLINGHAUSEN'S DISEASE

Three syndromes consisting chiefly of tumour formation of the
central nervous system have been entitled "phakomatoses" by
van der Hoeve (1932).[1] They are all of congenital origin and show
hereditary tendencies. They are the syndromes of Bourneville, of
von Hippel and Lindau, and of von Recklinghausen. The first is
mainly ectodermal and is limited to the cerebrum, the second mesodermal and found chiefly in the cerebellum, medulla, spinal cord and
retina. The one in which we are interested here is the third, which is
probably mixed in type (del Rio Hortega). It affects chiefly the cranial

---

[1] The exact value of van der Hoeve's classification is obscure. In these three diseases
he described each typical lesion as a phakos or "mother spot". To him a "phakos" is
a spot, congenital in origin, often hereditary and familial in appearance, which can be found
in different parts of the human body, either at birth or later on. Such spots vary in size,
enlarge by proliferation of any part of the tissue, grow to a real blastoma and even turn to
malignancy, but do not contain naevus cells. A phakos is a naevus without naevus cells,
a naevus is a phakos with naevus cells. van der Hoeve states: "As far as is known at
present real naevi are found in the skin only, whereas a phakos may be present in any part
of the human body." One wonders how this author would classify the telangiectases
that are found in the pons and, particularly, in the floor of the fourth ventricle. The
difference in site and the presence or absence of naevus cells are the characteristics that
separate the two types of lesions. It is of interest, however, that each type occurs in
association with congenital glaucoma, e.g. facial naevi and neurofibromata. Is there just
as little relationship between glaucoma and these conditions as between it and any one of
the other concomitant lesions, such as syndactyly and syringomyelia?

and the peripheral nerves and the sympathetic nervous system. While many pathologists class this tumour formation as a "Schwannoma", Penfield agrees with the original idea of von Recklinghausen that these tumours—molluscum fibrosum—grow from the endo- and peri-neurium and are therefore mesoblastic. The thickening of the nerves

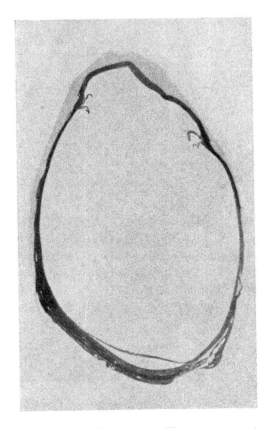

Fig. 80. Unpublished specimen II. × 3. Associated
with neurofibromatosis. Aged five weeks.

of the skin may be so great as to deserve the term plexiform neuroma, and the associated hypertrophy of surrounding tissues has led to the title of congenital elephantiasis of the lids.

Michel, who classified neurofibromata, gave as his third group those associated with complete unilateral facial hypertrophy and hydrophthalmia. The lesions appeared to be invariably on the same side and unilateral.

Generalised neurofibromatosis is a much more complex condition than was originally believed and described by von Recklinghausen (Macdonald Critchley, 1933).

In the great majority of cases it shows a decided familial and heredo-familial property. In Leclerc's family five generations were affected.

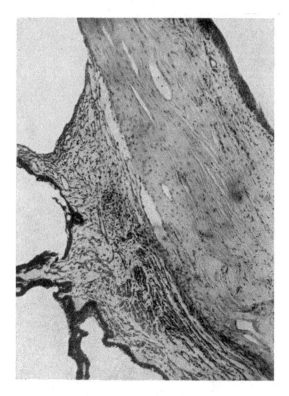

Fig. 81. ×80. The angle is closed—probably from failure of the iris to differentiate from the periphery of the cornea. There is no definite canal of Schlemm and no evidence of inflammation. There is neurofibromatous tissue in the ciliary muscle.

A completely negative family history may be regarded as exceptional. "This familial tendency escaped recognition for a considerable time, chiefly because the clinical manifestations are not usually homologous." The recognition of its familial tendency depends largely on the appearance of incomplete forms of the disease in several relatives of the one or more members of the family who exhibit the disease in its complete form. Sutherland's and Mayou's case of hydrophthalmia was of interest in this respect. The abdomen showed pigment patches and the cranial bones on the affected side were enlarged. The only signs of von Recklinghausen's disease in the family were similar pigment patches on both parents.

The clinical manifestations may be divided into five groups.

1. *Neurological findings.* Hard painless neurofibromatous masses may grow at any point in and upon the nervous system. If the terminal filaments are affected the condition of molluscum fibrosum arises. If the trunk and ramifications of one particular nerve are the seat of overgrowth, hypertrophy of the related skin and subcutaneous tissues may be found. This is the condition known as plexiform neuroma. An entire limb or half the face may be so hypertrophied that a form of hemihypertrophy is produced.

The cranial, spinal and autonomic nerve fibres may be affected. Of the first named the auditory nerves are the most vulnerable. Recently van der Hoeve emphasised the value of recognising as characteristic lesions the flat greyish-white masses found in the fundus at times in patients with neurofibromatosis. There is uncertainty regarding the relationship of the single neurofibromatous tumours that affect the spinal roots or the auditory nerves. The relationship of acoustic neuromata to von Recklinghausen's disease is obscure. No nerve fibres can be found entering the former though they may be found in the fibromata of the latter disease. Both types of tumour are composed of collagen fibres, and when the acoustic neuroma is bilateral, as it rarely is, it tends to be associated with the generalised form. The solitary form is identical with that found on the second and fifth cranial and other nerves. It has been suggested that von Recklinghausen's disease is a reaction to aberrant nerve fibres and that the tumours are simply fibromata growing upon a nerve.

2. *Cutaneous manifestations.* A uniform bronzing of various parts may occur. The most typical are circular or oval patches with sharply defined edges on the trunk. Naevoid formations of varying size are frequently found. An early neurofibromatous tumour in the deeper layers of the skin may appear as a "blue spot". Later they are raised above the surface of the skin and lose their characteristic colour.

3. *Skeletal changes.* Various forms of spinal curvature are probably the most important change. Exostoses, especially from the cranial bones, may be found or some thinning which is most commonly found under a plexiform neuroma. Other bony changes need not be mentioned here.

4. *Endocrine changes.* These are not frequently found and those due to pituitary disorders are most common. Acromegaly and other forms of hyperpituitarism have been recorded by several observers, but hypopituitarism has rarely been found. Disorders of the thyroid, adrenal and sex glands with skeletal and other defects have been reported.

5. *Psychotic changes.* Many of the patients are subnormal and a few are imbecile.

Incomplete forms. "The characteristic physical signs of von Recklinghausen's disease develop slowly and manifestations of one particular type, *e.g.* cutaneous, may antedate the onset of other signs by many years." Cutaneous changes are the commonest of the *formes frustes.* Parkes Weber's patient in 1905 showed areas of bronzing over her body and twenty-one years later developed a number of neurofibromata and a plexiform neuroma on the neck.

The disease is regarded as a congenital dysplasia and "this view is supported by the not infrequent co-existence of other anomalies, such as syringomyelia, spina bifida, and meningocele". In this way the disease is associated with the so-called status dysraphicus. Of the two other congenital dysplasias of the nervous system, hypertrophic interstitial neuritis and tuberose sclerosis, a brief reference to the latter disease will be made because of its similarity to neurofibromatosis.

Tuberose sclerosis, also known as epiloia, has been described recently by Macdonald Critchley and Earl (1932). Once unrecognised and described as epilepsy, this condition was first recognised as a pathological entity by Bourneville. The clinical picture consists of mental defect, epilepsy and cutaneous lesions. The affection, which is usually hereditary and familial and probably congenital, is rarely encountered outside an institution.

The characteristic skin lesion known as adenoma sebaceum occurs on the nose and cheeks. Various other skin lesions occur and these closely resemble those found in generalised neurofibromatosis. The pathological findings include circumscribed areas of sclerosis over the cerebral cortex, and multiple tumours consisting of an overgrowth of the primitive elements of the viscera, especially the kidneys and heart. The retinal tumours found in this disease have been discussed by Messinger and Clarke (1937).

Both this disease and generalised neurofibromatosis have a characteristic and striking cutaneous appearance, and naevi and various disorders of pigmentation are common to both. Both diseases are heredofamilial. Yet glaucoma has been described only with the latter.

The onset and distribution of ocular lesions in neurofibromatosis. The association with glaucoma was observed at birth or soon afterwards in all cases except those described by Rosenmeyer (1906), Komoto (1909), Pomplum (1921), Löb (1923) and Weber and Bode

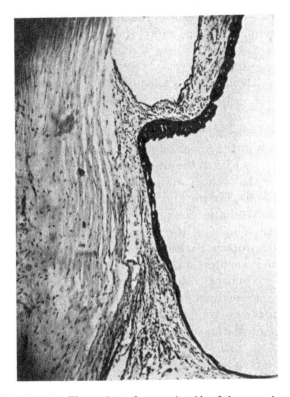

Fig. 82. × 80. The angle at the opposite side of the eye, where the presence of a synechia must be considered.

(1934). The specimen of the last observers was normal at birth and enlarged at the age of four years.

A description by Conrad Berens of the early history of a patient reported by Wheeler is of interest (1936). When the child was a day old the cornea on the same side as the palpebral neurofibromatosis was 11·5 mm. in diameter, and the other cornea was only 8·0 mm. There were vessels on each iris but chiefly on the affected side. During the first few weeks the cornea enlarged rapidly and a 2·0 mm. trephine operation was performed. Hypertension soon returned, and at the age of two years the globe and the orbit were greatly enlarged. After enucleation neurofibromatous changes were found in the ciliary body and the choroid. Tags of iris, ciliary body and connective tissue were present in the trephine opening and neurofibromatous tissue was adherent round it.

The situation in which plexiform neuromata are most frequently found is the subcutaneous tissue of the head and neck, in the distribution of the trigeminal and the superficial cervical nerves. They may, however, be met with anywhere throughout the sympathetic and peripheral cerebrospinal nervous systems. Of fifty-three cases collected by Alexis Thomson 33 % affected the temple, forehead and the upper lid and 24 % the posterior part of the neck and behind the auricle.

The favourite site for neurofibromata to occur when associated with glaucoma is in the upper lid and adjacent temple. Rosenmeyer referred to the upper lid as the site of the lesion. The adjacent temple or the skin over the orbit in addition to the upper lid was affected in the cases of Lezius, Collins and Batten, and Weinstein. Both lids were affected in the patients of Schiess-Gemuseus and Wheeler and, in addition, the temple in the following cases: Snell and Collins, Michelson-Rabinowitsch, Sachsalber (and bones of face), Achermann (and typical diffuse neuromata), Mintschewa (and body), and Verhoeff (and multiple neuromata). Merkulov (1935) described a ten-year-old girl with neurofibromatous nodules in the lids, the scalp, and hemi-hypertrophy of the same side of the head as the hydrophthalmic eye.

Hudson described the area affected in his case as that of the distribution of the fifth nerve. In the remaining cases half the face was affected and, in some, half the body and one arm or both legs as well.

It appears that the upper lid is always affected if hydrophthalmia is present.

Neurofibromatosis of the lids and orbit is not necessarily associated with hydrophthalmia. No ocular changes were described in the first six cases presented to the American Ophthalmological Society (Wheeler, 1936). Hydrophthalmia was absent in Kyrieleis's case (1927), with neurinoma at the limbus. Birch-Hirschfeld considered that hydrophthalmia or glaucoma occurred in approximately half the cases of orbital plexiform neuroma. De Schweinitz (1891), Snell and Collins (1903), Rockliffe and Parsons (1903), Knapp (1906),

Zentmayer (1912), Knapp (1916), Pomplum (1921), O'Brien and Leinfelder (1934) and others have reported neurofibromatous changes in the lids or the orbit and freedom of the eyeball from hydrophthalmia.

Achermann (1929) reported a father and son with von Recklinghausen's disease. The father, whose lids were affected, also had hydrophthalmia and the son, whose lids were normal, developed glaucoma in one eye at the age of thirty-four and in the other eye ten years later.

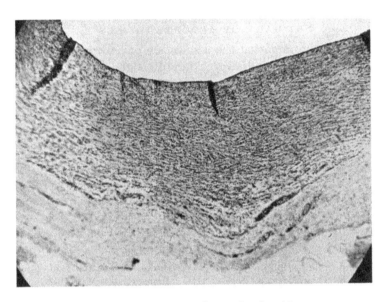

Fig. 83. ×40. Thickened posterior choroid.

Two points of clinical value deserve mention:

(1) The recognition of the hypertrophied nerves in the lids is aided by their characteristic resemblance on palpation to "knotted cords" "a bag of worms", "fiddle strings".

(2) When neurofibromata are present in the orbit a pulsation is not uncommonly found. Verhoeff considered this due to the tendency that these tumours possess of becoming vascular. Others thought that pulsation was transmitted from the brain to the globe through a defect in the wall of the orbit. The X-ray differentiation of this condition from sarcoma of the orbit is discussed by Le Wald (1933).

The association of von Recklinghausen's syndrome with congenital glaucoma suggests many problems. They will be considered as they arise in a discussion based on the following plan:

Neurofibromatosis with glaucoma$\Big\langle$ congenital
                                       adult
          ,   ciliary neurofibromata
          ,,   skull defects
          ,,   signs of intra-cranial disease
          ,,   hemihypertrophy
          ,,   other anomalies
          ,,   other ocular anomalies

SUMMARY OF REPORTED CASES

1. The following reported the association of hydrophthalmia and neurofibromatosis of the adjacent skin only (eight cases):

Schiess Gemuseus (1884)   Rosenmeyer (1906)
Lezius (1899) (Wagenmann)   Weinstein (1909)
Verhoeff (1903)   Hudson (1925)
Collins and Batten (1905) (Fig. 69)   Michel II (1908)

2. One instance has been reported of hydrophthalmia and neurofibromatosis of the uveal tract only:

Knight (1925).

3. The following reported in addition extensive facial involvement and even hemihypertrophy (twenty-one cases). Sixteen of these showed involvement of bone and, if all cases had been X-rayed, this number would probably have been greater.

Snell and Collins (1903)   Parkes Weber and Bode (1934)
Michelson-Rabinowitsch (1906)   Moore (two cases) (1936)
   (Siegrist, 1905)   Merkulov (1935)
Sutherland and Mayou (1907)   Sachsalber (1898)
Komoto (1909) (Murakami, 1913)   Verhoeff (1936)
Pomplum (1921)   Michel I (1908)
Vogt (1924)   Jaensch (1928)
Metzger (1925)   Wheeler (1936)
Wiener (1925)   Mintschewa (1926)
Awguschewitsch (1929)   Campbell (1937) (Figs. 109, 110)
Achermann (1929)

Vogt and Meeker (1936) reported the occurrence of secondary glaucoma with neurofibromatosis. Adequate information was not available concerning the cases of Löb (1923), and two others referred to by Michel.

Total: 32 cases of hydrophthalmia and facial neurofibromatosis.
       1 case of hydrophthalmia with uveal changes only.
All unilateral.

Ciliary neurofibromata. The choroid is richly supplied with nerve fibres. Salzmann found numerous nerve fibres in the stroma, especially in company with the arteries. Scattered ganglion cells are found in the inner strata of the vessel layer. The fibrillae show varicosities and spherical swellings in the vessel musculature. A fine plexus lies beneath the lamina vitrea.

The exact nature of the neurofibromatous tumours is uncertain. It has been suggested that they are allied to the fibroblastomata that grow in the arachnoid. This view is interesting in the light of the similarity in structure and function between the pia-arachnoid and the choroid.

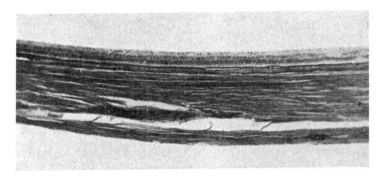

Fig. 84. × 40. Normal choroid from the same specimen.

Collins stated that all portions of the ciliary nerves supplying the eye may be affected by congenital neurofibromatosis, and that, in the uveal tract, as in the skin, there may be a general hyperplasia of the fibrous tissue of the part associated with the neurofibromatosis. The extent of the affection varies, however, in its distribution, sometimes being confined to one set of ciliary nerves and the part supplied by them, and sometimes to another (Collins, 1905).

Collins found an increase of peri- and endothelium of the ciliary nerves just posterior to the globe as well as in the uveal tract, sclera and cornea. The choroid may be much thickened by fibrous hyperplasia and will appear much less vascular than normal. Collins described small oval bodies showing nucleated capsules round a central core of convoluted nerve fibres. These he considered to be hypertrophied end-organs. Knight (1925) stated that they have been called Paccinian corpuscles but that they were, almost certainly, "hyalinised whorls of fibroblasts". They were present also in the specimens of

Wheeler (Figs. 90, 91) and Wiener. Wiener's patient had two pigment patches on the skin, one lying above the clavicle and the other above the groin. Wheeler's patient showed similar patches, mainly on the trunk.

As Knight stated, it is characteristic for the cells of these tumours to wrap themselves round each other or round collagen fibres and so form whorls (Fig. 85). Hyaline degeneration and calcification may take place in these formations. These ovoid bodies, that occur in the choroid

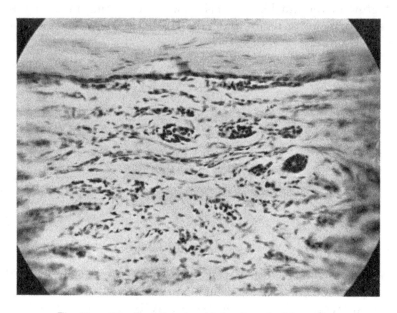

Fig. 85. × 200. Posterior choroid showing whorl formation
and linear strand of neurofibrillary tissue.

when affected by neurofibromatosis, are "structures similar to the psammoma bodies, or their hyaline *anlage*, in the so-called dural endothelium". Reese, in describing these bodies in Wheeler's specimen, referred to them as Meissnerian tactile corpuscles. Knight failed to trace any connection between these bodies and nerve fibres in her serial sections. Selective staining failed to reveal the presence of any nerve fibres within them. Ganglion cells were found in the specimens of Knight and Wheeler. Collins did not include them in his description and Sachsalber did not refer to ovoid bodies. Otherwise there was marked similarity between these four specimens and that of Murakami. The chief changes were a localised or a widespread replacement of the vascular tissue of the choroid by connective tissue, pigmented cells and hypertrophic nerve fibres.

Schiess Gemuseus (1884) appears to have been the first to describe the association with glaucoma. He described the ciliary nerves as showing peculiar constrictions. Signs of hypertrophy of these nerves were found by the following: Sachsalber (1898), Lezius (1899), Snell and Collins (1903), Collins and Batten (1905), Siegrist (1905), Michelson-Rabinowitsch (1906), Rosenmeyer (1906), Michel (1908), Komoto (1909), Murakami (1913), Wiener (1925), Moore (1936) and Wheeler (1936).

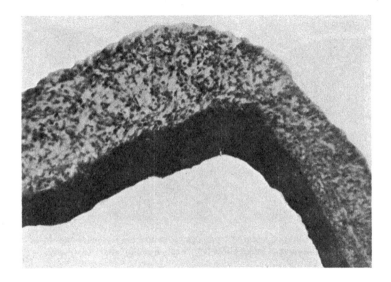

Fig. 86. × 155. Showing failure of iris to differentiate.

In some cases (Sutherland and Mayou, and Wiener) enlarged corneal nerve fibres were observed clinically. Hine and Wyatt (1928) described an almost continuous layer of groups of elongated cells lying under the anterior limiting membrane of the cornea, in a case of neurofibromatosis involving the upper eyelid and the orbit. These cells were more distinct at the limbus and numerous thickened nerves could be recognised. The presence of new growth around the nerve fibres in the cornea would suggest that the tissue in this disease developed from the cells of the sheath of Schwann (Collins, 1929).

Those who have reported cases without referring to the ciliary nerves are Weinstein, Hudson (1925), Mintschewa (1926), Awguschewitsch (1929), Metzger (1925), Löb (1923), Pomplum (1921), Weber and Bode (1934).

The tumour formation in Wheeler's specimen consisted of non-medullated nerve fibres and many foci of ganglion cells. Large areas of spindle-shaped cells containing pigment were also present. The choroid showed many round and oval laminated structures with laterally arranged nuclei. Temporally over the ciliary body the growth extended through the sclera to the external surface. Only in the pro-

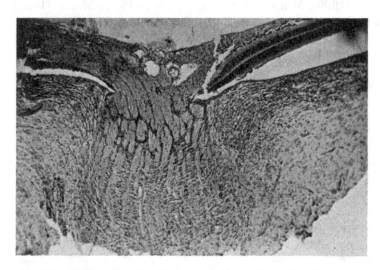

Fig. 87. ×45. Choroid replaced by avascular neurofibromatous tissue close up to the optic nerve (cut obliquely) which shows no sign of cupping.

lapsed tissue was intra-perineural fibrosis observed. The perforation of the globe in this specimen appears to be the only instance reported (see Figs. 88 to 91).

Verhoeff (1936) found that the choroidal changes varied considerably. In one place the structure might be typical, containing thickened nerves, and in others there might be so few nerves and so many vessels that one would be apt to diagnose angioma. He considered that there were two main types of choroidal involvement—the familiar type, with diffuse choroidal involvement and enlarged nerve endings and the presence of glaucoma, and secondly, that with nodular tumours, which though they can be traced to nerve fibres in some sections yet appear to be like spindle cell leucosarcomata. Callender and Thigpen (1930) have described the latter form. In their case, after enucleation on account of secondary glaucoma, two apparently separate neurofibromata were found. These tumours presented the typical palisade arrangement.   Phelan (1931) described multiple tumours on the naso-ciliary nerve. It has been suggested that the discrete form arises from the ciliary nerves and the diffuse form from the perivascular nerve plexus. Freeman and Knight emphasised the marked manner in which the vessels were affected in their specimens.

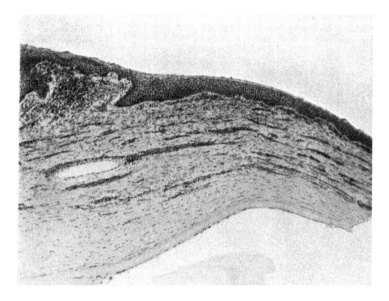

Fig. 88.   × 50. Section showing extensive neurofibromatosis throughout the cornea near the limbus. Descemet's membrane is greatly thickened (up to 50μ.).

A plexiform neuroma in the choroid was found by Meeker (1936) in a globe that had been removed because glaucoma supervened on iridocyclitis following a traumatic corneal ulcer. The choroid was thickened behind the equator and the normal stroma was largely replaced by nerve fibres, which were most numerous about the posterior ciliary vessels. Meeker considered that Freeman's case was the only previously reported one of choroidal neuroma in a non-hydrophthalmic eye. No other evidence of von Recklinghausen's disease was present. Verhoeff, however, referred to other specimens with choroidal and ciliary involvement and yet no hydrophthalmia. Michel (1908) also referred to a case where the only signs of neurofibromatosis were the fibromatous knots along the ciliary nerves.

Summary of histologically examined specimens with neurofibromatosis

Specimens examined	Age	Enlarged ciliary nerves	Choroid			Angle	Optic nerve or canal
			Diffuse changes	Ganglion cells	Ovoid bodies		
Unpublished specimen II (Moore's case I)	5 wks.	+	+	.	.	Closed by iris process	−
Michelson-Rabinowitsch (Siegrist's case)	23 mos.	+	+ Atrophy near disc	.	−	Partial synechia. Endothelial proliferation	−
Wiener	2 yrs.	+	+ +	−	+	Filled with foetal tissue	.
Wagenmann (Lezius's case)	2½ yrs.	+	.	.	.	Open. "pect. lig." full of pigment	.
Knight	5 yrs.	+	+ +	+	+	Iris and cornea adherent. D.'s membrane runs on to iris	? +
Snell and Collins	7 yrs.	+	+ Slight atrophic	? −	+	Iris and cornea united. No meshwork or spaces of Fontana. D.'s membrane runs round angle on to iris	−
Sachsalber	7 yrs.	+	+	−	−	Schlemm's canal closed by sclerosed tissue	?
Murakami (Komoto's case)	9 yrs.	+	+	?	?	Synechia. No meshwork	−
Wheeler	12 yrs.	+	+ +	+	+	Closed	+
Collins and Batten	16 yrs.	+	+ +	? −	+	Iris-like tissue. No spaces of Fontana or meshwork	? normal
Schiess Gemuseus	27 yrs.	+	Atrophic	?	?	Iris process	−

Cranial and intra-cranial lesions. Osseous changes, as characteristic of von Recklinghausen's disease as the skin tumours, are often due to the involvement of the bone by the growth of tumour tissue (Knapp, 1934).

Many skull defects have been reported in neurofibromatosis.

Winkelbauer (1927) classified these changes as lack of bilateral symmetry, thinning and defective development of cranial bones, and less often, thickening of bone. The osseous changes may extend to the posterior fossa and the base of the skull, as in Weber's and Bode's case.

Amongst these changes is the enlargement of the optic foramina due to diffuse thickening of the optic nerve (van der Hoeve, 1923). The optic nerve may be so enlarged that the foramen is six times as

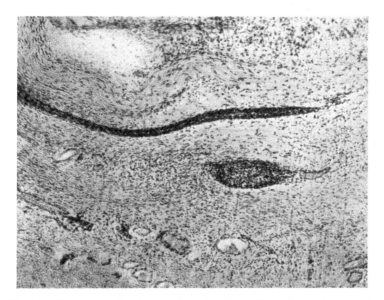

Fig. 89. × 50. Section showing the dense structure of the extra-ocular extension and two neurofibrillary strands (one cut transversely).

large as the other side (Berens). Michel found the involved orbits to be one-third greater than those on the normal side. The right optic canal in Wheeler's case was 8·0 × 11·0 mm. Moore (1936) described two patients with neurofibromatosis, hydrophthalmia, and defects of the orbital wall. In Komoto's patient the orbit was enlarged and pulsatile. The fontanelle was small and the ipsilateral mastoid, sphenoid and frontal bones were affected.

Jaensch (1928) reported a posterior orbital encephalocele with a greatly enlarged orbit and defects of the temporal bone in a fifteen-year-old boy with hydrophthalmia. The defect in the orbital wall may be so marked that a pulsatile exophthalmos is produced. This has been treated by ligation of the common carotid artery. A prominence in the temporal region is not uncommon, *e.g.* Pomplum (case II), and in one case the skull was trephined in this area (Foster Moore, 1930). In this case, that of Rockliffe and Parsons (1903), Snell's second case and at least two of Le Wald's patients (1933), there was absence of part of the orbital wall, definite signs of neurofibromatosis but none of hydrophthalmia. The orbits were extensively involved in two sisters reported by Holmström (1928) but without hydrophthalmia.

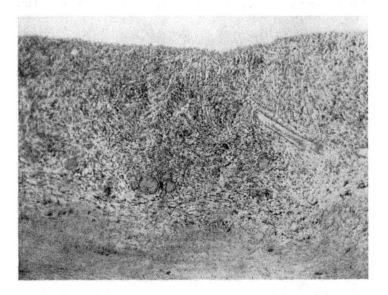

Fig. 90. × 50. Section showing whorls in the fibrosed choroid and the absence of a boundary between it and the sclera. Avascular.

Signs of intra-cranial disease. Vogt (1924) reported three female patients with what he considered to be a hitherto unknown disease. All showed unilateral elephantiasis of the upper lid with enlarged sella turcica. The right eye of the oldest patient, aged thirty-three years, had been removed because of secondary glaucoma and spontaneous intercalary staphyloma. The cornea took no part in the enormous distension. Fehr (1913) had previously described the association of a large sella turcica, though within normal limits, in a girl with elephantiasis of the left lid and normal eyes. The glial tumours of the brain that may occur with von Recklinghausen's disease have recently been described by van der Hoeve (1923).

An enlargement of the sella turcica is a relatively common accompaniment. It has been observed by Mintschewa, Metzger,

Awguschewitsch, Weber and Bode, A. E. Moore and Wheeler. In the case of the last named the sella measured 15·0 by 21·0 mm. and there was little evidence of a right anterior clinoid process. The middle fossa on the same side was enlarged. These findings are certainly suggestive of intra-cranial neurofibromatosis.

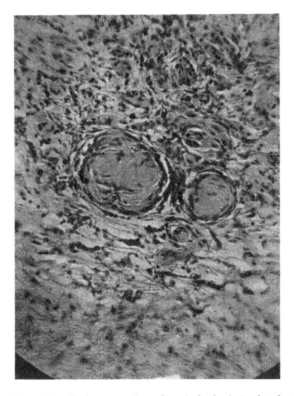

Fig. 91. ×220. High power view of typical whorls in the choroid, showing hyaline degeneration and palisade arrangement of the cells.

Association with hemihypertrophy. The form of hypertrophy that occurs with neurofibromatosis may lead to a most unsightly appearance. Half the face was affected in the cases of Sachsalber, Sutherland and Mayou, Michel, Pomplum, Wiener, Weber and Bode, Metzger, Mintschewa, Merkulov, Komoto, Moore (two cases) and Campbell (Figs. 109, 110). In addition half of the body and one or both legs were affected in Awguschewitsch's case. A patient described by Knapp (1933) had similar gross hypertrophy and a box-shaped sella turcica. His left eye, which had been removed in childhood, is not described, however, as being hydrophthalmic. Vogt stated that one complete side was hypertrophied and one foot acromegalic in his case. Metzger's case was described as being similar to that of Vogt. Of 768 cases of acromegaly from the literature, Atkinson found von Reckling-hausen's disease in only four (Reuben, 1934).

Metzger's and Mintschewa's cases showed an enlarged sella turcica with facial hemihypertrophy and hydrophthalmia on the same side. Awguschewitsch's case showed congenital glaucoma and hemihyper-trophy and an enlarged sella turcica on the same side. An elongated sella turcica without erosion and a unilateral enlargement of the orbit has been described (Weber and Bode, 1934). Avizonis found a normal pituitary body in an enlarged sella turcica associated with facial hemihypertrophy. Evidences of disordered pituitary function were found in Awguschewitsch's case, e.g. amenorrhoea, disturbed calcium metabolism, unilateral enlargement of lower extremities, and round shadows due to calcification of the hypophysis. However, one cannot attribute the enlarged sella turcica definitely to a diseased hypophysis, and one can only suggest a developmental defect of the former. The exact relationship of the pituitary disorders, the skull defects, the hemihypertrophy of the face, the hydrophthalmia, and the neurofibromatosis is yet to be disentangled.

Michel (1908) reported two cases of congenital hemifacial hyper-trophy, one of which was associated with hydrophthalmia. He also described three cases of neurofibromatosis with hydrophthalmia.

This form of hemihypertrophy which occurs with extensive neuro-fibromatosis must be distinguished from the true congenital form in which, in a typical case, all the structures of one side are enlarged, the limbs being longer as well as more developed. At times also a crossed condition is found, e.g. the leg on the one side and the arm on the other side. A central nervous origin is suspected but its nature is obscure.

The escape of the eye in hemihypertrophy and atrophy. The freedom of the organ of vision from involvement in cases of facial hemi-hypertrophy emphasises the influence that its different mode of origin may have. This organ is in the face but not of the face and, therefore, may escape when, from various causes, the facial tissues, from skin to bone, tend to undergo hypertrophy.

It is of interest also that the eye as a rule escapes in facial hemi-atrophy. At times pupillary disorders and heterochromia are found, and while these signs give further support to the contention that most cases of facial hemiatrophy are due to an involvement of the cervical sympathetic they show the slightness of the ocular upset. It is probable that the sympathetic lesion is partly destructive and partly irritative in type—the equivalent of the newer "release phenomenon", in which the destructive component probably predominates. "In

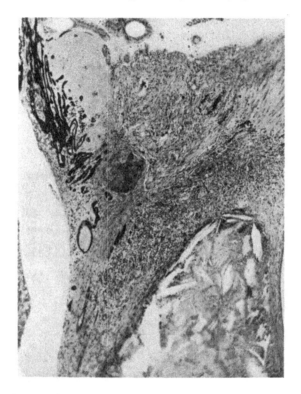

Fig. 92. ×50. Section of ciliary body showing (1) dense sclerosis of tissue containing one well-developed mass of metaplastic bone, (2) cyclitic membrane over shrunken ciliary processes and which runs into the vitreous, (3) masses of amorphous and crystalline debris containing spaces from which cholesterol crystals have been dissolved.

young dogs, section of the cervical sympathetic stunted the development of the face, cranium and ocular globe on the corresponding side. In congenital lesions of the cervical sympathetic heterochromia of the homolateral iris has repeatedly been observed in hemiatrophy in connection with infantile hemiplegias" (Archambault and Fromm, 1932).

There appears to be a tendency in some cases for the atrophy to become arrested and to remain within the limits of one or more of the divisions of the trigeminal nerve. The atrophy is sufficiently complete for bone to be involved in the majority of cases, particularly if the onset of the atrophy is in early life. The eye, however, tends to escape though enophthalmos has been described. A neuro-paralytic keratitis was present in a case carefully investigated by Stief (1933).

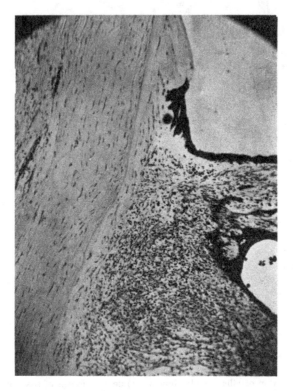

Fig. 93. ×50. Section showing wide open angle filled with a pigmented strand and proliferated hyaline material. Descemet's membrane extends far beyond the angle between the ciliary body and the sclera.

In addition to the right side of the face and neck, the right shoulder and lower extremity, certain internal organs were affected. Signs of sympathetic disturbance were present on the same side and, on examination, the right inferior cervical ganglion showed high grade degeneration and the superior ganglion was infiltrated. These changes were considered to be the cause of the cerebral vascular condition which was one of arteriosclerosis with ipsolateral dilatation and stasis and contralateral contraction of the terminal branch.

Other ocular changes in neurofibromatosis. Alterations in uveal pigmentation have been described by Goldstein and Wexler (1930). In their case the irides were very dark and studded with minute melanomata, and even the "ligamentum corneo-iridicum" was pigmented. Glaucoma, however, was not present. Coats (1912) referred to a similar iris as a "golf ball iris". Pigmentation of

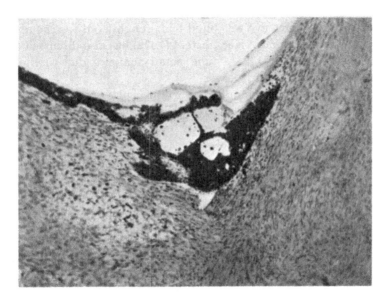

Fig. 94. × 50. Another view showing extension round the angle of pigmented tissue from the iris, and hyaline tissue from Descemet's membrane.

Schlemm's canal is shown in illustrations by Reese (1925) and others. The association with melanosis of the uveal tract is interesting since Masson suggested that the melanomata grow from naevus cells which are derived from cells of the sheath of Schwann. Neurofibromatosis may also grow from these cells. In a sixteen-year-old girl, who had not hydrophthalmia, Merkulov found nodules on both irides and facial neurofibromatosis. Vessels on both irides were found in the day-old infant examined by Berens.

In a patient with features of von Recklinghausen's disease on the chest, arms, legs and spine but not on the head, bilateral opaque retinal nerve fibres were reported by Copeland, Craver and Reese (1934).

They refer to Fischer's study of twelve patients with neurofibromatosis in which he found opaque nerve fibres in four (1924–5). Moravec (1924) referred to a patient with elephantiasis of the lids with colobomata of the retina and the iris and an orbital dermoid. Wiegmann's patient (1922) had bilateral optic atrophy and myopia. Brun's patient (1870) had an atrophic eye which probably had been hydrophthalmic. Shapland and Greenfield's patient (1935) presented an unusual association of three different types of slow growing and usually innocent tumours. They were neurofibromata of the cranial and spinal nerves, a psammoma of the meninges and gliomata of the spinal cord and right frontal lobe. One eye was blind but probably only as the result of the optic nerve tumour. Katzenstein (1932) has also discussed this association. Axenfeld (1925) found small tumours due to hypertrophied intrascleral ciliary nerves.

Apart from glaucoma the most important ocular changes are those retinal tumours and plaques described by van der Hoeve (1923 and 1932). These tumours are apparently built of the same fibres and cells as the lesions in tuberose sclerosis but at times they contain large vessels. They apparently originate in the nerve fibre layers.

HYDROPHTHALMIA AND FACIAL NAEVI

The co-existence of glaucoma with facial naevus flammeus has for long attracted attention. The glaucoma may be present at birth as hydrophthalmia, or it may arise at any stage during life in either an acute or a chronic form. It may be the simple or a secondary form of glaucoma, and several cases have been reported that may be classified as pseudo-glaucoma, as Ballantyne suggested. The relationship is probably not closer than that of a common underlying cause, but this point will be considered later. It must be mentioned that other ocular anomalies and particularly retinal detachment may occur with facial naevi, with and without glaucoma.

Schirmer (1860) was the first to report an example of the association of hydrophthalmia and facial naevus. Kaiser collected twenty-one cases of this association (Dettmering). Pi (1931) summarised thirty-five cases of facial naevus with glaucoma and of these ten showed hydrophthalmia. Dunphy (1935), when reporting two cases, referred to sixty-one cases of glaucoma and naevus in the literature. Of these sixty-three cases fourteen eyeballs had been examined microscopically.

The following summary forms the basis for this discussion:

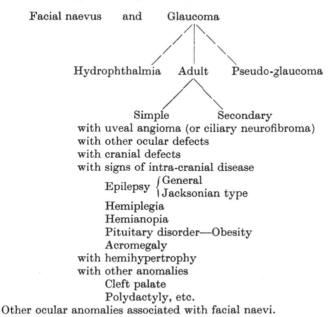

Facial naevus   and   Glaucoma

Hydrophthalmia   Adult   Pseudo-glaucoma

Simple   Secondary
with uveal angioma (or ciliary neurofibroma)
with other ocular defects
with cranial defects
with signs of intra-cranial disease
    Epilepsy { General
              { Jacksonian type
    Hemiplegia
    Hemianopia
    Pituitary disorder—Obesity
    Acromegaly
with hemihypertrophy
with other anomalies
    Cleft palate
    Polydactyly, etc.
Other ocular anomalies associated with facial naevi.

Nineteen instances of the simple association of unilateral hydrophthalmia and ipsolateral facial naevus have been reported by the following:

Galezowski	(1898)	Love	(1914)
Cuperus	(1909)	Freese	(1920)
Elschnig	(1918)	Dohme	(1920) (2 cases)
Zeeman	(1936)	Clausen	(1928)
Zaun	(1924)	Kostoulas	(1932)
Safar	(1929)	Gault	(1937)
Folk	(1935)	Jaensch (case XX)	(1927)
Panico (case I)	(1928)	Horay	(1929) (2 cases)
Stoewer	(1908)		

Nineteen cases of unilateral hydrophthalmia and unilateral facial naevus and other lesions.

Cabannes	(1909)	R. face	
Nakamura	(1922)	R. face	
Kiranoff	(1925)	L. face	. Osseous changes.
Padovani	(1935)	L. face	
Ballantyne I	(1930)	L. face	
Cushing II	(1906)	R. face. Epilepsy.	
Horrocks	(1883)	R. face. L. hemiplegia.	

van Rötth   (1928)   L. face. R. hemianopia and hemiparesis.
Voegele   (1928)   R. face. Enlarged posterior clivus.
Aynsley I   (1929)   L. face. R. hemiplegia.
  „   II   R. face. L. hemiplegia.
  „   IV   R. face. L. hemiplegia.
Weber   (1929)   L. face. R. hemiplegia.
Crouzon and   (1933)   L. face. Generalised epilepsy and intra-cranial an-
  others   gioma. X-ray (left side).
Vincent and   (1929)   L. face. R. hemiplegia and hemianopia.
  Heuyer II
Coppez   (1935)   L. face and Jacksonian epilepsy.
Joiris and   (1935)   L. face and L. hemiplegic attacks.
  Fauchamps I
O'Brien and   (1933)   L. face. ? R. Jacksonian epilepsy.
  Porter
Applemans   (1935)   L. face. Intra-cranial angioma.

Five cases of unilateral hydrophthalmia and bilateral facial naevus:

Vita   (1925)   R. eye. R. face, arm, chest and back and 0·5 cm. over
                            the mid-line of the nasal bridge. R. and L. lower
                            body and extremities.
Kaiser   (1927)   R. eye. R. and L. face.
Schirmer   (1860)   L. eye. R. and L. face. R. chest and back.
Safar   (1923)   R. eye. R. and L. face, trunk and limbs.
Pi   (1931)   L. eye. R. and L. face, chest.

Nine cases of unilateral hydrophthalmia, bilateral naevi and other changes (T.):

Krause   (1929)   L. eye. R. and L. face. R. Jacksonian epilepsy.
Kreyenberg I   (1935)   R. eye. R. and L. face, neck, etc. L. Jacksonian
  and Hansing   epilepsy, etc.
     „   II   R. eye. R. and L. face. Convulsions.
     „   III   R. eye. R. and L. head. R. epilepsy.
Sturge   (1879)   R. eye. R. and L. face. L. Jacksonian epilepsy.
Cushing I   (1906)   R. eye. R. and L. face. L. hemianopia and hemi-
                            plegia.
     „   III   R. eye. R. and L. face. L. hemiplegia, etc.
Aynsley   (1929)   R. eye. R. and L. face. L. hemiplegia, etc.
Unpublished   R. almost blind at thirty-eight years, L. contracted
  case. C.T.   field from simple glaucoma. R. and L. face, and
  (see Figs. 111, 112)   patches on all extremities and body. Epilepsy.
Kreyenberg and Hansing's case I had simple glaucoma in the other eye.

Eight cases of bilateral hydrophthalmia and facial naevus:

Horay (case   (1929)   R. and L. face.
  M.G.)
Beltmann   (1904)   R. and L. face and pharynx.
Marchesani   (1925)   R. and L. face and head.
Fleischer (case   (1918)   R. and L. face.
  XII)

Perera   (1935)   R. and L. face and scalp. R. arm bones thicker than
                           L. Intra-cranial haemangioma (X-ray).
Dunphy   (1935)   R. and L. face and body. L. Jacksonian epilepsy and
                           atrophy.
Santonastaso   (1936)   Only one side of face. L. upper lid.
  (case III)
Koyama   (1937)   R. naevus flammeus. L. naevus pigmentosus. Body
                           almost covered.

The association of unilateral simple glaucoma and ipsolateral facial
naevus has been reported by many, including the following:

Krause   (1929)   Onset puberty.
Duschnitz   (1923) R. Onset 11 years.
Zvereva   (1929)   Onset 25 years.
Steiner   (1932)
Derby, Waite   (1927)
  and Kirk
Dunphy   (1935) R. Onset 52 years (approx.).
Komoto   (1922) R. Onset (?).
Salus   (1923)
Horay I and II   (1929)   (Juvenile).
Löwenstein   (1923) L.
Corrado   (1933)   Onset 27 years.
Applemans   (1935)
Skydsgaard   (1935)
Evans   (1937)   Onset (? birth).

Unilateral simple glaucoma, facial naevi and other lesions:

Ginzburg   (1926) Onset 28 years. R. eye. R. face. L. hemianopia.
                                            Acromegaly, etc.
Hudelo   (1929) Onset 20 years. Hemiatrophy and hemiparesis, etc.
                                            Intra-cranial angioma (X-ray).
Tyson   (1932) Onset 26 years. L. eye. L. face, head (R. hemia-
                                            nopia). L. occipital angioma
                                            (X-ray).
Joiris and   (1935) Onset 24 years. R. lost after accident. L. glaucoma.
  Fauchamps II   R. and L. face. R. rigidity and
                                            tremor.

The association of secondary glaucoma and facial naevi has been
reported by:

Milles   (1884) R. Onset 15 years.
Lawford   (1885) L. Onset 8 years.
Snell   (1886) R. Onset 17 years.
Wagenmann   (1900)   L. eye always defective.
Steffens   (1902) L. Onset 19 years.
Quackenboss   (1908) R. Onset 7 years (approx.).
  and Verhoeff
Paton and   (1919) L. Onset 14 years.
  Collins

Bär   (1925)   Onset 23 years. R. and L. face. Unilateral
                                     secondary glaucoma.
Yamanaka   (1927)   R. Onset 21 years.
de Haas   (1928)   R.   Blind at 20 years.
Jahnke   (1930)   L. Onset blind at 11 years.
Granström   (1935)   L. Onset (?).

Bilateral glaucoma (other than congenital) bilateral facial naevi:

Biro   (1936)   Onset at 8 years at latest.
Knapp   (1927)   Onset 4 years. R. and L. face and body, and L.
                                   hemiplegia. (? mild hydrophthalmia.)
Horay (case   (1929)   Almost blind at 19 years.
  J.H.)
Mehney   (1937)   Onset 20 years. R. and L. face.

The association of pseudo-glaucoma and facial naevi has been reported by:

MacRae   (1929)   Age 13 years.   Naevus of face, arms and body. R.
                                                  upper extremity larger than L.
                                                  R. pseudo-cup.
Voegele   (1925)   Age 62 years.   Naevi of R. conjunctiva, sclera and
                                                  face. R. cup, but normal vision
                                                  and field.
Thomson   (1929)   Age 13 years.   R. temple, cheek and neck. R. cornea
                                                  2 mm. wider than L. Pseudo-cup.
                                                  Paralytic attacks L. arm and leg.
                                                  Mentally deficient.
Ballantyne II   (1930)   Age 29 years.   L. myopia, coloboma of disc and
                                                  facial naevi. L. facial bones slightly
                                                  larger than R.
Riser   (1936)   "Megalocornea" probably hydro-
                                                  phthalmia. The cornea was clear
                                                  and 14 mm. in diameter. The disc
                                                  and tension were normal. The
                                                  vision was only 20/100. So the
                                                  absence of glaucoma is disputable.

1. In the above summary the ages of onset are only approximate and in most cases give the age when the diagnosis was made. Even so they are sufficiently accurate to emphasise the early age of onset of glaucoma.

2. No attempt has been made to make a complete list of cases of senile glaucoma associated with facial naevi.

Twenty-one instances of bilateral naevus have been reported, and in fourteen of these hydrophthalmia was present on one side only. These were the cases of Schirmer, Krause, Sturge, Cushing (cases I and III), Aynsley (third case), Pi, Kaiser, Kreyenberg and Hansing

(I, II and III), Vita, Safar and unpublished case C.T. In the last case the affected eye was on the same side as the majority of the naevi. The following conditions were found with bilateral naevi: adult glaucoma (Biro, Knapp, unpublished case, Horay's case J.H.); Pseudo-glaucoma (MacRae, Voegele, Thomson, Ballantyne II, Riser). Knapp's case was probably an example of mild hydrophthalmia. In Vita's case the naevi involved half the face and passed $\frac{1}{2}$ cm. beyond the midline of the bridge of the nose. Both sides of the lower trunk and both legs were affected. It is of interest to note how this tendency to become bilateral in the lower extremities occurs also in neurofibromatosis.

In addition to the eight cases of bilateral naevi and hydrophthalmia, Clausen reported one of unilateral naevus with ipsolateral hydrophthalmia and a deep glaucoma cup in the other eye. Kreyenberg's and Hansing's first case and unpublished case C.T. were similar to this except that naevi were present on both sides. Vincent and Heuyer (1929) reported a four-year-old patient who had bilateral convulsions, mental deficiency, radiographic evidence of a right-sided occipital tumour and bilateral optic atrophy. Radiotherapy produced some improvement.

Apparently glaucoma is associated with a facial naevus only when it affects the lids or the conjunctiva.

Summary

52 {
19 cases of unilateral hydrophthalmia and unilateral naevus alone.
19 cases of unilateral hydrophthalmia and unilateral naevus with cranial lesions.
5 cases of unilateral hydrophthalmia and bilateral naevi alone.
9 cases of unilateral hydrophthalmia and bilateral naevi with cranial lesions.

8 {
5 cases of bilateral hydrophthalmia and bilateral naevi alone.
1 case of bilateral hydrophthalmia and unilateral naevus alone.
2 cases of bilateral hydrophthalmia and bilateral naevi with cranial lesions.

31 {
15 cases of unilateral simple glaucoma and unilateral naevus alone.
4 cases of unilateral simple glaucoma and unilateral naevus and cranial lesions.
12 cases of secondary glaucoma and facial naevi.

4 cases of bilateral glaucoma of various forms and bilateral facial naevi.

Bilateral hydrophthalmia has so far been found only with bilateral naevi, with the exception of Santonastaso's case.

Of sixty cases of hydrophthalmia associated with facial naevi

in 13 % the glaucoma was bilateral,

in 35 % the facial naevus was bilateral,

in 50 % cranial lesions were present.

Of thirty-five cases of other forms of glaucoma associated with facial naevi

in 12 % the glaucoma was bilateral, and

in at least 21 % additional lesions were present.

The angle of filtration. In an excellent summary of the histological examinations of fourteen globes, showing glaucoma or hydrophthalmia associated with facial naevi, Dunphy (1935) stated that a choroidal angioma was present in ten. One showed irregularities of Schlemm's canal and of the scleral spur, one an angiomatous change in the iris extending up to the angle, and in two no angioma or obvious angle obstruction was present. He agreed with Tyson that if the angle was free there was probably an excessive formation of aqueous from the intra-ocular capillaries, which, he considered, were usually dilated.

Vascular changes in the uvea. As a rule the iris is darker on the affected side—Ballantyne, Safar, O'Brien and Porter, Aynsley (4 cases). The stroma appeared to be denser than normal. In Clausen's patient telangiectasis of each iris was found. Krause (1929) in his specimen with glaucoma observed varicose iris vessels and very enlarged anterior choroidal vessels. Markus, who examined the hydrophthalmic globe removed from Weber's case, found no evidence of angiomatous formation but simply a partial heterochromia, the upper three-quarters of the iris being brown instead of blue. Pi's (1931) case of hydrophthalmia and naevus exhibited a spongy appearance of the iris surface. Knapp (1927) examined the hydrophthalmic eye of a boy who had a facial naevus of both sides of his face, upper trunk, and arms. He found the iris thickened and in an angiomatous state. The endothelial cells had proliferated and many newly formed blood vessels were found. As this change extended to the angle, Knapp thought that similar changes had blocked the angle.

Angioma of the choroid is a rare condition, but numerous reports of it are found in the literature. The majority appear to occur near the posterior pole of the globe, and like certain other developmental defects, particularly in the inferior temporal quadrant. If all eyes enucleated for glaucoma were examined microscopically haemangioma would be found more often.

Many instances of a choroidal angioma with a naevus and hydro-phthalmia have been reported by observers, including Galezowski (1898), Stoewer (1908), Love (1914), and Dunphy (1935). Galezowski's case (1898) was the first one of hydrophthalmia associated with a facial naevus in which the angioma was recognised clinically. Love (1914) examined a hydrophthalmic eye of a man aged twenty years with an ipsolateral naevus and he found a choroidal angioma, a retinal detach-ment, and the angle blocked by adhesions. A membrane was present on the anterior surface of the iris and it was continuous with and in every way similar to Descemet's membrane. In the cases of Milles (1884), Lawford (1885), Snell (1886), Steffens (1902), Wagenmann (1900), de Haas (1928), Jahnke (1931), and Granström (1935) no ocular enlargement was found. In Paton's and Collins's case (1919) acute glaucoma developed after ignipuncture for a retinal detachment. In Bär's case there were venous anastomoses near the disc and a naevus towards the periphery. Quackenboss and Verhoeff (1908) removed a blind glaucomatous eye from an eleven-year-old girl who had a naevus of the lower lid and cheek of the same side. Their findings resembled those of Love. On section a choroidal angioma, retinal detachment and blocking of the angle by the root of the iris were found. In this case hydrophthalmia was not present. The glaucoma was secondary in type and the disc was swollen. In the eye described by de Haas the posterior part of the choroid was three to four times the normal thickness. This was due to the presence of numerous distended vessels of varying calibre and thickness of wall.

Lindenmeyer (1932) analysed a series of forty-six cases of choroidal angioma. In five of these the diagnosis of choroidal sarcoma was made and in three others the symptoms were strongly suggestive of this condition. In the remaining thirty-eight cases the tumours were found accidentally in eyes that had been removed for absolute glaucoma.

Emory Hill and Dart (1936), when discussing five eyes containing haemangioma of the choroid, stated that these tumours were not recognised clinically, and that when a tumour was suspected a melanotic sarcoma was diagnosed. They considered that the patho-logist's report of "no tumour" may at times be made in error, for the smaller growths collapse to the point of invisibility when the eye is opened in the laboratory.

Ophthalmoscopic diagnosis of the choroidal angioma was made in Lawford's case of glaucoma, and in the case with retinal detachment and acute glaucoma following ignipuncture reported by Paton and Collins.

According to Brons (1936) only eleven cases of choroidal haemangioma have been accessible to ophthalmoscopy. His patient developed secondary glaucoma at the age of forty-six. Ludwig (1935) reported a woman with small temporal angioma which enlarged very considerably until she was twenty-eight years, when she developed a retinal detachment and other evidence of a choroidal angioma.

Some of these cases have been associated with glaucoma even in the absence of facial naevus, *e.g.* Guilini (1890), Meller (1907). Love (1914) collected twenty-two cases, and of these only seven were associated with facial naevi and four were described clinically. Fehr's case (1905) was observed for twenty years, and then as glaucoma developed after haemorrhage the eye was removed. The angioma was a greyish-white flat swelling, glistening in places and showing dark upper and lower edges. Since then Paton and Collins (1919) and Henderson (1920) have reported similar cases that developed glaucoma.

A choroidal angioma was assumed to be present in Paton's and Collins's case, because they found a retinal detachment with raised tension associated with an ipsilateral facial naevus. On histological examination a network of vascular spaces, as in a cavernous angioma, was found. Collins stated that a similar state had been found in all but one of the fourteen other cases examined microscopically. The exception was Deyl's case (1899), in which the growth had the appearance of a telangiectasis.

Wagenmann (1900) described one such lesion as a pure naevus vascularis or angioma cavernosum. It consisted mainly of close layers of various sized vessels. All transitory stages were found from capillaries to large spaces full of blood. Each large vessel consisted of a thin connective tissue wall with a simple regular endothelial layer.

Little is understood about the life history of angiomata. It seems probable that they tend to increase in size. There is evidence suggesting that the capillary form may not just grow *pari passu* with the body and may even take on an appearance resembling the cavernous type. The form that occurs in the orbit may certainly become neoplastic. Quackenboss and Verhoeff (1908) described a haemangioma that invaded the sclera, choroid and optic nerve. The spread along the posterior ciliary nerves of capillary-like vessels first, and later of cavernous structures, was of particular interest.

A condition sometimes described as a "naevus of the choroid" must not be confused with the tumour formation being discussed. It is a melanoma, which appears uniformly grey in colour. It has either a definite or a feathery edge. It shows little or no elevation, but has a tendency to become malignant (Johnston, 1929).

Other ocular changes. The retinal vessels (Schirmer, Yamanaka, Beltmann, Aynsley) and the choroidal vessels (Salus, Steffens, Krause), as seen with the ophthalmoscope, have frequently been described as being dilated and tortuous. The fundi were dark red in colour in the patients of Perera, Padovani and Sturge. Several instances of large tortuous retinal vessels in hydrophthalmic eyes not accompanied by facial naevi have been reported. In Grimsdale's case (1917) the arteries were tortuous and much larger than the veins. Instances of tortuous retinal vessels, particularly in the neighbourhood of the disc on the same side as facial naevi in non-hydrophthalmic patients have been referred to by Collins (1917), Hartridge (1901), Voegele (1925), Yamanaka (1927), Work Dodd (1901) and others. It is not surprising that some of such patients have also a naevoid state of the nasal mucous membrane. The man reported by Collins had recurrent epistaxis. Such cases constitute a link with the syndrome of facial and intra-nasal naevi which is commonly hereditary and is known as Osler's disease. See Goldstein (1936) and McArthur (1937).

Bär (1925) described a case of glaucoma with naevus of the eyeball and numerous tortuous anastomosing retinal veins in the fundus. A clearly defined patch in the retina was found, and Bär considered it to be haemorrhagic in origin. O'Brien and Porter described an unusual pigmented patch near the temporal periphery of the affected eye in their patient. Enlarged choroidal vessels surrounded this area but the neighbouring retinal vessels were reduced in size. These patches, like other retinal anomalies, appear to be most commonly found in the inferior temporal quadrant. Compare anterior dialyses, falciform fold, cysts, and vascular tumours of the retina.

The association of a facial naevus, hydrophthalmia, contralateral convulsive seizures and probably a hepatic haemangioma was found by Krause (1929). The conditions in Bär's, and O'Brien's and Porter's cases, and in those with wide and tortuous retinal vessels, are sufficiently like v. Hippel's disease to make brief reference to it and to Lindau's syndrome worth while (see below). The haemangiomatous tumours and cysts present in Lindau's syndrome have a widespread and characteristic distribution and are of congenital origin. This syndrome may also be associated with facial naevi (Collins, 1917), and with a late secondary glaucoma.

Other ocular anomalies than hydrophthalmia have been described in association with facial naevi. MacRae (1929) and Thomson (1929) each described a child with facial naevi and anomalous optic discs on the side of most or all of the naevi. The eye described by MacRae was of normal size, but the right upper extremity was larger than the left. Thomson considered that the ocular distension in his patient was not hydrophthalmic but possibly the result of birth injury. Paralytic attacks of the contralateral limbs had been described.

SUMMARY OF SPECIMENS WITH FACIAL NAEVI

Specimen Examined	Age (years)	Choroid			Angle
		Angioma	Bone forma-tion	Pigment	
Stoewer (1908)	9	+	⊥	?	Closed near angioma
Love (1914)	20	+	+	?	Closed by union of iris and cornea
Dunphy (1935)	21	+	+	+ + (sclera too)	Closed. Meshwork sclerosed
Safar (1929)	28	−	−	+ + (both eyes)	Poor and posterior canal. Separated from angle by pigmented sclerosed framework
Cabannes (1909)	6	−	−	−	Normal. An atypical case
Specimens of other forms of glaucoma with facial naevi					
Lawford (1885)	8	+	−	−	Blocked
Jahnke (1930)	11	+	−	−	Closed by connective tissue
Quackenboss and Verhoeff (1908)	11	+	+	.	Blocked by iris root
Collins and Paton (1919)	14	+	−	−	Blocked
Milles (1884)	15	+	+	.	
Snell (1886)	17	+	.	.	
de Haas (1928)	20	+ (3–4 × normal)	.	.	
Weber (1929)	22	−	−	.	Angle and canal appeared normal
Clausen (1928)	.	.	.	.	Angle and canal appeared normal

A facial naevus has been found in association with retinal detachment. In some of the reported cases no glaucoma was found, *e.g.* Milles, Salus (1923), Onken (1928), and a probable instance by Ballantyne. A choroidal angioma was reported in the cases of Milles and Salus. Both retinae were detached, a tear was found in one retina, and a unilateral naevus was present in Onken's patient, aged forty-five years. In other cases with this association a choroidal angioma was present also and secondary glaucoma ensued: Lawford, Snell, Steffens, Paton and Collins, Wagenmann. Glaucoma was absent in the specimen associated with facial naevi reported by Wagenmann (1900).

Oguchi (1933) found in a hydrophthalmic eye a mixed growth— a "haematoma"—made up of tissue resembling that of an angioma, myoma, lipoma and fibroma. It was situated behind and temporal to the entrance of the optic nerve.

Angiectasia solely of the eyeball have been described by Leber, A. Fuchs, Henderson (1920), James and others. The patient of the last named developed glaucoma.

Cranial and intra-cranial lesions. The following instances of unilateral hydrophthalmia and facial naevi with involvement of the skull bones in addition have been reported:

> Cabannes, enlarged right orbit and temporal region.
> Nakamura, thickened bones of head, arm, trunk.
> Kiranoff, exostosis over left brow.
> Padovani, dense mastoid and temporal bone.
> Ballantyne, enlarged superior alveolar ridge.
> Suglian reported an instance of simple glaucoma in association with a facial naevus and radiographic facial asymmetry.

Intra-cranial lesions. There are several symptoms which suggest the presence of an associated intra-cranial angioma. These are localised and general epileptiform seizures, hemiplegia, hemianopia and mental deficiency.

Contralateral homonymous hemianopia was found in the cases reported by van Rötth (1928), Cushing (first case), Ginzburg (1926) (simple glaucoma), Tyson (1932) (simple glaucoma), and Foster Moore (1929) (no glaucoma).

In approximately half of the reported cases the lesions have been detected by X-rays and in several they have been examined at operation or autopsy. The means of diagnosis of an intra-cranial angioma is indicated in the following summary. It must be remembered that not all meningeal angioma show signs of calcification by X-rays. The examination may have been made before much calcium had been deposited in the vessel walls, or in the underlying cortex. The latter appears to be a common site. The calcification may commence in early life. Symmonds reported calcification in a child of ten years.

Unilateral hydrophthalmia and facial naevi and evidence of intracranial lesion:

Horrocks	R. face. L. hemiplegia.
van Rötth	L. face. R. hemianopia, hemiparesis. ? L. occipital calcification. (X-rays.)
Cushing II	R. face. ? epilepsy. Naevoid condition of dura. (Operation.)
Voegele	R. face. Hypothyroidism. Enlarged posterior clivus. (X-rays.)
Aynsley I	L. face. R. hemiplegia. Calcified meningeal angioma. (X-rays.)
„ II	R. face. L. hemiplegia. Calcified R. cerebellar angioma. (X-rays.)
„ IV	R. face. L. hemiplegia. Meningeal.
Weber	L. face. R. hemiplegia. R. face and limbs poorly developed, etc. R. fossa small. (X-rays.)
Coppez	L. face. ? Jacksonian epilepsy. Meningeal. (X-rays.)
Joiris and Fauchamps I	L. face. L. hemiplegic attacks. (X-rays.)
O'Brien and Porter	L. face. R. Jacksonian epilepsy of head and arms. Occipital calcification. (X-rays.)
Applemans	L. face. Intra-cranial angioma. (X-rays.)
Sturge	R. and L. face. L. twitching, fits and weakness.
Cushing I	R. and L. face. L. spastic hemiplegia and epilepsy. R. hemisphere small and meninges vascular (autopsy).
„ III	R. and L. face, etc. L. spastic hemiplegia, epilepsy, idiocy. Flat area R. skull. (X-rays.)
Aynsley III	R. and L. face, etc. L. hemiplegia. R. cerebellar calcification. (X-rays.)
Kreyenberg and Hansing I	R. and L. face, etc. L. epilepsy; moderate mental deficiency. Calcification frontal areas. (X-rays.) (Autopsy: R. half-brain smaller than L., dural and pial vessels greatly enlarged, especially on R.)
„ „ II	R. and L. face, etc. Convulsions. Backward mentally. Thickened supraorbital ridge. (X-rays.)
„ „ III	R. and L. face, etc. R. epilepsy, facial palsy. Nystagmus on looking to R.
Krause II	R. and L. face. R. Jacksonian epilepsy. Mentally deficient. Enlarged liver. (? angioma.) (X-rays.)

Bilateral hydrophthalmia, facial naevi and evidence of intra-cranial lesion:

Perera	R. and L. face, etc. Intra-cranial haemangioma. (X-rays.) R. arm bones thicker than L.
Dunphy I	R. and L. face, etc. L. Jacksonian epilepsy with atrophy. Mentality poor. (X-rays.)

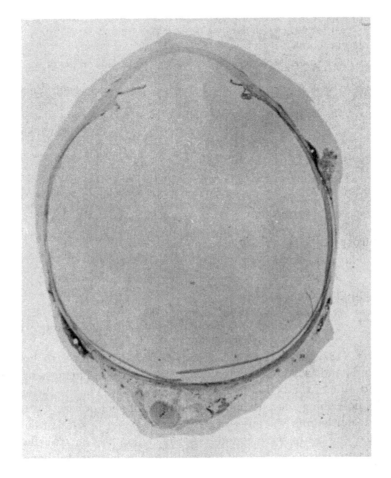

Fig. 95. Unpublished specimen III. ×3. Observe peripheral synechia and that the centre of the cornea is thinner than the periphery. Observe, too, the atrophic ciliary region. Aged twenty-one years.

In the above list, with one exception (Coppez), the signs suggesting the presence of an intra-cranial lesion indicated its presence on the same side as the affected eye. The limitation of the ocular, meningeal

AH   13 and the main facial manifestations to one and the same side is re-markably constant.

Schwartz's patient (1926) with hydrophthalmia was subject to epileptiform seizures preceded by aura of severe ocular twitching. No naevi were described in this patient.

Simple glaucoma has been found in patients with facial naevi and evidence of an intra-cranial angioma. The following are some of the reports:

Simple glaucoma:

Dunphy	Glaucoma at 57 years.	L. epilepsy. L. side of body atrophic with diminished reflexes.
Ginzburg	Onset 28 years.	L. temp. Hemianopia. Acromegaly. Enlarged sella turcica, etc.
Hudelo	Onset 20 years.	Hemiatrophy of one side of body and hemi-paresis of other. Intra-cranial angioma. (X-rays.)
Tyson	Onset 26 years.	R. homonymous hemianopia. L. occipital angioma. (X-rays.)
Knapp	Onset 11 years.	L. hemiplegia (transient). This may have been a mild example of congenital glaucoma. Vision was defective at 4 years. At 11 years he had 6 D. of myopia and each cornea was 13·0 mm.
Joiris and Fauchamps	Onset 25 years.	R. limbs slightly rigid and muscular tremor.

Secondary glaucoma:

Jahnke	No symptoms.	Tortuous diploic veins.

Pseudo-glaucoma:

Thomson	R. < 6/60.	Large cornea. Deep cup. Naevus R. face. L. hemiplegia and mental deficiency. Mentality impaired.

Sturge (1879) and Horrocks (1883) found in addition to hydro-phthalmia and facial naevi a tendency to epileptiform attacks on the opposite side of the body. To Kalischer (1897, 1901) is due the credit of first describing the post-mortem findings of such a case, but in it no hydrophthalmia was present. Extensive naevi of the left side of the face and scalp were found. In the region of the glabella the naevus spread 1–2 cm. beyond the midline. The left frontal bone was greatly thickened and the affected area extended across the midline underlying the cutaneous lesion. In some areas the frontal bone was more than three times the thickness of its fellow. Right-sided Jacksonian epilepsy commenced at the age of six months. The signs spread to the other side and unconsciousness supervened. Later a right hemiparesis appeared, and at the age of eighteen months the child died from bronchopneumonia. The left occipital bone was found to be very thin. The left hemisphere was considerably smaller than the right. It was 3 cm. shorter and correspondingly smaller in other dimensions. The pia mater on this side was dark and covered with very tortuous vessels. The whole area supplied by the middle cerebral arteries was affected and particularly that corresponding with the

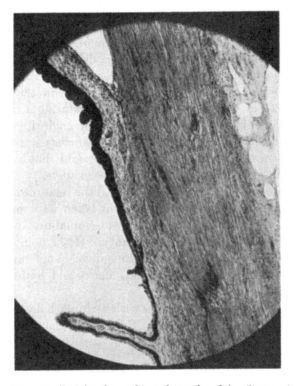

Fig. 96. × 60. Peripheral synechia and atrophy of the ciliary region.
The canal of Schlemm is blocked with pigment, etc.

site of origin of the seizures, viz. right side of the lower face. Aynsley (1929) reported four similar cases showing cerebral disorders and hydrophthalmia. He collected at least five others from the literature. They were reported by Cushing (1923), Krause (1929), and Parkes Weber (1929). Tyson's patient (see below) probably had a congenital venous angioma undergoing calcification. It was the fourth that had been recognised before operation, and few have been recognised even during operation.

Applemans (1935) described a hydrophthalmic eye associated with facial and intracranial angiomata and suggested the title "neuro-cutaneous angiomatosis".

Joiris and Fauchamps (1935) reported a 4½-year-old girl with hydrophthalmia of the left eye and a left facial angioma, who developed convulsions at seven months and transient palsies of her limbs. H. Coppez, in discussion, reported Jacksonian epilepsy in association with a left-sided naevus of the face and hydrophthalmia.

A meningeal angioma was found by X-ray in a case of Foster Moore, in which no hydrophthalmia was found. Slight dislocation of each lens and a coloboma of the left optic disc were present on the side of a large facial naevus. In addition to a facial naevus and glaucoma Tyson's patient had vascular changes in the iris and a calcified growth in the left occipital globe, producing a right homonymous hemianopia. Gonioscopy showed an angle free from any adhesions and the fluorescein test showed increased permeability of the vessels in the affected eye. Tyson thought that hypertension was due to the plasmoid aqueous blocking the angle.

Aynsley appears to have over-emphasised the relationship between meningeal and ocular angiomatous lesions when he wrote "that it is probably in the cases where there is intra-cranial involvement that eye defects are likely to arise". As Ballantyne (1930) points out, there are many cases of associated facial and meningeal angiomata without ocular lesions and of associated facial naevi and hydrophthalmia without meningeal lesions.

A considerable number of patients with hydrophthalmia and extensive naevi are mentally defective. Congenital glaucoma has been described with idiocy in the absence of facial naevi (Brissot and Delsuc, 1936).

Disorders of growth. Disorders of growth suggesting pituitary disturbance were present in Weber's patient in the form of obesity, defective sexual development, and a small sella turcica. Voegele's patient (1925) with pseudo-glaucoma had dystrophia adiposo-genitalis. His patient (1928) with hydrophthalmia had slight hypothyroidism and a large clivus posterior. Ginzburg (1926) reported a patient who developed simple glaucoma at twenty-eight and had acromegaly and an enlarged sella turcica. No sella turcica was present in one of Brushfield's cases with hemiplegia and a meningeal naevus. An angioma was present on the same side as the naevus but no mention of glaucoma is made. He and Wyatt described a syndrome consisting of facial naevi, hemiplegia, and mental deficiency (1927–8). Two of these cases were later found by Aynsley to have hydrophthalmia.

Hemihypertrophy. Reliable information is difficult to obtain concerning the association of this disorder with facial naevi and hydrophthalmia. It is not always possible to determine whether the condition is one of hemihypertrophy of one side or atrophy or arrested development of the opposite side. Macrae found the contralateral

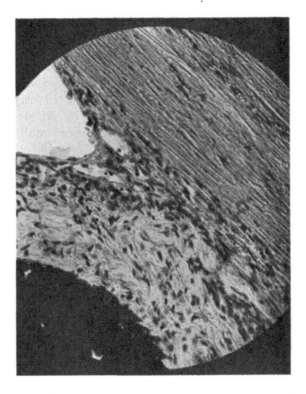

Fig. 97. ×260. Observe the new vessels in the tissue that unites the cornea and sclera.

hand and arm to be noticeably larger than the ipsolateral in a thirteen-year-old girl with pseudo-glaucoma and widespread naevi (face, limbs and body). Parkes Weber confirmed radiographically the presence of a meningeal angioma, on the opposite side to hemiplegia and hemihypertrophy of face and limbs, and on the same side as a hydrophthalmic eye, in a patient with widespread naevi of face, body and limbs. Kaiser's eight-month-old child (1927) showed an enlargement of the ipsolateral half of the body with negative X-ray findings.

Hudelo's young man (1929) had adolescent glaucoma and facial naevus, hemiatrophy of one side of the body, hemiplegia of the opposite side and X-ray evidence of an intra-cranial angioma. The cerebral hemisphere underlying the angioma is frequently found to be reduced in size. Kreyenberg's and Hansing's first patient had congenital glaucoma of the right eye and simple glaucoma of the left eye, bilateral naevi of face, parts of head and neck, palate, the whole of the tongue, etc. In addition left-sided Jacksonian epilepsy was present with moderate mental deficiency. X-ray revealed a shadow in the frontal region. Autopsy disclosed that the right half of the brain was smaller than the left and had greatly increased dural and pial vessels.

Ocular enlargement does not appear to be included in the description of true hemihypertrophy. Gesell (1921) collected forty cases and found the right side involved in twenty-seven. Nineteen showed skin abnormalities, chiefly naevi. Thirteen were mentally deficient. In a series of the larger group of partial and crossed hypertrophies sixteen out of thirty were right sided, in five both sides were affected. Skin complications and mental deficiency were common. In Gesell's own case the palpebral fissure was wider but the eyes were symmetrical. This condition must be distinguished from the false state of hypertrophy, in which enlargement is due to an extensive naevoid or lipomatous growth and the bones are not involved. Such a case was described by Cabannes (1909). In it hydrophthalmia was associated with facial hemihypertrophy and a large angioma in the temporal region. The enlargement of the eye was considered to be the result of hypernutrition, though no sign of a choroidal angioma was detected. In true hypertrophy all structures are involved and the limbs are lengthened as well as increased in girth. In rare cases the cerebral hemisphere on the opposite side has been reported as being smaller than that on the same side.

Meningo-cutaneous angiomatosis. The Sturge-Kalischer disease or meningo-cutaneous angiomatosis or syndrome neuro-cutane is the combination of a capillary naevus of the skin, especially when of trigeminal distribution, with contralateral spastic hemiplegia or seizures developing in early life. The latter are probably sometimes due to an intra-cranial haemorrhage from the abnormal vessels of a diffuse lepto-meningeal angioma lying on the same side as the main facial naevus. It is at times associated with naevi of the body, limbs and one or both eyes, with or without hydrophthalmia. Other associations are those of (1) syringomyelia and syringobulbia with cutaneous naevi, (2) a haemangioma of the spinal meninges and of the skin of the same metamere (Cobb, 1915; Chaput, 1904). Berenbruch's case, according to Weber (1929), had an angioma of the renal capsule as well.

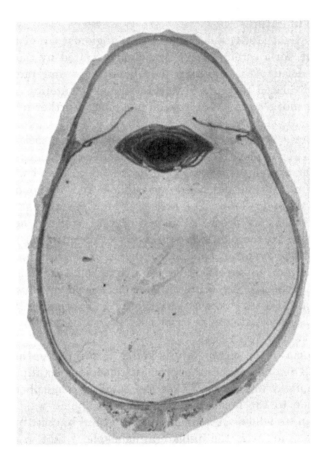

Fig. 98. Unpublished specimen IV. × 3. Marked peripheral thinning of the cornea. Compare the relation of the iris and the cornea in this specimen with that in unpublished specimen III. Aged twenty-eight years.

These wide associations suggest kinship with Lindau's disease or neuro-retinal angiomatosis—a disease characterised by vascular tumours and cysts of the cerebellum and the retina and occasionally of other parts of the central nervous system, the kidneys, the pancreas, and suprarenal organs, etc. It is frequently familial and hereditary.

Lindau's complete syndrome is rare, but it is surprising how many instances of it have been described since 1926–7 when this author drew attention to its characteristic lesions.

Lindau believed that haemangioblastomata do not occur in the cerebrum. Cushing was inclined to agree with this view, for he had not observed such a case in his practice nor was he able to find a proven case in the literature.

Isnel's patient (1934) was of interest, if angiomatosis of the retina was present, for a cerebral lesion was demonstrated by the presence of intense headaches, vomiting, left hemiplegia and radiographic evidence of dilated tortuous vessels in the right anterior convexity. The child's mother presented a facial angioma. Further reference to it will be made shortly.

Since Sturge first described hydrophthalmia in association with facial naevi and evidences of an intra-cranial disorder, many instances of the latter combination have been described with and without an ocular lesion. It was described by Lannois and Bernoud without hydrophthalmia in 1898. The first post-mortem findings made by Kalischer (1901) are described above. Parkes Weber, who in 1922 first described the radiographic appearance of such a lesion, suggested (1936) that the syndrome should be known as the Sturge-Kalischer disease. Other examples of this disease with radiographic confirmation have been reported by Dimitri, Marque, Sheldon, Rawling and Symonds (also Foster Moore's case). Nothing abnormal was detected by X-rays in two patients described by Worster-Drought (ages six years and twenty-two years).

An angioma of the meninges was found at autopsy in the cases of Vincent and Strominger. In the former the haemangiectatic condition of the meninges was marked over the cerebral hemisphere on the opposite side to the facial naevus. This hemisphere was definitely smaller than its fellow. A similar state appeared to exist in Weber's case. It was, however, the ipsolateral hemisphere that was reduced in size.

Hugo's (1927) case was similar to Lindau's syndrome in that the tumours, which were described as angio-endotheliomata, were present in brain, the kidneys and the liver but not in the meninges. In Greig's (1922) case instead of a facial naevus bilateral multiple adenoma sebaceum of the face were found. Operation revealed a unilateral meningeal angioma. In the majority of these cases idiocy or imbecility was present.

Haemangioma of the meninges may occur with other ocular anomalies than hydrophthalmia, viz. heterochromia iridis (Parkes Weber, 1929, and others); coloboma of the disc, and high refractive errors (Foster Moore, 1929). Facial naevi have been described in association with haemangioma of the meninges in the absence of hydrophthalmia (Foster Moore, 1929). Indeed the only combination of facial, uveal and meningeal naevi that appears not to have been described is that of uveal and meningeal naevi without facial involvement.

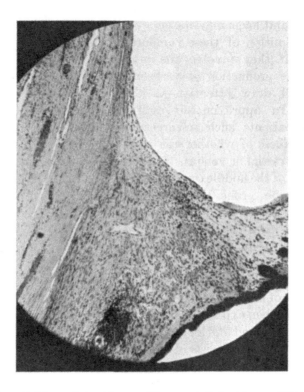

Fig. 99. × 60. The angle is wide open. There are indistinct traces of Schlemm's canal and perivascular infiltration in the ciliary region.

Foster Moore, Aynsley and others have suggested that all cases exhibiting facial naevi, hydrophthalmia or retinal haemangiomatosis (v. Hippel's disease) should be examined neurologically and by X-rays with a view to excluding the presence of intra-cranial lesions. Even so a tumour may be missed because of its lack of calcification or its situation in a silent area. In addition, all cases of cerebellar tumours should have a careful examination made of the periphery of each retina.

Intra-cranial angiomatous malformations that may be associated with facial naevi and glaucoma

Cushing and Bailey classified venous and arterial angiomata as angiomatous malformations rather than true tumours. Until the pathology of these and of kindred disorders is better understood there is no need to exchange the old title of angiomata for the possibly more exact names tele- and haemangiectasia.

The recognition of these tumours is facilitated if they involve the motor area, for the production of Jacksonian seizures will draw attention to their presence. In approximately half of Cushing's patients such seizures were found regardless of whether the angiomata were arterial or venous. The wide distribution of the middle cerebral artery makes it more prone than the other cerebral arteries to malformations, and so the paracentral convolutions are the most common site for such disorders (Cushing). Venous angiomata in blind areas may easily escape recognition. They consist of masses of dilated cortical veins, which, when exposed at operation, contain venous blood and do not pulsate. An arterial angioma consists of a mass of veins with a direct connection with an arterial trunk which is usually abnormally large. The veins, however, contain arterial blood and they pulsate. A systolic bruit is frequently heard.

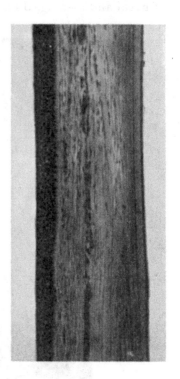

Fig. 100. ×90. Periphery of the cornea. Descemet's membrane appears to be thicker than in the centre of the cornea where the substantia propria is thicker.

The venous type may show signs of calcification by radiography. Though Dimitri's and Marque's cases were unverified they probably were venous in type because of their association with facial naevi (Cushing).

Only the venous type appears to be associated with facial naevi. When associated in this way the facial naevus is capillary in type and the angioma is almost always in the pia. Cushing collected the following cases, some of which had unproven meningeal lesions, though epilepsy was present: Kalischer (1897, 1901), Lannois and Bernoud (1898), Cassirer (1902), Naecke (1905), Strominger (1905), Cushing (1906), Broeckaert (1908), Volland (1912), Hebold (1913), Oppenheim (1913), Sachs (1915), Spiller (1919), Dimitri (1923),

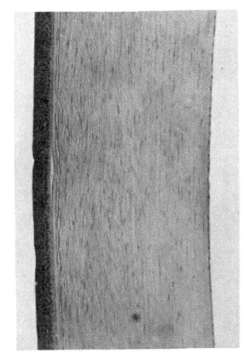

Fig. 101. × 90. Centre of the cornea.

Marque (1927). Krabbe (1934) has discussed his own cases and summarised others reported since 1927. His own cases showed either hemiplegia or epilepsy and facial naevi. One autopsy revealed calcification in the outer layers of the cortex, not of the pia mater. Though abundantly vascular no true angioma was found.

"Should a naevus of the face happen to be present in a patient with contralateral Jacksonian epilepsy or a cerebral palsy of some form, the presence of a pial angioma, even without its betrayal by calcification, is sufficiently probable to justify the diagnosis" (Cushing and Bailey). In the absence of a naevus and without exploration a clinical diagnosis is hardly possible.

The arterial angiomata, however, are rarely if ever associated with facial naevi. Steinheil's (1895) and Bregman's and Mesz's (1927) are unproven instances. These anomalies, however, may be associated with enlarged and pulsating scalp arteries and other evidence of

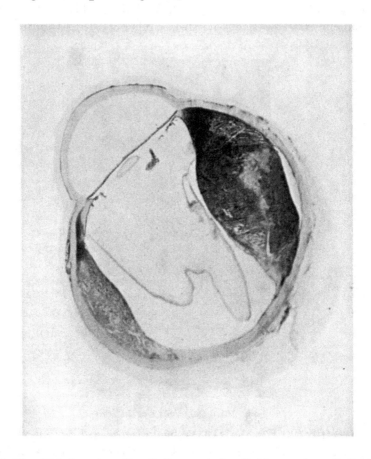

Fig. 102. Unpublished specimen V. ×3. Large sub-choroidal haemorrhage dividing the ciliary body from the sclera. There has been unusual resistance to distension at the limbus. Aged twelve years.

increased extra-cranial vascularity. The presence of such external associations may depend on the different stages at which the venous and the arterial lesions arose (Cushing).

The venous angiomata are rarely accompanied by raised intracranial pressure and papilloedema, while this condition and unilateral exophthalmos are common in the arterial group. Epilepsy is frequently present with the venous type. Referring to an example of the arterial group, Cushing and Bailey wrote: "Here is a lesion which takes up room, not because of its size as a foreign body, nor because it causes cerebrospinal fluid stasis, but because it actually increases the amount of blood in the intra-cranial chamber by pumping arterial blood directly into the cerebral veins, a condition which is, in the nature of things, more marked in the vicinity of the lesion." This quotation is of interest when we ask the question, "Which of the two types of

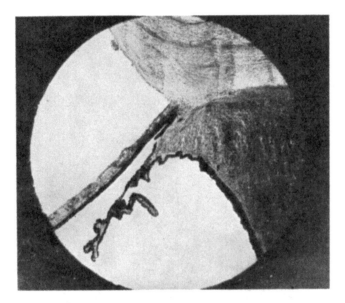

Fig. 103. × 22. Sclerosis of the tissues near the iris base. Deposit on the corneal surface.

angioma is associated with congenital glaucoma?" Apparently the type that is associated with facial naevi, viz. the venous angiomata.

It is difficult to ascertain what proportion of the venous type is limited to the area of trigeminal nerve distribution. The majority appear to be so, particularly if we exclude a group not encountered by Cushing at operation. This is the racemose type, which is wedge-shaped and extends deeply into the brain. It is possible that the true venous type may become known as part of the manifestation of trigeminal haemangiomatosis.

Schiötz (1935) described a man aged forty-four years with epilepsy and a facial naevus that corresponded to the first branch of the contra-lateral trigeminal nerve. Radiography revealed gyriform shadows in the neighbourhood of the occipital lobe. He had collected eighty-six cases from the literature and of these fifty-three were men. The diagnosis was made as a probability in twenty-nine cases, was verified at autopsy in thirteen other cases, by X-ray in thirty-four, by X-ray and autopsy in one, by operation in six and by X-ray and operation in four. He found that the calcification was in the cortex and not in the pia and that a glio-angiomatosis of the brain was

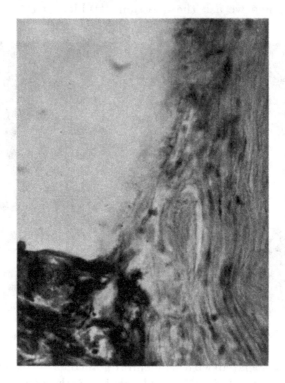

Fig. 104. × 180. The angle is wide open but there is no canal of Schlemm. Hyaline tissue forms an oval mass. The iris is richly pigmented.

present under the teleangiectasis of the pial vessels. This supports Krabbe's views (1934). Further support for them is supplied by Moniz and Lima (1935) who by arteriography and phlebography convinced themselves that the calcification was not a calcified angioma.

Contrast with neuro-retinal angiomatosis. It is of value to associate facial and meningeal naevi, neurofibromatosis and congenital glaucoma as extra-neural vascular disorders and to contrast them with the intraneural vascular anomalies such as neuro-retinal angiomatosis or haemangioblastomata.

It is well to remember that the retina and the optic nerve are simply an extension of the central nervous system and that just as the latter has two separate and unrelated systems for blood supply, so the retina has two, viz. the central retinal artery and the choroidal

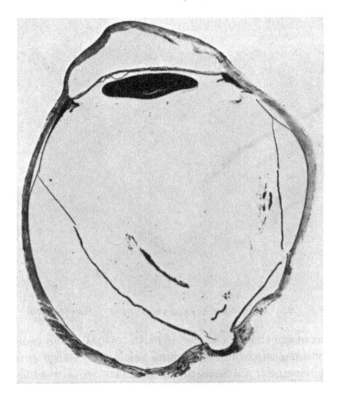

Fig. 105. Unpublished specimen VI. × 3·5. Observe peripheral thinning of the cornea, and the wide open angle. Aged ten years.

network. The latter structure then appears as the meninges of the retina. When considered in this way there is ample reason why there should be two separate entities: angiomatosis of the meninges, viz. the meningo-uveal form, and angiomatosis of the internal blood system of the brain as seen in neuro-retinal angiomatosis or Lindau's disease.

The angiomata are excluded from the group of true neoplasms of blood vessels, because, even in the most intricate examples, more or less well-preserved traces of glia are found between the vascular channels. The true neoplasms—the haemangioblastomata—may be highly vascularised, almost avascular, or simply a small nodule in the wall of a large cyst. They are "composed of the same elements that enter into the development of the primordial blood channels".

The angiomata are much more frequent in the cerebrum than in the cerebellum (7 to 1), but the true neoplasms are probably confined, or almost so, to the cerebellum.

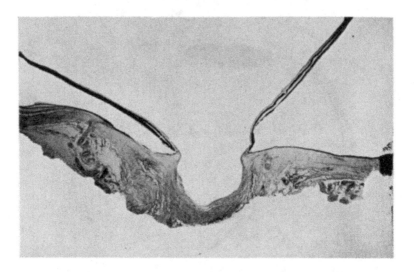

Fig. 106. × 4·5. Marked cupping and atrophy of the optic disc.

The percentage that is associated with retinal tumours is difficult to gauge, because the interest of the physician-in-charge in the retina varies and because a microscopical examination is essential before one can exclude a retinal haemangioma. Lindau (1927) reported one such tumour of microscopic size.

Cushing and Bailey considered that Lindau overestimated the frequency with which retinal lesions occurred with cerebellar tumours of this type. They considered that the position of retinal lesions is comparable with the acoustic tumours in relation to von Reckling-hausen's disease. Isolated acoustic tumours occur much more frequently than those with this disease. However, the finding of a retinal angioma with the signs of a cerebellar tumour permits a pre-operative diagnosis of the condition. Cushing and Bailey commented on the surprisingly late average ages at which tumours with a congenital "anlage", such as acoustic neuromata and cerebellar angiomata, first produce symptoms, viz. thirty-nine years and thirty-four years.

For an explanation of the angiomatous malformations of brain, meninges and skin we must go back to the stage when blood vessels are developing from the primordial endothelial blood-containing channels which are neither arterial nor venous in character. The works of Sabin (1917) and particularly that of Streeter (1918) help one to understand the mode of origin of such anomalies. Streeter described

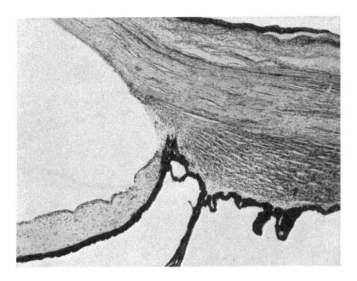

Fig. 107. ×45. The angle is torn open. Schlemm's canal is closed. Hyaline tissue is stretched round the angle and there is a cyst behind the root of the iris.

five periods in the development of the intra-cranial vascular system. Each would be a special adaptation to the requirements of the time. At first the primordial vascular plexus is established. This slowly resolves into arteries, veins and capillaries. In the next stage as dura mater and cranium are developing the vascular system breaks up into a superficial, a dural, and a pial circulatory supply. In the fourth period a series of changes in the arrangement of the vascular trunks occurs, and finally the histological changes necessary for the development of mature arteries and veins are completed. It is during the third stage—a period of rearrangement—that a maldevelopment of a vascular area might lead to a vascular naevus of the scalp, to varices of the dura or to a venous angioma of the pia or to all three simultaneously, whereas an interference with the normal development during the second period might lead to the tumour formation known as Lindau's disease or retino-cerebellar haemangioblastoma.

Lindau considered that the characteristic lesions of his syndrome were the result of a mesodermal disturbance in the third foetal month. Cushing suggested that this would explain the prevalence of haemangioblastomata in the posterior fossa, for Karlefors (1924) has shown that at this stage in this area there is a very rich capillary network which later enters into the formation of the vascular plexus of the choroidal tufts of the fourth ventricle.

It is of interest here to recall the fact that the arteria centralis retinae is just recognisable at the 100 mm. stage (fourth month),

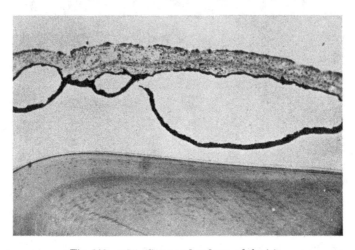

Fig. 108.   × 35.   Cysts and oedema of the iris.

having vascularised a small area of the nerve-fibre layer around the disc. The branches, however, do not reach the ora serrata till the eighth month, at which period the development of the retinal system is complete.

During the third month the chorio-capillaris becomes visible and some larger tributaries of the venae vorticosae appear. Approximately at the fourth month branches of the middle layer of vessels are first seen spreading from the region of supply of the short ciliary arteries. They are arterial in nature. It may be at this age that neuro-cutaneous and uveal angiomatoses arise. By the fifth month the choroid shows all the layers present in the adult but differs in having a much more richly nucleated stroma. At this stage pigment-bearing cells are first recognisable.

*Causes of hydrophthalmia in association with
facial naevi and neurofibromatosis*

Our main concern here is to attempt to ascertain why the conditions of hydrophthalmia, naevi and neurofibromatosis are associated. To do this let us first of all consider the causes of raised tension as suggested by various observers.

In doing so, one finds a variety of causes. The actual conditions vary greatly, and it is unlikely that one explanation will prove satisfactory for them all.

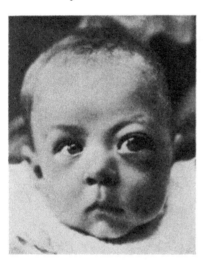 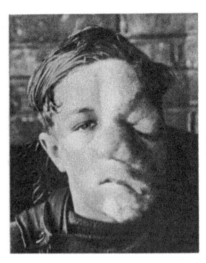

Figs. 109 and 110. Photographs of Dr Glen Campbell's patient when six months and fifteen years old. The great enlargement of the left eye and the evidence of early facial hemi-hypertrophy are evident in the first photograph. The eye was removed three years later.

1. *Mechanical theories.*

(*a*) *Cause as in hydrophthalmia in general.* **Naevus.** In some specimens the hypertension can be accounted for by the presence of the lesions that occur in hydrophthalmia in general, These are chiefly, persistence of the uveal meshwork, the complete or partial obliteration of Schlemm's canal, and the posterior position of this canal and the scleral spur. Such findings were made by Safar (1923). He described the meshwork as being thick and pigmented. No angioma was present.

Only three typical specimens with naevi have been examined histologically: those of Stoewer, Love and Dunphy. They each showed more or less complete peripheral synechiae, and marked atrophy of the iris and ciliary body and a choroidal angioma with bone formation. In addition Dunphy described an absence of Schlemm's canal and sclerosis of one section of the meshwork. Unfortunately all these specimens were old.

Neurofibromatosis. The majority showed tissue, that is best described as an iris process, filling the angle. As a rule neither meshwork nor Schlemm's canal was found. Collins and Snell stated that the cornea and the iris had failed to separate at the angle. The iris root was everywhere intimately adherent to the cornea at its periphery.

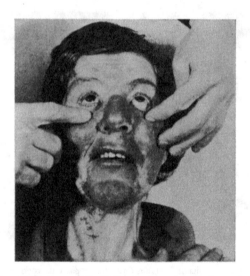

Fig. 111. Unpublished case C.T. Patient with generalised naevi, epilepsy and hydrophthalmia of the right eye. Observe the corneal asymmetry.

Descemet's membrane curved round on to the anterior surface of the iris and became incorporated in its tissues, instead of splitting up into fibres at the angle. Seefelder found in one carefully examined globe persistent foetal tissue blocking the angle.

Treacher Collins, Snell, Batten and Seefelder considered that the glaucoma was not part of the elephantiasis even though ciliary neurofibromatosis was present. They attributed it to the presence of the malformations at the angle of the anterior chamber, that usually account for congenital glaucoma.

(b) *Cause due to special conditions.* **Naevus.** It has been suggested that either the choroidal angiomatous changes spread so far forwards, or the iris changes extended so close to the periphery, that the escape of fluid at the angle was interfered with. This was possible in the specimens of Stoewer and Dunphy and those with glaucoma described by Knapp and Jahnke.

In these, either the anterior portion of the choroid or the iris showed pathological changes. The iris may be more vascular than normal or have thickened stroma or be darker in colour from excessive pigment. Dunphy considered that the angle might be blocked by peripheral synechiae due to the toxic action of degenerative changes, such as those that had led to bone formation in his own case.

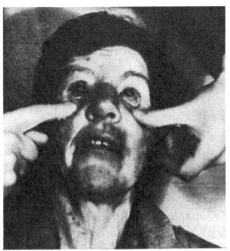

Fig. 112. Photograph of the same patient taken with infra-red light.

In those cases in which a choroidal angioma is present, the mere increase in bulk of the intra-ocular contents may account for hypertension. In this respect a choroidal angioma acts as a choroidal sarcoma does.

Such an angioma was found in the cases of Snell, Stoewer, Jahnke (secondary glaucoma) and de Haas (secondary glaucoma), and a similar condition was suspected in the cases of Galezowski and O'Brien and Porter. de Haas, in his case of glaucoma, described the choroid as being three or four times its normal thickness.

The ocular state was of great interest in Cabannes' case. In it a large angioma in the temporal fossa was associated with marked hypertrophy of the same side of the face, tongue, facial bones and orbit. Though the eyeball was greatly enlarged, the tension was not raised and no cupping and no obstruction at the angle were found. If over-nutrition were the direct cause and the actual condition was one of hypertrophy, an explanation is still required for the cases of hydrophthalmia in which no angioma exists within or close to the eye. Neither will this theory of hypertrophy explain the cases of pseudo- and simple glaucoma.

Neurofibromatosis. Michel considered that a fibromatosis in the neighbourhood of the angle led to obstruction of the passage of fluid. In this connection the finding of minute nerve fibres accompanying the arterioles in this area is of great interest.

2. *Neuro-vascular theories.*

Many authors have sought to explain those cases that have choroidal angiomatosis, on a vascular basis. They have assumed an increased transudation of fluid through the thin-walled vessels (Beltmann), a slowing of the choroidal blood stream from pressure (Bär and Zaun), and some interference with outflow as a result of the great increase in number of choroidal veins.

As the tumour is vascular, variations in its size may occur and may markedly affect intra-ocular tension. One must remember that as a rule naevi have no vasomotor nerve supply, and so probably have none in the choroid. Therefore, in the choroid these tumours will not be as susceptible to nervous stimuli as some authors have considered. The size of the angioma, however, would vary with the pulse pressure and particularly with any obstruction situated further on in the blood stream. Just as facial naevi can vary with psychic stimuli, similar changes may occur in the choroid. It is of value to remember Zaun's observation that an increase of the corneal opacity and of the ocular tension accompanied an increase in the fullness and redness of the facial naevus.

Though their views are not identical, the following have supported, to a certain extent, a vascular theory: Ginzburg, Beltmann, Elschnig, Clausen, Nakamura, Yamanaka, Krause, Vita and Oguchi. Elschnig considered, that as compression of the carotid artery lowered the intra-ocular pressure, the hypertension was probably the result of a plethora of the choroid. He stated that though glaucoma accompanied naevus flammeus it did not appear with angiomata of the face.

Hudelo held that the cerebral angioma, which he believed was almost always present and frequently in a silent area, was the anatomical link between facial naevus and the glaucoma. The angioma probably interfered with the cavernous sinus and so tended to lead to obstruction of the ocular venous circulation.

Biro thought that hypertension followed intra-ocular vascular dilatation and hypersecretion. At first this was balanced by an increased absorption, but later the telangiectasis led to an obstruction of the outflow of aqueous. He agreed with van Rötth that the naevus probably arose from the vasomotor system, and that hyperaemia might easily produce an effusion owing to the sieve-like character of the vessels' walls being influenced by the sympathetic system.

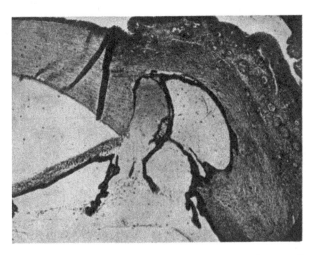

Fig. 113. Hydrophthalmic eye at ten months. This illustrates the dangers of a posteriorly situated trephine-wound in a hydrophthalmic globe. A cyst-like space is seen into which some ciliary processes have prolapsed. The space is lined by uveal tissue. (Jaensch, 1927.)

Tyson considered that increased vascular permeability and the production of plasmoid aqueous were the important factors in raising the tension. Applemans held that a neurovascular origin was probable. Granström (1935), after a review of the literature, stated that the reported anatomical examinations showed the presence of uveal vascular changes of a telangiectatic nature. He held that the facial naevi were the result of a developmental vascular disorder which might be limited to the facial vessels or involve the uveal and intra-cranial vessels as well. The rise in tension, he thought, was due to the presence of the uveal telangiectasis. Senile glaucoma has been found associated with telangiectasis of the iris in diabetic patients (Salus, 1923; Gallino, Arruga and others).

Marchesani held that if a naevus is an anomaly of cutaneous vessels, hydrophthalmia is probably a related disorder of a part, the blood supply of which is also from the internal carotid artery.

Neurofibromatosis. Most interest has been taken in the presence of the ciliary neurofibromatosis that is so frequently found in these cases. It was certainly absent in Seefelder's case, and probably so in one or two others.

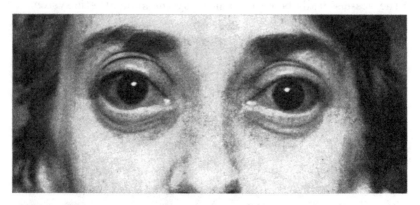

Fig. 114. Photograph to show enlarged cornea and bluish sclerae of adult patient with arrested hydrophthalmia.

Komoto and Murakami believed that stasis and hypersecretion followed the enormous increase of connective tissue which involves the ciliary nerves and the vessels of the choroid, and that obliteration of Schlemm's canal and the closure of the angle is the result rather than the cause of the hypertension.

Sachsalber held that the trophic nerves of the choroid were upset and as a result a fibrosis developed which impeded the lymph circulation of the choroid.

Michelson-Rabinowitsch postulated a paralysis of the vasomotor branches of the ciliary nerves which produced hyperaemia, and the excess fluid led to a thickening and sclerosis of the tissues at the angle of filtration.

Verhoeff, in 1903, was so struck by the fact that in the only three instances of this association of which he knew, the glaucoma was ipsolateral, that he considered the hypertension resulted from a metabolic disorder due to the affection of the ciliary nerves. He wrote

(1937) that if the ciliary nerves are affected, even behind the globe, they may promote hypersecretion of aqueous. If, however, neurofibromatosis of the choroid is present glaucoma may follow increased pressure in the choroidal vessels, "just as in cases of sarcoma of the choroid".

Michel held that the association was not accidental and that the hydrophthalmia in the absence of other stigmata may be the only sign present of a unilateral facial hypertrophy. Is the enlargement of the ocular globe a sign of hypertrophy? Wiener suggested that the condition is that of an enlarged eyeball lying in an enlarged orbit. Such tissues as the lid and the skull bones are certainly hypertrophied

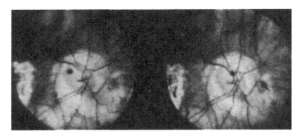

Fig. 115. Stereoscopic view of optic disc of patient with arrested hydrophthalmia.

in some of the reported cases. Wiener was unduly influenced by the absence of hypertension in his case, which is a very common state in hydrophthalmia. Hypertrophy will not produce the glaucoma cup as found in many specimens including his own.

3. *A nervous origin.*

Naevus. It was in 1863 that von Baerensprung brought forward a theory that naevi developed in an area that corresponded to the distribution of a spinal nerve, the spinal ganglion of which was affected by intra-uterine disease. Love and Verhoeff suggested that congenital absence or a destructive lesion of the vasoconstrictor fibres supplying the area was the cause of the naevus. They held the view that dilatation of the vessels led to a local increase in capillary tension and that a compensating hypertrophy followed, which was manifested by a new growth of capillaries rather than a thickening of the vessel walls.

Quite recently Verhoeff stated that without doubt vascular naevi of the skin follow the distribution of the nerves and that angiomata of the choroid may also have a neurogenic association. He considers that the latter are capillary and not cavernous in type.

A tendency for the naevus to be delimited by the distribution of one or more branches of the trigeminal nerve is suggestive of an underlying nervous influence.

Lenthal Cheatle (1906) reported the distribution of a cutaneous naevus according to a segmental nerve area, viz. that of the third cervical nerve. It is of interest, therefore, to summarise the findings when glaucoma is present.

BRANCHES OF TRIGEMINAL NERVE CONCERNED

	R.	L.
Beltmann	1, 2, 3	1, 2, 3
Marchesani	1, 2, 3	1, 2, 3
Perera	1, 2, 3	1, 2, 3
Joiris and Fauchamps	1, 2, 3	
Coppez		1, 2, 3
Schirmer	2	1, 2, 3
Pi	3	1, 2, 3
Sturge	1, 2, 3	1 (patches)
Cushing I	1, 2, 3	3
,, III	1, 2, 3	(patches over 1, 2, 3)
Vita	1, 2	
Ballantyne	1, 2	L. upper jaw and small naevus. L. occipital region
Applemans		1, 2
Tyson		1, 2 (Glaucoma)
Joiris and Fauchamps		1, 2 (Glaucoma)
Voegele	1, 2	(Pseudo-glaucoma)
O'Brien and Porter		1
Cushing II	1	
Granström		2 (Glaucoma)
Ballantyne	2	(Pseudo-glaucoma)

It must also be remembered that the meninges that appear to be chiefly affected by angiomatous changes in these cases are supplied mainly by the trigeminal nerve. The meningeal branch of the tenth, and the recurrent branch of the twelfth, cranial nerves and the sympathetic system constitute the remaining nerve supply.

4. *Other theories.*

As for so many other conditions, an endocrine origin has been attributed to hydrophthalmia in association with facial naevus. The findings of a pituitary disturbance in Ginzburg's case and of acromegalic changes in Vogt's case of neurofibromatosis and hydrophthalmia is insufficient evidence to justify a belief in these conditions being primary rather than merely associations.

5. "Birth injury could not...account for a fully developed buphthalmos or congenital malformation of the disc" (Ballantyne). It may, however, solve the problem of those cases of pseudo-glaucoma described by Macrae (Thomson and Ballantyne). In these, histories

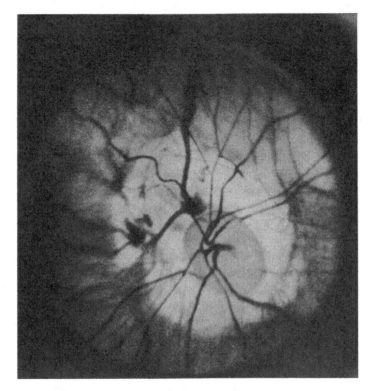

Fig. 116. Glaucoma cup of the above patient.

of maternal injury in the seventh month of pregnancy, of instrumental delivery with facial injuries, and of a difficult birth, were reported.

6. Many writers have considered that the association is merely coincidental. The glaucoma may be present at birth as hydrophthalmia, or it may arise at any stage during life in either an acute or chronic form. In Dunphy's second case glaucoma did not appear till fifty-eight years of age, and then only on the side of the naevus. The other eye survived an attack of ulcerative keratitis at this age without developing hypertension.

It is most likely that the relationship is not closer than a common underlying cause. Possibly "either a toxin, or, as Unna suggests, some trauma to the branchial clefts, acts to produce naevi of the cerebral vessels; then the mesoblastic structures of the developing eye may be affected, and this may lead either to imperfect formation of the filtration angle or canal of Schlemm, or to a coloboma of the disc or choroid; or to a telangiectatic condition of parts of the intra-ocular vascular system which may sooner or later, through growth, sclerosis, transudation, or haemorrhage, lead to a disturbance of balance of the intra-ocular fluids and the production of increased tension" (Aynsley, 1929).

The development of glaucoma in aged patients with facial naevus suggests that though an anomaly may be the commonest cause in early life, it is of diminishing importance in later cases, and in middle and old age it plays no part. The influence of the naevus is then purely on a vascular basis.

It is well to consider the wide range of lesions that may occur. It includes facial naevi, coloboma of various ocular structures, telangiectasis, neurofibromatosis, meningeal angiomatosis, cleft palate, polydactyly, and hypertrophy of soft and bony tissues. The fact that any of these conditions may occur alone or in any combination suggests not only their mutual independence but a common dependence on some influence that may excite the production of developmental defects.

One may conclude, therefore, that the association of cutaneous naevi and hydrophthalmia is due to some ill-understood influence acting in very early embryonic life, and that the actual cause of the hydrophthalmia is as a rule either an anomaly such as is found in hydrophthalmia in general, or the uveal angiomatous changes producing an increase in the intra-ocular fluid which proves too much for either normal channels of escape, or those that are defective from sclerosis, adhesions, or angiomatous changes.

Neurofibromatosis. The drainage of fluid in the affected eye is impeded just as it is in the facial tissues, but we do not know whether the choroidal hyperplasia, or a primary fibromatosis of the angle (Michel), or a paralysis of the vasomotor branches of the ciliary nerves with hyperaemia and a thickening round the angle (Rabinowitsch), or the anomalies described by Collins and Seefelder, are the actual causes of the glaucoma. In some specimens so little neurofibromatosis is present that in them at least the developmental defects found in hydrophthalmia in general are most probably the concomitant anomalies and the cause of the glaucoma.

SUMMARY

1*a*. Thirty-two cases of hydrophthalmia and facial neurofibromatosis have been studied. The glaucoma was unilateral in every instance, though congenital glaucoma in general is bilateral in approximately 70 % of cases. The facial changes appear also to have been unilateral. The upper lid on the same side was always affected. The associated changes varied from local tumours in the lids to facial and even general hemihypertrophy and evidence of intra-cranial neurofibromatosis.

1*b*. Eleven specimens have been examined histologically. Hypertrophied ciliary nerves and a diffuse thickening of the choroid appear to be constant changes. The characteristic change in the angle is the presence of an iris-like sheet of tissue.

2*a*. Sixty cases of hydrophthalmia and facial naevi have been studied. The glaucoma was unilateral in 87 % and the naevi were unilateral in 65 %. Thirty-five instances of other forms of glaucoma are also discussed. The upper lid on the same side was always affected. The associated changes varied from a small palpebral naevus to hemiplegia of the other side of the body. Evidences of a cranial or an intra-cranial lesion were found in 50 %.

2*b*. Five specimens have been examined histologically. An angioma in the choroid with the presence of osseous tissue was found in the majority of these. All of them except one exceptional specimen (Cabannes) showed the changes at the angle that are characteristic of congenital glaucoma.

3. The association of neurofibromatosis and naevi with hydrophthalmia is probably coincidental, but the result of a common cause. The main cause of hypertension is most probably an anomalous state of Schlemm's canal and the adjacent meshwork. The involvement of the ciliary nerves and the ciliary veins and the choroid probably plays an important part in certain cases.

4. The choroid may be considered as the meninges of the retina. The time of origin of angiomatous malformations in the choroid and in the meninges is probably during the third stage of development—a period of rearrangement (Streeter).

REFERENCES

THE PATHOLOGY OF CONGENITAL GLAUCOMA

INTERFERENCE WITH FUNCTION

1912 GILBERT, W. *Arch. f. Ophthal.* **82**, 396.
1920 PARSONS, J. H. *Brit. Jl. Ophthal.* **4**, 211.
1929 HÜHN, K. *Klin. Monatsbl. f. Augenheilk.* **82**, 254.

ALTERATIONS IN STRUCTURE: ORBIT, GLOBE, SCLERA

1896 CROSS, F. R. *Trans. Ophthal. Soc. U.K.* **16**, 340.
1905 AXENFELD, TH. *Klin. Monatsbl. f. Augenheilk.* **43**, 157.
1910 BLAIR, C. *Trans. Ophthal. Soc. U.K.* **30**, 228.
1911 HÖEG, N. *Zeitschr. f. Augenheilk.* **25**, 191.
1912 CORONAT and AURAND. *Clin. Ophthal.* **18**, 498. Quoted by Elliot.
1913 BEHR, C. *Klin. Monatsbl. f. Augenheilk.* **51**, 2, 281.
1913 TAKASHIMA, S. *Klin. Monatsbl. f. Augenheilk.* **51**, 2, 180.
1914 ZENTMAYER, W. *Ophthal. Year Book*, **11**, 204.
1917 BRONSON, E. *Edinburgh Med. Jl.* **18**, 240.
1920 WESSELY, K. *Arch. f. Augenheilk.* **83**, 99.
1922 BALL, J. N. *Interstate Med. Jl.* **17**, 47. Quoted by Elliot. *A Treatise on Glaucoma*, p. 439. London: Frowde.
1923 BUCHANAN, L. *Trans. Ophthal. Soc. U.K.* **43**, 352.
1925 BOREL, G. *Bull. et Mém. Soc. franç. d'Ophtal.* **38**, 426.
1928–31 FISCHER, F. P. *Arch. f. Augenheilk.* **98**, 41; *Klin. Monatsbl. f. Augenheilk.* **86**, 298.
1934 CASANOVAS, J. *Zentralbl. f. ges. Ophthal.* **31**, 580.
1934 FRIEDBERG, C. K. Quoted by Krause, *Biochemistry of the Eye*. Baltimore: Johns Hopkins Press.
1936 RANGARCHARI, V. *Proc. All India Ophthal. Soc.* **4**, 136. Abst. *Amer. Jl. Ophthal.* **19**, 1134.
1936 RADOS and ROSENBERG. *Arch. of Ophthal.* **16**, 8.
1936 WIRTH and VOGT. Quoted by Rados and Rosenberg.

CORNEA

1884 GRAHAMER. *Arch. f. Ophthal.* **30**, 265.
1891 ARNOLD, TH. *Beitr. z. Augenheilk.* **3**, 16.
1899 HAAB, O. *Zeitschr. f. Augenheilk.* **2**, 235.
1904 PARSONS, J. H. *Trans. Ophthal. Soc. U.K.* **24**, 128.
1905 REIS, W. *Arch. f. Ophthal.* **60**, 1.
1907 COATS, G. *Trans. Ophthal. Soc. U.K.* **27**, 48.
1909 RUMSCHEWITSCH, I. *Klin. Monatsbl. f. Augenheilk.* **46**, 1, 435.
1910 LANDOLT, M. *Arch. d'Ophtal.* **30**, 666.
1910 MAYOU, M. S. *Trans. Ophthal. Soc. U.K.* **30**, 128.
1915 STÄHLI, J. *Arch. f. Augenheilk.* p. 141.
1918 STÄHLI, J. *Klin. Monatsbl. f. Augenheilk.* **60**, 721.
1918 VON HIPPEL, E. *Arch. f. Ophthal.* **92**, 2, 307.
1918 WIRTHS, M. *Klin. Monatsbl. f. Augenheilk.* **61**, 625.
1920 GUIST, W. *Klin. Monatsbl. f. Augenheilk.* **65**, 114.

1921 Vogt, A. *Atlas of Slit-lamp microscopy*, p. 57. Berlin: Springer.
1922 Clausen, W. *Arch. f. Augenheilk.* **91**, 198. Quoted by Peters.
1923 Meisner, M. *Arch. f. Ophthal.* **112**, 433.
1924 Clapp, C. A. *Johns Hopkins Hosp. Bull.* **35**, 85.
1924 Elschnig, H. H. *Klin. Monatsbl. f. Augenheilk.* **73**, 395.
1925 Gallemaerts, E. *Bull. et Mém. Soc. franç. d'Ophtal.* **38**, 201.
1931 Hoffman, R. *Arch. f. Augenheilk.* **105**, 162. Abst. *Arch. of Ophthal.* **7**, 310. 1932.
1934 Crvaric, L. *Klin. Monatsbl. f. Augenheilk.* **92**, 413.

Changes in the Uveal Tract

1877 Brünhuber. *Klin. Monatsbl. f. Augenheilk.* **15**.
1888 Pflüger, E. *Ber. d. deutsch. Ophthal. Gesell. Heidelberg*, **7**.
1890 Lembeck. Dissert. Halle. Quoted by Seefelder, *Kurzes Handb. der Ophthal.* **1**.
1891 Collins, E. T. *Ophthal. Review*, **10**, 101.
1892 Wagenmann, A. *Arch. f. Ophthal.* **38**, 2, 91.
1895 Cabannes, C. *Ann. d'Ocul.* **5**, 115.
1900 Collins, E. T. *Lancet*, **1**, 439 and 441.
1902 Venneman, E. *Soc. Belge d'Ophtal.* April.
1902 Halben, R. *Arch. f. Augenheilk.* **49**, 220.
1903 Wiener, A. *Arch. f. Augenheilk.* **48**, 51.
1903 Pagenstecher, A. H. *Arch. f. Ophthal.* **55**, 75.
1909 Seefelder, R. *Arch. f. Ophthal.* **70**, 65.
1912 Stimmel and Rotter. *Arch. f. Ophthal.* **28**, 114.
1916 Meller, J. *Arch. f. Ophthal.* **92**, 34. Abst. *Klin. Monatsbl. f. Augenheilk.* **7**, 418.
1919 Zeeman, W. P. C. *Amer. Jl. Ophthal.* **2**, 145.
1920 Axenfeld, Th. *Ber. d. deutsch. Ophthal. Gesell. Heidelberg*, **38**, 301.
1920 Guist, G. *Zeitschr. f. Augenheilk.* **44**, 242.
1921 Clausen, W. *Klin. Monatsbl. f. Augenheilk.* **67**, 116.
1921 Hudson, A. C. *Trans. Ophthal Soc. U.K.* **41**, 274.
1921 Weekers, L. *Bull. de la Soc. Belge d'Ophtal.* **43**; *Amer. Jl. Ophthal.* **4**, 757.
1922 Gloor, A. *Klin. Monatsbl. f. Augenheilk.* **69**, 126.
1922 Somogyi, Z. *Klin. Monatsbl. f. Augenheilk.* **69**, 853.
1923 Krauss, F. *Amer. Jl. Ophthal.* **6**, 495.
1923 Licsko, A. *Klin. Monatsbl. f. Augenheilk.* **71**, 456.
1924 Mann, Ida. *Trans. Ophthal. Soc. U.K.* **44**, 171.
1926 Denis. *Arch. of Ophthal.* **45**, 527.
1927 Collins, E. T. *Trans. Ophthal. Soc. U.K.* **47**, 155.
1927 Duggan and Nanavati. *Brit. Jl. Ophthal.* **11**, 447.
1927 Jaensch, P. A. *Arch. f. Ophthal.* **118**, 1, 27.
1927 Würdemann, H. V. *Amer. Jl. Ophthal.* **10**, 761.
1930 Friedenwald, J. S. *The Pathology of the Eye*, Fig. 116. London: Kimpton.
1930 Penman, G. G. *Brit. Jl. Ophthal.* **14**, 232.
1933 Chowdbrury, A. *Proc. All-India Ophthal. Soc.* **3**, 145.
1933 Mann, Ida. *Brit. Jl. Ophthal.* **17**, 458.
1933 Remky, E. *Zeitschr. f. Augenheilk.* **81**, 48.

The Lens, Retina and Optic Nerve

1891 Dub, B. *Arch. f. Ophthal.* **37**, 4, 26.
1904 Dalen, A. Ref. *Nagel's Jahresber.* **35**, 303.
1913 Löhlein, W. *Arch. f. Ophthal.* **85**, 393.
1916 Fleischer, B. *Arch. f. Augenheilk.* **80**, 248.
1924 Marshall, J. *Trans. Ophthal. Soc. U.K.* **44**, 176.
1930 Urbanek, J. *Zeitschr. f. Augenheilk.* **54**, 164.
1931 Kunz, E. *Klin. Monatsbl. f. Augenheilk.* **87**, 433.
1934 Belskiy, A. A. *Sovet. Vestnik, opft.* **5**, 579. Ref. *Abl. Ophthal.* **33**, 599.
1937 Gault, E. L. Personal Communication.

The Anterior Chamber

1897 Gros, E. L. Thèses de Paris. Abst. *Ann. d'Ocul.* **118**.
1908 Schmidt-Rimpler, H. *Graefe-Saemisch Handb.* **6**, ch. 7, p. 57.
1916 Lindstedt, F. *Arch. f. Augenheilk.* **80**, 104.
1922 Cucco, A. *Ann. di Ottal.* **50**, 621. Abst. *Ophthal. Year Book*, 1924, p. 175.
1929 Herbert, H. *Brit. Jl. Ophthal.* **13**, 337.
1933 Fischer, F. *Arch. f. Ophthal.* **131**, 318.

The Association of Hydrophthalmia with other anomalies

1903 Marlow, F. W. *Arch. of Ophthal.* **32**, 470.
1905 Reis, W. *Arch. f. Ophthal.* **60**, 1.
1910 Mayou, M. S. *Trans. Ophthal. Soc. U.K.* **30**, 124.
1915 Böhm, K. *Klin. Monatsbl. f. Augenheilk.* **55**, 556.
1929 St Germain, A. J. *Amer. Jl. Ophthal.* **12**, 126.
1930 Penman, G. G. *Brit. Jl. Ophthal.* **14**, 232.
1933 Oguchi, C. *Arch. f. Ophthal.* **130**, 432.
1934 Waardenberg, P. J. *Klin. Monatsbl. f. Augenheilk.* **92**, 29.
1936 Lacroix, A. *Bull. et Mém. Soc. franç. d'Ophtal.* **49**, 313.
1937 Brown, Edgar. Personal Communications.

Hydrophthalmia and Neurofibromatosis

1870 Bruns, H. D. *Virchow's Arch.* **50**. Quoted by Murakami.
1884 Schiess Gemuseus. *Arch. f. Ophthal.* **30**, pt. 3, p. 195.
1991 de Schweinitz, G. *Trans. Amer. Ophthal. Soc.* **6**, 48.
1898 Schiess Gemuseus. *Arch. f. d. ges. Ophthal.* **20**, 195.
1898 Sachsalber, A. *Beiträge z. Augenheilk.* **3**, pt. 27, p. 523.
1899 Lezius. Inaug. Dissert. Jena. Quoted by Reis.
1903 Snell and Collins. *Trans. Ophthal. Soc. U.K.* **23**, 157.
1903 Verhoeff, F. H. *Trans. Ophthal. Soc. U.K.* **23**, 176.
1903 Rockliffe and Parsons. *Trans. Path. Soc.* **55**, 27.
1905 Collins, E. T. *Trans. Ophthal. Soc. U.K.* **25**, 256.
1905 Collins and Batten. *Trans. Ophthal. Soc. U.K.* **25**, 248.
1905 Siegrist, A. *Ber. d. deutsch. Ophthal. Gesell. Heidelberg,* **32**.
1906 Michelson-Rabinowitsch. *Arch. f. Augenheilk.* **55**, 245.
1906 Rosenmayer, L. *Zentralbl. f. prakt. Augenheilk.* **30**, 70.
1906 Knapp, H. *Trans. Amer. Ophthal. Soc.* **6**, 48.
1907 Sutherland and Mayou. *Trans. Ophthal. Soc. U.K.* **27**, 179.
1908 v. Michel, J. *Klin. Monatsbl. f. Augenheilk.* **46**, 2, 191.

1909 Komoto, J. *Klin. Monatsbl. f. Augenheilk.* pt. 1.
1909 Weinstein, A. *Klin. Monatsbl. f. Augenheilk.* **47**, 2, 635.
1912 Coats, G. *Trans. Ophthal. Soc. U.K.* **32**, 165.
1912 Zentmayer, W. *Trans. Amer. Ophthal. Soc.* **13**, 205.
1913 Fehr, O. *Zentralbl. f. prakt. Augenheilk.* **37**, 233.
1913 Murakami, S. *Klin. Monatsbl. f. Augenheilk.* **51**, 514.
1916 Knapp, A. *Trans. Amer. Ophthal. Soc.* **14**, 534.
1921 Pomplum, F. *Klin. Monatsbl. f. Augenheilk.* **67**, 242.
1922 Wiegmann, E. *Klin. Monatsbl. f. Augenheilk.* **68**, 395.
1923 Löb, C. *Arch. f. Augenheilk.* **93**, 1-2, 73.
1923 van der Hoeve, J. *Trans. Ophthal. Soc. U.K.* **43**, 536.
1924 Fischer, H. *Dermat. Zeitschr.* **42**, 143. Quoted by Copeland, Craver and Reese.
1924 Moravec, Z. *Cas. Lek. Cesk.* **63**, 1082. Abst. *Jl. Amer. Med. Ass.* **83**, 654.
1924 Vogt, A. *Klin. Monatsbl. f. Augenheilk.* **72**, 507.
1925 Axenfeld, Th. *Ber. d. deutsch. Ophthal. Gesell. Heidelberg*, **43**, 266.
1925 Metzger, E. *Klin. Monatsbl. f. Augenheilk.* **75**, 248.
1925 Wiener, Alfred. *Arch. of Ophthal.* **54**, 481.
1925 Hudson, A. C. *Proc. Roy. Soc. Med.* p. 12, Dec.
1925 Knight, M. S. *Amer. Jl. Ophthal.* **8**, 791.
1925 Reese, W. S. *Amer. Jl. Ophthal.* **8**, 865.
1926 Mintschewa, M. *Klin. Monatsbl. f. Augenheilk.* **76**, 403.
1927 Winkelbauer, A. *Deutsch. Zeitschr. f. Chir.* **205**, 230.
1927-8 Kyrieleis, W. *Arch. f. Ophthal.* **119**, 119.
1928 Jaensch, P. A. *Ber. d. deutsche Ophthal. Gesell. Heidelberg*, **46**, 455.
1928 Holmström, M. *Acta Ophthal.* **6**, 403.
1928 Hine and Wyatt. *Brit. Jl. Ophthal.* **12**, 256.
1929 Awguschewitsch, P. L. *Klin. Monatsbl. f. Augenheilk.* **83**, 91.
1929 Achermann, E. *Zeitschr. f. Augenheilk.* **67**, 141. Abst. *Brit. Jl. Ophthal.* **13**, 411.
1929 Collins, E. T. *Trans. Ophthal. Soc. U.K.* **49**, 166.
1930 Foster Moore, R. *Trans. Ophthal. Soc. U.K.* **50**, 451.
1930 Goldstein and Wexler. *Arch. of Ophthal.* **3**, 288 and 374.
1930 Callender and Thigpen. *Amer. Jl. of Ophthal.* **13**, 121.
1931 Phelan, H. V. *Arch. of Ophthal.* **5**, 800.
1932 Critchley, Macdonald. *Medical Annual*, p. 323.
1932 Critchley, Macdonald and Earl, C. J. *Brain*, **50**, 311.
1932 Katzenstein, R. *Virchow's Arch. f. Path. Anat.* **286**, 42.
1932 van der Hoeve, J. *Trans. Ophthal. Soc. U.K.* **52**, 391.
1932 Archambault and Fromm. *Arch. of Neurol. and Psychol.* **27**, 529, March.
1933 Knapp, A. *Jl. Amer. Med. Assoc.* Feb. p. 18.
1933 Le Wald, Léon. *Amer. Jl. Roentgenology*, Dec. p. 756.
1933 Critchley, Macdonald. *Medical Annual*, p. 511.
1933 Stief, A. *Zeitschr. f. d. ges. Neurol. und Psychiat.* **147**, 573.
1934 Weber and Bode. *Proc. Roy. Soc. Med.* **27**, 638, April.
1934 O'Brien and Leinfelder. *Trans. Amer. Ophthal. Soc.* **32**, 324.
1934 Knapp, A. *Medical Record*, **139**, 62.
1934 Reuben, M. S. *Arch. of Ped.* **51**, 522.
1934 Copeland, Craver and Reese. *Arch. of Surgery*, **29**, 108.
1934 Freeman, D. *Arch. of Ophthal.* **11**, 641.
1935 Shapland and Greenfield. *Trans. Ophthal. Soc. U.K.* **55**, 257.

1935 MERKULOV, A. Awerbach Jubilee Volume, p. 280. Abst. *Amer. Jl. Ophthal.* **19**, 830, Sept.

1936 WHEELER, J. M. *Trans. Amer. Ophthal. Soc.* **34**, 152.

1936 MEEKER, L. H. *Arch. of Ophthal.* **16**, 152.

1936 VERHOEFF, F. H. *Arch. of Ophthal.* **16**, 898.

1936 MOORE, A. E. *Aust. and New Zealand Jl. of Surgery*, **5**, 314.

1936 FRIEDENWALD, J. S. *Arch. of Ophthal.* **16**, 65.

1937 VERHOEFF, F. H. Personal Communication.

1937 CAMPBELL, GLEN. Personal Communication. (Case reported also by E. Stier. *Deutsche Zeitschr. f. Nervenheilk.* **44**, 1912.)

1937 MESSINGER and CLARKE. *Arch. of Ophthal.* **18**, 1.

HYDROPHTHALMIA AND NAEVUS

1860 SCHIRMER. *Arch. f. Ophthal.* **7**, 119.

1879 STURGE. *Trans. Clin. Soc.* **12**, 162.

1883 HORROCKS. *Trans. Ophthal. Soc. U.K.* **3**, 106.

1884 MILLES. *Trans. Ophthal. Soc. U.K.* **4**, 168.

1885 LAWFORD, J. B. *Trans. Ophthal. Soc. U.K.* **5**, 136.

1886 SNELL, S. *Brit. Med. Jl.* **2**, 68.

1890 GUILINI. *Arch. f. Ophthal.* **36**, 247.

1897 KALISCHER, S. *Berlin. Klin. Wochenschr.* **48**, 1059.

1898 GALEZOWSKI, X. Abst. Love, *Amer. Jl. Ophthal.* **43**, 607.

1899 DEYL, J. *Wiener Klin. Rundschau.* Quoted by Collins.

1900 WAGENMANN, L. *Arch. f. Ophthal.* **51**, 533.

1901 KALISCHER, S. *Arch. f. Psychiat. und Nervenk.* **34**, 171.

1901 HARTRIDGE, G. *Trans. Ophthal. Soc. U.K.* **21**, 83.

1901 WORK DODD, H. *Trans. Ophthal. Soc. U.K.* **21**, 82.

1902 STEFFENS. *Klin. Monatsbl. f. Augenheilk.* **40**, 113.

1904 BELTMANN, J. *Arch. f. Ophthal.* **59**, 502.

1905 FEHR, O. *Zentralbl. f. prak. Augenheilk.* **29**, 161.

1906 CUSHING, H. *Jl. Amer. Med. Ass.* **47**, 178.

1907 MELLER, J. *Zeitschr. f. Augenheilk.* Jan. p. 50.

1908 QUACKENBOSS and VERHOEFF. *Trans. Amer. Ophthal. Soc.* **11**, 510.

1908 STOEWER, P. *Klin. Monatsbl. f. Augenheilk.* **46**, 323.

1909 CUPERUS, N. J. *Klin. Monatsbl. f. Augenheilk.* **47**, 334.

1909 CABANNES, C. *Arch. d'Ophtal.* **29**, 368.

1914 LOVE, J. M. *Arch. of Ophthal.* **43**, 607.

1917 COLLINS, E. T. *Trans. Ophthal. Soc. U.K.* **37**, 173.

1917 GRIMSDALE, H. *Trans. Ophthal. Soc. U.K.* **37**, 175.

1918 ELSCHNIG, A. *Zeitschr. f. Augenheilk.* **39**, 188.

1918 FLEISCHER, B. *Klin. Monatsbl. f. Augenheilk.* **61**, 152.

1919 PATON and COLLINS. *Trans. Ophthal. Soc. U.K.* **39**, 157.

1920 FREESE. *Klin. Monatsbl. f. Augenheilk.* **65**, 922.

1920 DOHME, B. *Klin. Monatsbl. f. Augenheilk.* **65**, 923.

1920 HENDERSON, E. E. *Brit. Jl. Ophthal.* **4**, 373.

1921 GESELL, A. *Arch. Neurol. and Psychiat.* **6**, 4, 400.

1922 KOMOTO, J. P. *Klin. Monatsbl. f. Augenheilk.* **69**, 158.

1922 NAKAMURA, B. *Klin. Monatsbl. f. Augenheilk.* **69**, 312.

1923 CUSHING, H. *Modern Medicine*, **6**, 250.

1923 SAFAR, K. *Zeitschr. f. Augenheilk.* **51**, 501.

1923 DUSCHNITZ, L. *Klin. Monatsbl. f. Augenheilk.* **70**, 404.
1923 SALUS, R. *Klin. Monatsbl. f. Augenheilk.* **71**, 303.
1923 LÖWENSTEIN, A. *Klin. Monatsbl. f. Augenheilk.* **70**, 540.
1924 ZAUN, W. *Klin. Monatsbl. f. Augenheilk.* **72**, 57.
1925 VOEGELE, J. *Klin. Monatsbl. f. Augenheilk.* **74**, 755.
1925 KIRANOFF. *Klin. Monatsbl. f. Augenheilk.* **74**, 502.
1925 VITA, A. *Atti d. Cong. d' Oftal. Roma,* Oct.
1925 MARCHESANI, O. *Wien. Med. Wochenschr.* Abst. *Ophthal. Lit.* 1927
    p. 118.
1925 BÄR, C. *Zeitschr. f. Augenheilk.* **57**, 628. Quoted by Yamanaka.
1926 GINSBURG, G. *Klin. Monatsbl. f. Augenheilk.* **76**, 298.
1926 SCHWARTZ, V. T. *Amer. Jl. Ophthal.* **9**, 447.
1927 KNAPP, A. *Trans. Amer. Ophthal. Soc.* **25**, 154.
1927 YAMANAKA, T. *Klin. Monatsbl. f. Augenheilk.* **78**, 372.
1927 DERBY, WAITE and KIRK. *Trans. Amer. Ophthal. Soc.* **25**, 154.
1927 KAISER, J. H. *Klin. Monatsbl. f. Augenheilk.* **79**, 547.
1927 JAENSCH, P. A. *Arch. f. Ophthal.* **118**, 21.
1927–8 BRUSHFIELD and WYATT. *Brit. Jl. of Children's Diseases.*
1928 DE HAAS, H. L. *Klin. Monatsbl. f. Augenheilk.* **80**, 830.
1928 VOEGELE, J. *Klin. Monatsbl. f. Augenheilk.* **81**, 393.
1928 VAN RÖTTH, A. *Klin. Monatsbl. f. Augenheilk.* **80**, 405.
1928 ONKEN, TH. *Klin. Monatsbl. f. Augenheilk.* **81**, 651.
1928 PANICO, E. *Boll. d'Ocul.* **1**, 5.
1928 CLAUSEN, W. *Klin. Monatsbl. f. Augenheilk.* **81**, 393.
1929 SAFAR, K. *Klin. Monatsbl. f. Augenheilk.* **82**, 534 and 825.
1929 HORAY, G. *Zentralbl. f. d. ges. Ophthal.* **20**, 793. Quoted by Biro.
1929 AYNSLEY, T. B. *Brit. Jl. Ophthal.* **13**, 612.
1929 KRAUSE, K. *Zeitschr. f. Augenheilk.* **68**, 244. Abst. *Klin. Monatsbl. f.*
    Augenheilk. **83**, 698.
1929 ZVEREVA, V. *Moscow. Zentralbl. f. d. ges. Ophthal.* **20**, 847. Quoted by
    O'Brien and Porter.
1929 HUDELO, A. *Ann. d'Ocul.* **166**, 889.
1929 MACRAE, A. *Brit. Jl. Ophthal.* **13**, 63.
1929 THOMSON, E. *Brit. Jl. Ophthal.* **13**, 127.
1929 JOHNSTON, K. B. *Brit. Jl. Ophthal.* **13**, 498.
1929 FOSTER MOORE. *Brit. Jl. Ophthal.* **13**, 252.
1929 VINCENT and HEUYER. *Revue Neurol.* p. 361.
1929 WEBER, PARKES. *Proc. Roy. Soc. Med.* Neurol. Sect. **22**, 25.
1930 BALLANTYNE, A. J. *Brit. Jl. Ophthal.* **14**, 481.
1930 JAHNKE, W. *Zeitschr. f. Augenheilk.* **72**, 354. Quoted by Tyson.
1931 PI, H. *Nat. Med. Jl. China,* **17**, 95.
1932 LINDENMEYER, O. *Klin. Monatsbl. f. Augenheilk.* **88**, 339.
1932 KOSTOULAS, A. *Ann. d'Ocul.* **169**, 341.
1932 STEINER, K. *Dermat. Wochenschr.* **1**, 851. Abst. *Zentralbl. f. d. ges.*
    Ophthal. **27**, 767.
1932 TYSON, H. H. *Arch. of Ophthal.* **8**, 365.
1933 CORRADO, M. *Rassegna Ital. d'Ottal.* **2**, 553. Abst. *Amer. Jl. Ophthal.*
    1934, **17**, 272.
1933 CROUZON and others. *Revue Neurol.* p. 509.
1933 O'BRIEN and PORTER. *Arch. of Ophthal.* **9**, 715.
1933 OGUCHI, C. *Arch. f. Ophthal.* **1**, 3 and 4, p. 432.

228   REFERENCES TO CHAPTER IV

1935 Dunphy, E. B. *Amer. Jl. Ophthal.* **18**, 714.
1935 Padovani, S. *Atti Cong. Soc. Oftal. Ital.* p. 689. Abst. *Zentralbl. f. Ophthal.* 1936, **35**, 547.
1935 Ludwig, A. *Klin. Monatsbl. f. Augenheilk.* **95**, 160.
1935 Granström, K. O. *Acta Ophthal.* **13**, 1–2, p. 115.
1935 Skydsgaard. *Acta Ophthal.* **13**, 273.
1935 Perera, C. A. *Arch. of Ophthal.* **14**, 626.
1935 Kreyenberg and Hansing. *Zentralbl. f. d. ges. Neurol. und Psych.* **152**, 751.
1935 Applemans. *Arch. d'Ophtal.* **52**, 835.
1935 Joiris and Fauchamps. *Bull. et Mém. Soc. Belge*, **70**, 92.
1935 Coppez, H. *Bull. et Mém. Soc. Belge*, **70**, 96.
1935 Folk, M. L. *Amer. Jl. Ophthal.* **18**, 903.
1936 Riser, R. O. *Amer. Jl. Ophthal.* **19**, 155.
1936 Zeeman, W. P. C. Personal Communications.
1936 Biro, J. *Zeitschr. f. Augenheilk.* **88**, 80. Abst. *Amer. Jl. Ophthal.* **19**, 540.
1936 Emory Hill and Dart, R. O. *Arch. of Ophthal.* **16**, 897.
1936 Brons, C. *Klin. Monatsbl. f. Augenheilk.* **97**, 3.
1936 Goldstein, H. I. *Brit. Med. Jl.* April, p. 721.
1936 Brissot and Delsuc. *Ann. Méd. Psychol.* **94**, 62, June.
1936 Santonastaso, A. *Ann. di Ottal. e Clin. Ocul.* **64**, 405, 437.
1937 Gault, E. L. Personal Communications.
1937 McArthur, G. A. D. *Med. Jl. of Austral.* May 22, p. 780.
1937 Mehney, G. H. *Arch. of Ophthal.* **17**, 1018.
1937 Evans, P. J. *Arch. of Ophthal.* **18**, 193.
1937 Koyama, A. *Chuo-Ganka Iho*, **29**, 12; Abst. *Klin. Monatsbl. f. Augenheilk.* **99**, 565.

Meningo-Cutaneous and Retino-Cerebellar Angiomatoses

1895 Steinheil. Inaug. Dissert. Würzburg. Quoted by Cushing and Bailey.
1897 Kalischer, S. *Berlin. Klin. Wochenshr.* **48**, 1059.
1898 Lannois and Bernoud. *Nouvelle Iconig. de la Saltpétrière*, **11**, 446. Quoted by Weber.
1901 Kalischer, S. *Arch. f. Psychiatr. und Nervenk.* **34**, 171.
1902 Cassirer, R. *Neurol. Zentralbl.* **21**, 32.
1904 Chaput. *Bull. et Mém. de la Soc. chirurgie.* Quoted by Weber.
1905 Naecke, P. *Neurol. Zentralbl.* **24**, 30.
1905 Strominger, L. *Spitalul* (Bucaresti), **25**, 147. Quoted by Weber.
1906 Cushing. *Jl. Amer. Med. Ass.* **47**, 178.
1908 Broeckaert, J. *Bull. Acad. Roy. de Méd. de Belge*, **22**, 360.
1912 Volland, R. *Zeitschr. f. d. Erforsch. und Behandl. d. jug. Schwachsinns*, **6**, 130. Quoted by Cushing.
1913 Hebold, O. *Arch. f. Psychiatr.* **51**, 445.
1913 Oppenheim, H. *Neurol. Zentralbl.* **32**, 3.
1915 Cobb, S. *Annals of Surgery*, **62**, 641.
1915 Sachs, E. *Amer. Jl. Med. Sc.* **150**, 565.
1917 Sabin, F. R. *Anat. Record*, **13**, 199.
1918 Streeter, G. L. *Carnegie Publications*, **271**, 5. Quoted by Cushing.
1919 Spiller, W. G. *Arch. Neurol. and Psychiatr.* **2**, 50.
1922 Greig, D. M. *Edinburgh Med. Jl.* **28**, 105.

1922 WEBER, F. PARKES. *Jl. of Neur. and Psychopath.* **3**, 134.

1923 DIMITRI, V. *Rev. assoc. méd. Argent.* **36**, 63. Quoted by Cushing.

1924 KARLEFORS, J. *Die Hirnhauträume des Kleinhirns.* Stockholm. Quoted by Cushing and Bailey.

1927 BREGMAN, L. E. and MESZ. *Rev. Neurol.* **342**, 191.

1927 HUGO, H. J. *Jl. Med. Ass. South Africa.*

1927 MARQUE, A. M. *Revista Oto-N.-Oftal. y de Cirurgía Neurol.* (Buenos Aires), **1**, 202. Abst. *Klin. Monatsbl. f. Augenheilk.* 1928, **80**, 136.

1927 LINDAU, A. *Acta Ophthal.* **4**, 193.

1929 WEBER, F. PARKES. *Proc. Roy. Soc. Med.* Neurol. Sect. **22**, 25.

1929 FOSTER MOORE, R. *Brit. Jl. Ophthal.* **13**, 252.

1934 ISNEL, R. *Bull. Soc. d'Ophtal. de Paris*, Dec. p. 652.

1934 KRABBE, K. *Arch. Neurol. and Psychiatr.* **32**, 737.

1935 SCHIÖTZ, E. H. *Norse mag. f. laegevidensk*, **96**, 737. Abst. *Zentralbl. f. d. ges. Neurol. und Psych.* **78**, 352.

1935 MONIZ and LIMA. *Soc. de Neurol. Paris*, **2**, 5. Abst. *Zentralbl. f. d. ges. Neurol. und Psych.* **78**, 93.

1936 WEBER, F. PARKES. *Brit. Med. Jl.* April 4, p. 708.

CAUSES OF HYDROPHTHALMIA IN ASSOCIATION WITH FACIAL NAEVI AND NEUROFIBROMATOSIS

1903 VERHOEFF, F. H. *Trans. Ophthal. Soc. U.K.* **23**, 176.

1906 CHEATLE, L. *Brit. Med. Jl.* August, 18.

1923 SAFAR, K. *Zeitschr. f. Augenheilk.* **51**, 301.

1923 SALUS, R. *Klin. Monatsbl. f. Augenheilk.* **71**, 303.

1929 AYNSLEY, T. B. *Brit. Jl. Ophthal.* **13**, 618.

1935 GRANSTRÖM, K. O. *Acta Ophthal.* **13**, 1, 2, p. 115.

1937 VERHOEFF, F. H. Personal Communication.

CHAPTER V

PATHOGENESIS

THE THEORIES OF ORIGIN OF HYDROPHTHALMIA

A survey of the foregoing summary of the morbid anatomy of early specimens reveals two types of disorder in the ocular tissues. Firstly, one detects developmental defects due to an arrested or an otherwise faulty growth. Secondly, undoubted evidences of inflammatory changes are found.

It is difficult to divide with certainty all the changes into one or other of these types. The distension of the globe has led in most cases to so much distortion that it is not always possible to visualise the state of the affected tissues before they were stretched and affected by late or secondary degeneration and even inflammatory changes. One must be constantly asking whether the signs of inflammation in the iris, for example, are due to intra-uterine infection or to a relatively late postnatal process that developed with ease in an already over-stretched and disordered structure.

Even when one has decided that the main changes in a certain globe are such that one can label them as congenital anomalies, one has not definitely excluded them as ravages of intra-uterine infection.

One must remember that, even in such true examples of the developmental type as Seefelder specimens II and III, traces of an almost vanished intra-uterine iridocyclitis were found. This suggests that the initial cause was inflammation, and that the direct cause of hydrophthalmia was the developmental defect that resulted from the inflammatory state. Therefore, when we state that a certain specimen is of the developmental type we do not deny an initial rôle to an earlier inflammation. We simply mean the direct cause was an arrested or defective development of some structure. Possibly, however, in such an eye the filtration apparatus, though developmentally defective, was adequate until a mild attack of inflammation developed. Then the albuminous aqueous blocked the restricted means of escape and hydrophthalmia ensued.

The finding of such traces of iridocyclitis and the more obvious signs of secondary iridocyclitis tends to obscure the picture and make the recognition of the direct cause of hypertension very difficult.

Numerous difficulties arise when one attempts to summarise the reports of others concerning the findings and the theories that relate to congenital glaucoma. So often one man's summing up is influenced by his own interpretation of structural defects. This might be quite different from that of another with a different viewpoint. The interpretation made by any observer may depend on his previous training, particular interests, or the system of thought prevailing in his city or his country at the particular time when he received his training or when he is writing.

This may help us to understand why Seefelder, after his extensive embryological studies, emphasises developmental defects, why all the early cases reported by French oculists and none by any other observers are attributed to phlebitis of ocular veins, and why so much was written of "ulcus corneae internum" during last century and yet so little during the present one.

Therefore, where possible, the author has endeavoured to rely on the published microphotographs and the reports of findings rather than on the ideas of any one observer. It must also be remembered that some observers have changed their viewpoint from time to time and their later interpretation was different from the first they adopted. The change in the opinions of Collins will be referred to shortly.

If we confine ourselves to a consideration of the earliest histological examinations made on hydrophthalmic globes we shall have a better chance of evading the influences of prolonged distension and superadded inflammation.

Though the suggested causes are numerous, they can be conveniently grouped according to the emphasis placed on either a developmental, a post-inflammatory, or a nervous explanation of the disease.

1. THE DEVELOPMENTAL THEORY

Introduction.

The significance of ocular anomalies.

Association with other ocular anomalies.

Association with non-ocular anomalies.

1. The significance of persistent and aberrant mesoblastic tissue in and round the anterior chamber.

The variations in the meshwork at the angle.

The meshwork in the angles of the earliest specimens.

    ,,   ,,   specimens with neurofibromatosis.

    ,,   ,,   ,,   .,   naevi.

The meshwork in the specimens with aniridia.

,,   ,,   ,,   ,,   microphthalmia.

2. The significance of obliteration or the absence of Schlemm's canal.

3. The significance of iris processes.

4.   ,,   ,,   peripheral synechiae.

5. The significance of congenital pupillary synechiae and congenital corneal defects—"ulcus corneae internum".

When considering the part that a developmental defect may play in tissues at the angle, it is well to recall certain embryological facts. In early life "the angle is blocked by mesodermal tissue continuous with the pupillary membrane and this mesodermal tissue shares in the process of atrophy which involves so much of the embryonic mesoderm associated with the optic cup". "The canal of Schlemm is deeply embedded in mesoderm at the 65·0 mm. stage. The open mesh of the spaces of Fontana is formed by atrophy of this mesoderm between the canal and the angle of the anterior chamber. This atrophy is probably only completed during the eighth month" (Mann). This atrophy coincides with, and appears to be a similar process to, the atrophy of the lateral and the anterior portions of the tunica vasculosa lentis.

There is no single aetiology for all cases of hydrophthalmia (Reis, Seefelder, Takashima and others). In any series, particularly of early cases, there is, however, a striking resemblance. The majority show the presence of some abnormality in or near the angle that would impede the escape of fluid. Though the angle itself may be either blocked or wide open, one of several forms of obstruction is nearly always present. There is evidence in many cases that such is a primary change. The remarkable absence of inflammatory signs in early cases and the resemblance of the lesions to earlier normal embryonic conditions are points that strongly support one's belief in the theory that explains hydrophthalmia by defective development.

THE SIGNIFICANCE OF OCULAR ANOMALIES

Seefelder concluded that a defective development of the filtration channels was the primary cause of most cases of simple congenital hydrophthalmia. Inflammatory processes as well as vasomotor disturbances, due either to the trigeminal or the sympathetic nerve, in his opinion, are entitled only to secondary consideration.

Parsons in England, Siegrist in Switzerland, and Lagrange in France arrived at similar conclusions. "Developmental defects such as absence of Schlemm's canal and a 'soudure de Knies', lessening the escape of fluid at the angle, are the essential anatomical findings to which, to a very great extent if not exclusively, the pathogenesis of infantile glaucoma must be attributed", wrote Lagrange.

Even in some of the late specimens evidence of a developmental defect was found. Consider, for example, Dürr and Schlegtendal specimen I. The angle was wide open in each eye and only traces of a canal of Schlemm were found. Not only was the condition bilateral but two of the patient's brothers were affected and the parents were first cousins.

Resemblance to hydrocephalus. Terson (1920, 1925) stated that hydrophthalmia is simply hydrocephalus of the eye. Pesme (1934) found the two conditions associated in one patient. After anatomical examination he concluded that the retention of the cerebro-spinal fluid and of the aqueous was in both the result of aplasia of the drainage channels concerned.

Lagrange, when emphasising hypoexcretion as the essential condition, compared infantile glaucoma and congenital hydrocephalus. The latter condition is due to the imperforate state of the communicating apertures between the ventricular and the meningeal spaces. This obstruction prevents the passage of the cerebro-spinal fluid which arises principally from the choroid plexus.

"In infantile glaucoma, we believe we are right in suggesting a mechanism analogous to that which provokes hydrocephalus by obliteration of the aqueduct of Sylvius. The canal of Schlemm, and the trabecular region of Fontana are often maldeveloped, often absent. Here there is no 'soudure de Knies', such as develops secondarily in the adult, and which may lead to identical functional disturbance, but the cause is a congenital malformation of the excretory channels" (Lagrange).

THE SIGNIFICANCE OF THE ASSOCIATION
WITH NON-OCULAR ANOMALIES

Very important support for the developmental theory comes from the not infrequent combination of congenital glaucoma with facial naevi and neurofibromatosis. The latter anomalies are most probably errors in development. It is unlikely that maternal sepsis is their underlying cause. The characteristic lesions of congenital glaucoma are found in the majority of the specimens associated with either naevi or neurofibromatosis. In some of these either an angiomatous or a neurofibrillary state of the uveal tract may be the main cause of glaucoma.

THE SIGNIFICANCE OF PERSISTENT AND ABERRANT MESOBLASTIC TISSUE IN AND ROUND THE ANTERIOR CHAMBER

We have seen that defects in development may be evident in the following ways:

1. Variations in the state of the meshwork of the angle. This may appear either as dense sclero-corneal trabeculae or as persistent uveal meshwork, with or without a poorly developed and posteriorly situated canal of Schlemm.

2. Such meshwork may be absent, when there is either a sheet of iris-like tissue filling the angle or a state of union between the iris and the sclero-corneal junction.

3. Apparent hypoplasia of Descemet's endothelium and membrane and of the iris stroma, with, at times, an adhesion between the two that may vary from a delicate strand to so wide a union that gross deformity or even microphthalmia ensues.

The actual cause of hypertension in the great majority of specimens is an interference with the escape of fluid from the angle of the anterior chamber. This is, as a rule, due to one of a variety of developmental and post-inflammatory lesions that produce obstruction of the canal of Schlemm. This is the common direct cause of congenital glaucoma. Other direct causes, such as absence of drainage through the iris tissues, are conceivable, but their exact nature is uncertain. Their existence is suggested by the patency of Schlemm's canal in quite late cases, e.g. several described by Gallenga. Little also is known of the state of the venules into which the canal of Schlemm drains. These may be undeveloped or occluded by disease. The frequently described new circumcorneal vessels may be an attempted collateral circulation or the result of repeated inflammatory attacks.

In the following attempt to analyse the causes of glaucoma in our series of specimens we will first consider those that show developmental defects that either tend to obstruct the canal of Schlemm or by their presence and close relationship to the canal suggest its inclusion in the disorder of growth.

Once again a considerable doubt exists when we are dealing with most of the later specimens. A close study of the earlier ones gives some guide, however, to the probable initial conditions that existed in the former.

Obstruction at the angle. The defects in the neighbourhood of Schlemm's canal are more or less constant and various theories to explain these have been put forward. They attribute the defects to (1) a primary inflammation of the uveal tract, (2) a congenital malformation, (3) a disordered intra-ocular circulation due to a defect of the ciliary nerves.

"Horner (1889) first put forward the idea that buphthalmia might be due to some congenital abnormality of the angle of the anterior chamber."

Raab, some years before (1876), had stressed the importance of an obstruction at this site, but had assumed it was cyclitic in origin. Numerous investigations have shown that though the angle may be apparently open, it may still differ widely from the normal condition.

Landolt stated that a congenital atresia of the filtering angle was the cause of all his cases of infantile glaucoma. The condition found in these eyes is similar to that in the adult form of glaucoma in which obstruction is offered to the escape of fluid. Hypertension results whether the obstruction is due to peripheral synechiae ("soudure de Knies"), an absence of Schlemm's canal, or other lesion that may arise from various forms of disease. De Wecker explained the frequent association of glaucoma and trachoma in the East by deep limbal cicatrisation. A similar state can be produced experimentally by cauterisation, or "colmatage" at this point. More recently Cucco, Jaensch and Lagrange supported these views.

Reis and Seefelder concluded that the drainage defects where the angle is open cannot be attributed to any single cause. Takashima's comment concerning his own specimens would apply to many others— the inflammation was probably secondary, for the structure of the anterior uveal tissues was comparatively good.

Reis (1905) summarised his findings as follows: "The displacement of the filtration channels of the angle of the anterior chamber, which is probably a necessary preliminary condition for congenital hydrophthalmia and which may be present in various forms, can be brought about through various causes and in various ways. It must be left to further anatomical investigations, especially in the early stages of the disease, to decide what change is the cause of individual cases, and to throw light on the frequency with which certain forms of filtration blockage occur." It was chiefly his specimen IV that convinced Reis of the importance of an obstructed canal of Schlemm, for in it no other defect and no sign of inflammation was present.

In 1910 Seefelder wrote that his views and those of Reis regarding the importance of congenital disturbances in the angle were almost universally accepted at any rate in Germany.

Though there are no constant histological findings to throw light on the cause of hydrophthalmia, yet there is sufficient resemblance between the findings in the great majority of cases to prove that conditions at the angle of the anterior chamber are abnormal. Though the angle may be open, yet drainage is interfered with by a displacement of the filtration channels or a simple obstruction of Schlemm's canal due to chronic inflammation or an anomaly. Particularly important are those eyes in which absence of the chief drainage channels are the only anatomical changes to be found.

THE SIGNIFICANCE OF THE MESHWORK IN THE ANGLE

Collins (1893), Cross (1896) and others were struck by an apparent union of iris and cornea at the angle and were inclined to explain this as an imperfect separation of the two structures. Collins referred to such a lesion as a congenital anterior synechia. Gros agreed with this view.

Later, however, Collins was inclined to consider that a persistence of the prenatal condition of the "ligamentum pectinatum" was a more likely explanation. This means that the inner looser part or uveal meshwork had failed either to differentiate or almost to disappear at the normal time, viz. the sixth month of intra-uterine life.

Cross (1891, 1896) strongly supported the view that the essential cause of hydrophthalmia was the imperfect condition of the filtration angle. He found that in some specimens the angle appeared to be closed and contained either fine trabeculae or pigmented connective tissue. In other eyes the angle was blocked by an adhesion of the iris root to the periphery of the cornea.

Collins held that the findings in this region resembled those in the prehuman stage in phylogeny. In man there is much less cavernous tissue and the anterior chamber angle is prolonged farther outwards than in lower mammals. The cornea is smaller in relation to the size of the globe in man than in mammals. The escape of aqueous in man is aided by simplification of the meshwork and the outward extension of the angle. If the condition in this region is almost normal at birth in an eye that is otherwise fully developed it may be able to carry on till teething, or some inflammatory or other upset embarrasses the channels of exit and tension rises and the eye becomes distended.

Mann (1926) found an interesting state in the left eye of an eight-year-old child with infantile glaucoma. Defective vision had been discovered one year previously. The base of the iris in the outer half of its circumference was imperfectly separated from the cornea. The angle was filled with loose meshwork of tissue containing a few very fine blood vessels. The structure of this tissue resembled the stroma of the iris. The angle of the right eye showed no definite abnormality, though the anterior chamber was shallow. Each eye showed a deep cup and slightly raised tension.

This case is of great interest, for it shows how certain developmentally defective eyes can carry on for a number of years before they are sufficiently embarrassed by some upset which may, indeed, be trivial, teething for example, and a rise of tension occurs. The incidence of this upset will determine whether glaucoma is congenital, infantile or even adolescent in type. This case also helps us to understand the occasional good results from operation at a relatively late age, *e.g.* six years and over.

It is possible also that the distension of the globe may lead to stretching, attenuation of such a meshwork and even the formation of a channel of exit for fluid. This will be considered later as an explanation of some of the instances of spontaneous arrest.

Taking these findings into consideration it appears likely that a defect in the meshwork of the angle is the most common cause of interference with the function of the canal of Schlemm. This may be either an absence, undue persistence, or an aberrant growth of the sclero-corneal trabeculae or of the uveal meshwork. It must be added that the exact effect of the defect is often obscure. Our methods of investigation are very imperfect, even serial sections providing a poor means of investigating function.

Let us now consider the state of the angle in the specimens that are reported in the literature or make their first appearance in this work.

The high percentage of defects in the meshwork amongst the early specimens is of great significance.

The meshwork in the angle of the earliest specimens (under one year)

In Seefelder's week-old specimens II and III the abnormally persistent uveal meshwork filled the angle. It ran as a hook of tissue towards the end of Descemet's membrane. The sclero-corneal meshwork was well developed and, as is normal, formed the inner wall of the narrowed and posteriorly situated canal of Schlemm. It is very instructive to compare the illustrations of these with that of the normal foetal eye at the ninth month. They are remarkably similar, but very different from the normal angle at birth. The iris root in specimen III sent out a very well-developed process to the posterior end of Descemet's membrane. This is probably similar to those already discussed instances described by Barkan, Troncoso and Salzmann. The distance between the iris root and Descemet's membrane was smaller than normal, so that the approach for aqueous to the canal of Schlemm was narrowed. The lumina of this canal lay behind the angle, as in an early stage of foetal life. Seefelder, finding evidence of an inflammatory process in each of these eyes, considered that the anomalous filtration apparatus was able to fulfil its task as long as it had only the normal quantity of aqueous to cope with, but the increased quantity and the higher albumen content of the aqueous, when inflammation appeared, led to hypertension and ocular distension. If death had not interfered with the development of changes at the filtration angle one probably would have found later the following appearances: the breaking-free of the iris root from the sclero-corneal trabeculae or Descemet's membrane, and further obliteration of the angle. "Had not the process been so early brought to an end by the death of the child, it is very possible that in time the continual stretching at the limbus, which was as yet only slight, would have led to a complete breaking free of the iris root from the sclero-corneal network or Descemet's membrane, and that the venous circle would have been still further obliterated and we would have got the same picture that we know well enough in the description of old hydrophthalmic eyes" (Seefelder).

Meller's eight-day-old specimen exhibited a foetal condition at the angle. The "pectinate ligament" had a compact structure. In Clapp's ten-day-old specimen the iris was described as being adherent to the cornea to an extent that was greater than is present in a six months' foetus. The specimens of Cosmetattos, von Hippel and Mayou (7 days, 4 weeks, 7 weeks) presented central anterior synechiae, and the meshwork was described as indefinite and imperfectly formed.

The unpublished specimen II, aged five weeks, showed a sheet of iris-like tissue filling the angle and no sign of meshwork.

Seefelder's specimen VIII, later described by Stimmel and Rotter (I), showed a more persistent framework than is normal at the age of two months.

Würdemann stated that in his three-month-old specimen the "ligamentum pectinatum" was in an embryonic state. In Spielberg's five-month-old specimen, two months premature, the angle was filled with foetal tissue.

The sclero-corneal meshwork in Kalt's six-month-old specimen was described as a thick mass containing cells.

In Juler's ten-week-old specimen the corneal perforation and iris prolapse rendered the initial state of the angle obscure.

In Magitot's ten-month-old specimen I the exact state of the meshwork is not described.

Seefelder's ten-month-old specimen I was a typical example of an angle that has persisted in a foetal state. The outer layers of the sclero-corneal meshwork were dense and compact, rich in cellular elements with spindle-like nuclei and only distinguishable from the sclera with difficulty. The inner layers were displaced because of the posterior situation of the poorly developed scleral spur. Schlemm's canal was also in a foetal position. The meshwork contained pigment and corpuscles.

The meshwork in the angle of specimens associated with neurofibromatosis and naevi

Hydrophthalmia and neurofibromatosis. Of the thirty-two instances of this association in the literature there are histological reports by the following:

*Michelson-Rabinowitsch (also Siegrist).	Snell and Collins.
	Sachsalber.
*Wagenmann.	Murakami (also Komoto).
*Wiener.	Knight.
*Unpublished specimen II.	Schiess Gemuseus.
Collins and Batten.	Wheeler.

* Not over $2\frac{1}{2}$ years of age.

With one exception the meshwork in these specimens was denser than normal. It was sometimes difficult to decide whether the condition was one of an abnormal development of meshwork or of a peripheral synechia. Murakami stated that in his nine-year-old specimen a peripheral synechia was present and no meshwork was visible.

In certain specimens the meshwork contained proliferated endothelium and pigment, and in others it was described as being "iris-like tissue" filling the angle.

There was a small canal of Schlemm in Michelson-Rabinowitsch's case. No reference was made to its presence by Schiess Gemuseus. In all the others it was absent.

Almost without exception the choroid contained neurofibromatosis, and in all the specimens the ciliary nerves were definitely affected. As a rule the choroid was dense, but that described by Schiess Gemuseus was atrophic and contained "nerve constrictions".

The similarity of the meshwork in these cases is very remarkable. The characteristic findings and the absence of signs of inflammatory changes are very strong support of the developmental theory.

Hydrophthalmia and facial naevi. Of sixty instances of hydrophthalmia and facial naevi histological examinations of the five following specimens were made:

> Safar. Thickened extensive meshwork, containing pigment, separates the angle from a small and posteriorly situated canal of Schlemm.
>
> Love and Stoewer each found an extensive peripheral synechia.
>
> Dunphy reported a sclerosed "pectinate ligament" and a peripheral synechia on one side.
>
> Cabannes's specimen was atypical and does not concern us here.

It is of interest to consider here two other conditions in which one may find a persistence of uveal meshwork, viz. aniridia and microphthalmia.

Aniridia. Frequently aniridia appears to be simply one of many defects present in an eye that must have been submitted to some harmful influence early in prenatal life. For example we find:

1. Aplasia of the fovea with amblyopia and nystagmus, as described by Seefelder (1909), Holm (1921), Velhagen (1923), Vogt (1924) and others.

2. Cataract.

3. Immature ciliary processes.

4. Peripheral corneal opacities. Engelbrecht (1908) described an opacity to which delicate threads proceeded from the anterior surface

of the iris. Since then numerous instances have been described: Axenfeld, Kayser, Thier. Axenfeld (1920) described the strands in his case as being a "ligamentum pectinatum in man". See also embryotoxon corneae posterius and hypoplasia of iris stroma.

5. Certain associations that directly concern us here are:

(a) Persistent uveal meshwork (van Duyse, 1907; Rieger, 1934).

(b) Adhesion of iris stump with cornea (Clausen, 1921).

(c) Iris process (Seefelder, 1909).

These explain the frequent association of congenital or adult glaucoma with aniridia.

Rieger considered that many cases of aniridia were due to persistent strands of mesodermal tissue that projected from the angle and normally underwent atrophy. He disagreed with Mann's view that they were due to persistent vascular branches. When the strands persist they are in the form of either a projecting layer filling part of the angle, a flat layer on the posterior corneal surface, a more or less regular network of varying thickness on the anterior surface of the iris, or strands which connect the periphery of the anterior surface of the iris to the cornea. They then may run even along the iris towards the pupil.

In a specimen with incomplete aniridia van Duyse (1907) found that in front of the most rudimentary part of the iris root there lay a cilioscleral space, which was homologous to that found in quadrupeds and representative of the period in foetal life when the iridian angle in man is filled with cilio-scleral trabeculae. Whereas these trabeculae, which limited the intercommunicating lacunae—the spaces of Fontana—remained in a foetal state, the sclero-corneal trabecular system had developed normally. The author held the view that the tissue in the angle in this specimen corresponded to a late period of development, after the seventh month.

In the lower part of Seefelder's specimen (1909) of aniridia a well-defined process of mesodermal tissue was attached to the end of the scleral meshwork and by this attachment the entire stroma of the iris was drawn forwards. This attachment appeared entirely to block the communication between the well-developed canal of Schlemm and the angle. Hopf's specimen (1900) was similar and showed several strands of tissue connecting the iris root and the scleral meshwork.

Microphthalmia. In three of six congenitally microphthalmic eyes Collins (1893) found the canal of Schlemm external to the angle and a well-marked cavernous zone of meshwork. Concerning his case II we read: "The fibres of the ligamentum pectinatum below are numerous and widely separated." In one of the others the "ligamentum pectinatum" resembled that found in ungulata and he wrote: "In some sections portions of the fibrous tissue from the anterior part of the iris seem to pass forwards to the posterior surface of the cornea in the position where Descemet's membrane ends and the ligamentum pectinatum begins. Externally to this prolongation forwards of iris tissue are some irregular trabeculae with large spaces between them, and anteriorly and externally to this cavernous zone are the laminated fibres of the ligamentum pectinatum with slit-like spaces between them." In these eyes the structure of the meshwork and the relation of parts about the angle of the anterior chamber seem to have remained in their foetal condition and to have simulated that met with in lower mammals. Probably on account of the smallness of the eyeballs these abnormalities in the filtration area did not cause sufficient obstruction to the exit of the aqueous humour to give rise to increase of tension.

THE SIGNIFICANCE OF AN "ABSENT" CANAL OF SCHLEMM

The state of Schlemm's canal has been considered of great import-ance when attempting to ascertain the cause of congenital glaucoma. Lagrange wrote: "The primary lesion is the defective development in the region of the canal of Schlemm and of this canal itself." The canal can close or be closed by such a variety of causes that the interpretation of this finding is probably more difficult than other authors believed. For example, it may never have developed; it may have closed as a result of the stretching of the surrounding tissues or from involvement in inflammation; it may have closed because its function was interfered with by atrophy of the ciliary muscle or by obliteration of the spaces that open into it, as a result of maldevelopment or of the products of inflammation.

Of course in many of the specimens showing persistent or abnormal uveal meshwork as the main lesion the cause of hypertension was not this *per se*, but its influence as an obstruction to the entrance of fluid into Schlemm's canal.

An absence of Schlemm's canal appears to be at times the only lesion present that might produce hypertension, *e.g.* specimens of Christel. Schlaefke, Reis II and VII, Takashima II.

Take, for examples, Reis II and IV (ages $5\frac{1}{2}$ and 4 years) (Figs. 56, 61, 62). In each no signs of inflammation were present, the iris and ciliary muscle were normal. In Reis's specimen II the uveal meshwork was well developed and showed open and empty spaces. The inner scleral lamellae lying lateral to the meshwork were very compact. In sections 220–280 no trace of a canal was found. In section 280, only on the temporal side was a lumen found and it disappeared very soon. In many sections between 120 and 200 no lumen was present, but it, or more probably a capillary, was represented by a narrow cord of parallel nuclei. In some such specimens the canal is not annular, for it appears only in certain sections of the eye. In some cases the absence of Schlemm's canal is associated with other developmental defects that probably share the responsibility of rendering filtration inadequate, and sometimes the absence of the canal is due to inflammation, as shown by round cell infiltration at its site.

If Schlemm's canal is incomplete it may prove adequate, as already stated, until some such cause of congestion as teething, measles, etc. arises and the embarrassment at the angle leads to a rise in tension. Particularly if the canal is defective the passage of excessive fluid or of inflammatory products may promote an induration of the canal and the meshwork.

The canal of Schlemm and the adjacent equatorial fibres that largely determine its shape and its extent are features that appear relatively late in evolution and in the development of the human foetal eye.

The variation in the estimates of the first appearance of this canal in the foetus are probably due not simply to differences in histological technique but also to an individual variation in the time of its appearance—a characteristic of structures that have recently emerged. Compare the following estimates:

Seefelder and Wolfrum: end of fourth month (85·0–100·0 mm.) "a vascular lumen in some places".

Mann: in 65·0 mm. stage but not in 48·0 mm.

Fischer: Possibly in 80·0 mm. stage and in many sections of 105·0 mm. a small single lumen was found.

In some instances the late development of Schlemm's canal may not lead to glaucoma unless other anomalies, such as a cryptless iris, are present, or there is undue congestion promoting an embarrassment at the exits for the intra-ocular fluid. Otherwise the canal goes on to complete though retarded maturity.

After the same manner a defect in the regression of the uveal mesh-work may arise. This structure, too, is a late development. The meshwork may be persistent or aberrant in growth.

In our study of morbid anatomy we have shown that

(1) The canal was present, although sometimes small and in a posterior position, in 45 % of specimens not over $2\frac{1}{2}$ years.

(2) A similar state existed in only 25 % of specimens over this age.

(3) The canal was almost or entirely absent in 75 % of specimens over $2\frac{1}{2}$ years.

THE SIGNIFICANCE OF IRIS PROCESSES

An interesting structure that may be found in the angle of specimens with congenital glaucoma is that which, for lack of a better term, is known as an iris process. It is in direct continuity with the iris and its structure is so similar to that of iris stroma that this term has been adopted. It consists of a hook-shaped process of tissue which curves round the angle to become attached to the end of Descemet's membrane or some point on the sclero-corneal trabeculae. Such a process is an annular sheet of tissue, and not an isolated strand across the angle, such as is found not infrequently in normal eyes. Seefelder wrote that analogous changes, between the root of the iris and Descemet's membrane (called the continuation of the iris or Hueck's pectinate ligament), are known in various animals' eyes, e.g. the ox, pig, rabbit, etc. In these, however, it does not appear to be analogous, for it is not so directly part of the iris or so extensive, and in addition uveal meshwork is present. Neither in the human foetus do we find a corresponding structure, though, of course, there is more tissue in the angle than in the adult state. Consequently, when it is found in a grown eye it should not be regarded as a "pectinate ligament" persisting in an abnormal manner, but rather as a variation of it. Possibly it is aberrant tissue laid down on the framework of the uveal meshwork which has failed to undergo the normal process of atrophy. In this case it will grow from the anterior fibro-vascular sheath which normally becomes the anterior layers of the iris (see "Anatomy of involved tissues").

In the eye at birth delicate trabeculae are sometimes found, which cross the area that later becomes the angle of the adult eye. These are comparable with the innermost trabeculae of the uveal meshwork in the chimpanzee, which bend across to be attached to the root of the iris (Collins). Thomson (1911), when describing the normal state of the meshwork, wrote: "Around the bottom of the iridial angle the fibres which pass to the substance of the iris display, in well-stained specimens, a direct continuity with the muscular radial fibres of the iris." It is of interest that in practically all of the specimens of congenital glaucoma associated with neurofibromatosis an iris process is present. As in all these no signs of uveal meshwork were present the question arises, whether such an iris process is an abnormal development of the tissue that normally becomes meshwork and then atrophies?

It is possible that the iris processes under discussion are similar to the adhesions found between the root of the iris and the cornea in some specimens with aniridia (Collins, 1893).

A patient with an early onset of glaucoma reported by Fisher (1901) is of great interest. At the age of twenty-seven years acute hypertension developed after the use of a mydriatic. On examination a narrow crescent of pigmented iris was found adherent to the periphery of the cornea. Delicate strands of iris tissue passed from the anterior surface of the iris on to this detached slip. The whole anterior surface of the iris was rugged and irregular with excavations. No congenital pupillary membrane was present, and though the pupil was slightly eccentric it acted normally. The other eye was normal and responded normally to the mydriatic. Fisher considered that there was a congenital imperfect separation of the iris from the back of the cornea.

The very extreme degree of aberrant iris formation present in Mann's patient, aged eight years (1926), with bilateral infantile glaucoma, has been discussed already.

THE SIGNIFICANCE OF PERIPHERAL ANTERIOR SYNECHIAE

Various factors may play a part in the narrowing of the filtration angle in primary glaucoma. Apart from peripheral synechiae they include a disproportion between the size of the lens and the size of the globe, any cause of congestion or inflammation of the uveal tract and possibly some structural defect that has just permitted filtration to carry on until other factors closed the channels for the escape of fluid. Such a defect in structure might help to explain the inherited and familial tendencies of glaucoma.

Priestley Smith contributed more than anyone else to our knowledge of the part that closure of the filtration angle plays in the production of glaucoma. He considered that at first there was merely a mechanical obstruction due to the base of the iris being pushed against the cornea. Later, as a result of exudation, the opposed surfaces became adherent. As these adhesions developed the adjacent iris became compressed, so that its spaces were closed and fluid could no longer find its way through the iris stroma and thence to the canal of Schlemm. The compression of the iris later led to atrophy. Hamburger emphasised the seriousness of this state in his writings, for to him the iris was an absorptive sponge.

The following is a summary of the evolution of peripheral synechiae in adult glaucoma. Can a similar process occur in the early stages of hydrophthalmia?

The ciliary processes contain more veins than any other ocular structure and so, in a congestive state, they may become so swollen that the root of the iris may press against the sclero-corneal junction and close the sinus of the angle. Agglutination leading to firm union may then occur between the opposed surfaces. Later the whole of the uveal tract may atrophy and the iris become narrowed and fibrous and the walls of its vessels thickened. The atrophy tends to be most marked in that part which adheres to the cornea, and nothing but the retinal pigment layer may persist. Schlemm's canal may disappear and the sclero-corneal meshwork may become denser and indistinguishable from sclera. Later the ciliary muscle may shrink away from the iris root (see unpublished specimen III, Fig. 96) and become flat, and the processes may almost disappear.

The significance of these peripheral synechiae is established. "The one common feature in the morbid anatomy of secondary glaucoma is the apposition or adhesion of the periphery of the iris to the cornea, first described by Knies and Weber" (Parsons, 1905). This view is supported by a considerable amount of experimental work.

Knies originally considered that the peripheral adhesions were due to a circumscribed inflammation of the meshwork at the angle and the adjacent tissues. This view was held also by Birnbacher and Azermak. It lost favour when signs of congestion only and not of true inflammation were found.

Inflammation of the meshwork. It must not be forgotten, however, that the meshwork is live tissue and apt to respond to any influence that is capable of affecting the remainder of the tissues of which it is a part—the uveal tract. The meshwork will not become simply clogged with pigmented cells and other inflammatory products, but its own fibres will be inflamed and will tend to show the fibrosis that usually follows in the train of inflammation. Fortin described under the name of "pectinitis" the inflammation of the meshwork, or more exactly of the endothelium lining the meshwork, whether accompanied or not by Descemetitis, cyclitis or iritis.

It is difficult in many specimens to decide whether the union of the periphery of the cornea and of the iris is a developmental defect—lack of separation—or a peripheral synechia and the result of inflammation. In the former state as a rule there is little or no sign of either Schlemm's canal or a scleral spur. On the other hand, either a narrowed lumen or a collection of cells and pigment will mark the site of the canal and the atrophic remnant will be adjacent to the spur if a true peripheral synechia is present. See illustrations of unpublished specimen III. Descemet's membrane is more likely to extend beyond the angle when inflammation has been present. Evidences of either arrested development or of inflammation in adjacent tissues may facilitate a diagnosis.

A developmental origin was suggested for the following specimens: Seefelder VIII (Stimmel and Rotter's early case, six weeks old, Fig. 63), and Lagrange's IV, VII. If the adhesions were synechial and due to intra-uterine inflammation all traces of this had vanished. The three specimens examined by Cross and Treacher Collins had closed angles and adhesions between the iris and the cornea. Their first explanation, as we have seen, was that the cornea had imperfectly separated from the iris. Later they considered that there was a persistence of foetal meshwork.

The inflammatory signs present vary greatly in degree. In case II of Reis's series they were minimal. In Stimmel and Rotter specimen III, though there was evidence of a chronic iridocyclitis, "congenital changes in the angle" were held responsible. Pesme considered that malformation was the cause of glaucoma in his case, but the presence of extensive synechiae and of closed spaces of Fontana and canal of Schlemm suggested that inflammation was the probable cause. Gallenga considered that his second, third and fourth specimens, which had "closed spaces of Fontana" and anterior synechiae, were inflammatory in origin. In Lagrange's ninth specimen the synechiae were described as being secondary to a corneal staphyloma.

An attack of glaucoma developed in Lagrange's case VII. This occurred during an attack of measles at $2\frac{1}{2}$ years and afterwards a corneal scar was found. The peripheral synechiae may have been associated with this attack but probably were the result of intra-uterine inflammation.

Böhm's first three specimens had extensive peripheral anterior synechiae, and the first in addition had a posterior synechia which was almost conclusive evidence of inflammation.

Summary. The absence of peripheral synechiae in early specimens certainly suggests that these lesions do not play a primary part. They do not produce congenital glaucoma. They arise as a secondary development. It is a little difficult to understand how such adhesions can develop once the angle is widely separated and the ciliary body is atrophic and incapable of much congestion. Compare unpublished specimens III and IV (Figs. 95, 96, 98, 99). Adhesions probably usually develop in those eyes that have iris processes. Such formations may be used as a first step in the development of synechiae. It is conceivable that synechiae may form in the absence of an iris process if fibrous tissue binds the iris and the adjacent cornea together after an exudation or haemorrhage.

THE SIGNIFICANCE OF CONGENITAL PUPILLARY SYNECHIAE AND CONGENITAL CORNEAL DEFECTS— ULCUS CORNEAE INTERNUM

In addition to the opacities associated with tears in Descemet's membrane there are two kinds of congenital corneal opacities, those due to faulty development and those which are inflammatory in origin. The former are more common, and Peters described them as being due to defective development of Descemet's membrane and the inner corneal surface. The developmental corneal defects are almost always bilateral and a central corneal opacity of parenchymatous appearance is found with more or less involvement of the endothelium. The opacity may vary in form and intensity, but it will be characterised by its deep and central position. The opacity may be so dense as to be classed as a leucoma and may at first even obscure the tendency to glaucoma. It may be associated with ectasia, and there occur all gradations from a simple leucoma, with or without synechiae, to the advanced forms of congenital staphyloma (see later). Sometimes there is a corneal opacity in one eye and a staphyloma in the other. Of course not all these cases are associated with congenital glaucoma, but it is difficult to draw a sharp line of separation.

The form of hydrophthalmia with a deep anterior chamber and a clear cornea must be separated from that with a shallow or absent anterior chamber and congenital corneal opacities.

Reis wrote: "I have now been able to examine numerous cases of the so-called secondary type (of hydrophthalmia) in very young children: these differ from the pure congenital type with a deep anterior chamber in that they have none or a very shallow one. But they cannot be classed as congenital staphyloma because there is only an internal layer of the iris, on which there is a slightly clouded, globular, but certainly not perforated cornea, and there is also a central, narrow but perfectly rounded pupil. It is clear that owing to continual increase of pressure and the development of ectasia, the original congenital changes may disappear completely. One then finds this picture—a highly distended cornea and an iris, which is bound up with the posterior surface of the cornea. There is no doubt that this is a characteristic case of defective development."

The primary lesion—corneal or lenticular. von Hippel entitled this condition "ulcus corneae internum"—a term not found in current literature. He considered that, as a result of foetal disease, an ulcer of the posterior corneal surface appeared, which produced an iridocyclitis and a sclerosis of the canal of Schlemm. May (1902) traced the origin of the ulcer to a foetal uveitis and Terrien (1907) reported a "healed" internal ulcer of the cornea in an eight-day-old child which he considered due to this cause. He found iridocyclitis without corneal involvement in another child of the same age.

von Hippel's views were modified later, but he still maintained that the initial defect was corneal and that the lens was involved secondarily. Peters (1926) and Wirths (1918), however, strongly opposed this view. They considered that the lens defect was fundamental. They held that a very early defect in differentiation of the mesoderm, which lies between the ectoderm and the lens vesicle, caused the corneal changes, and that a defect in the position of the ectoderm was the primary change. The lens was absent in the specimens of Meisner III (1923), Mohr III (1910), von Hippel IV (1918), Wirths (1918), Schlaefke and others. The chief objection to Peters's theory is the not infrequent absence of any lenticular lesion. Seefelder agreed with von Hippel that the primary cause is a defect in the endothelium of the posterior corneal surface, but he thought it was developmental as a rule, rather than of inflammatory origin. In certain animals (sheep, pig, rabbit) the pupillary membrane develops fully before the endothelium does. In man, cat and possibly dog, the endothelium is present when the pupillary membrane is limited to its marginal parts (Seefelder). Mans (1933), more recently, has written that a congenital weakness of the surface ectoderm is probably the cause.

As these defects probably represent arrested growth at various stages, or an aberration of the mesoblast which intrudes between the surface epithelium and the lens vesicle, a brief résumé of the normal development of this tissue will be made here.

Descemet's endothelium is formed from mesoderm cells, which appear to grow into the tissue that separates the lens and the surface ectoderm. Descemet's membrane is produced by these endothelial cells about the fourth month. The substantia propria is formed from a further ingrowth of mesodermal cells from the region of the edge of the optic cup (Wolff). About the 18·0 mm. stage vacuoles form in this mesoderm, which, coalescing, lead to a split which widens to form the anterior chamber. The posterior part of this ingrowth is vascular. Its central portion forms the pupillary membrane and its peripheral portion unites with the rim of the optic cup to form the iris. The pupillary membrane forms at approximately the same time as Descemet's membrane. Its peripheral portion persists as the superficial stroma lying outside the collarette of the iris. The central portion, however, begins to disappear in the eighth month of intra-uterine life. Remnants of it are frequently found adherent to the collarette (circulus iridis minor).

The iris begins to form about the fourth month. For a time it is hidden by the limbus, as in aniridia. The ectodermal part of the iris appears as a small blunt margin just anterior to the folds of the primitive ciliary processes, at the end of the third month. This margin extends steadily forwards over the anterior surface of the lens and by the eighth month it is practically complete.

Hypoplasia of Descemet's endothelium and of the iris stroma. The part played by the iris in the escape of aqueous from the eye must not be forgotten. Fuchs claimed that tension appeared to remain normal in many eyes with peripheral synechiae of long duration, until the iris became sclerosed. Therefore it is of interest not only to recall Meller's early specimen and certain others with few or absent crypts, but also those cases with an apparent secondary sclerosis and filling of the crypts with pigment and a covering of the surface with hyaline material. Is it possible that aqueous can escape adequately, even though the canal of Schlemm is imperfect, until sclerosis of the iris occurs?

Hypoplasia of a large portion or even the whole of the iris stroma or of its anterior part is uncommon. Such a condition may be associated with lacunae or holes and is falsely called polycoria. It has been described by Axenfeld (1920), Kayser (1922), Gloor (1922), Thier (1921), Thye (1903), Engelbrecht (1908), Rübel (1913), Lindberg (1923) and others.

Such a defect of the iris stroma may be associated with anomalous tissue in the angle, and with a corneal adhesion that may vary from a fine strand to a broad area of union. For example:

Doyne (1921) described a specimen with the following features: (1) absence of the anterior layers of the iris in many places, (2) filling of the angle with a whitish substance, (3) peripheral corneal opacities, (4) strands running from the posterior surface of the sclero-corneal junction to the anterior surface of the iris. Rieger (1935) described such tissue in the angle as "membrana corneoscleralis persistens" and discussed its relationship with various forms of embryotoxon.

Hypoplasia of the iris may be found with glaucoma in adults. Frank-Kamenetzki (1925) found many cases amongst peasants, near Irkutsk, with hypoplasia of the iris and glaucoma that developed in early old age. The relationship is easier to demonstrate in congenital glaucoma.

Central corneal defects with adherent iris. The following ocular lesions of increasing severity have been recognised:

1. Deep central leucoma with superficial iris defect.
2.   ,,   ,,   with anterior synechia.
3.   ,,   ,,   with anterior synechia and lens defect.
4. Types of anterior staphyloma.
5. A type of microphthalmia.

1. Central deep leucoma with superficial defect of the iris.

These might not be recognised as associated lesions but for the fact that they have been found in one eye and a more advanced state with synechia in the other. Seefelder held that the centre of the cornea was its weakest part. Only gradually by the growth of the mesoderm cells from the periphery and later by local proliferation does it attain the thickness of the periphery. A delay or defect in development throws light on the formation of staphyloma and hydrophthalmia and keratoconus.

Waardenberg (1923) operated on both eyes of an infant with porcelain-white congenital corneal opacities, glaucoma and no distension of the anterior segments. The corneal diameter was 11·25 mm. He suggested that there was a very rigid sclera, poor in vessels. Miosis was present and the irides did not bleed after iridectomy.

2. Leucoma with synechia of:

(a) Pupillary membrane (Mohr IV, Seefelder, Ballantyne, 1905, Collins, 1907). The adherent tissue runs from the collarette to the margin of (Reis, Peters), or to the surface of, the defect in Descemet's endothelium (Seefelder). The former state is more frequent. In Collins (1894) and Ballantyne's case the adhesion was to Descemet's membrane, but in Collins (1907) and von Hippel's (1905) there was a larger defect, with union between the substantia propria and the pupillary membrane.

(b) Iris (Peters, Reis, Mohr III).

(c) Sphincter iridis (Reis, Peters, von Hippel's fourth case).

As a result of stretching the muscle fibres ran perpendicularly to the surface of the iris and not in a circle (Reis).

The type of adhesion will depend on the extent of the corneal defect and the stage of regression of the pupillary membrane, etc. The sphincter can only be adherent to the cornea if the pupillary membrane, which separates these structures, has almost completely atrophied. This condition therefore probably arises late in intra-uterine life.

Consideration must be given to the stage in development of the lesion in any specimen. In the early stage, as a result of imbibition of aqueous, the cornea may be very swollen and opaque. Later, when the defect is closed, the corneal lesion may appear much less. The defect in Descemet's membrane may have become healed (von Hippel, Meller). In Mohr's first specimen the synechia had broken down in one eye and was attenuated in the other. Reparative changes also may be found, as in Seefelder's specimen (1920), in which connective tissue had formed from the cornea, and not from the synechiae at all. This new tissue filled the defect in Descemet's endothelium.

3. Leucoma with synechia and lens defects.

In Mohr II an adherent lens with lenticonus was present and in Wirths' I an anterior and posterior polar cataract. In Schlaefke's specimen and Wirths' III the lens was absent.

In others a meshwork of tissue lies near the lens and is connected with the cornea and the ciliary region (Meisner II, Pinkus, Reis, Böhm). In others a mass of tissue is found close to the cornea (Wirths; von Hippel IV, glial tissues; Meisner, ? lenticular derivatives).

Mayou described a typical example of congenital glaucoma, with congenital anterior synechiae (1910). The eye had been removed from a child of seven weeks. The cornea was 14·0 mm., clear, and its only defect was an absence of Descemet's membrane centrally within the area surrounded by its adhesions; the angle was blocked from lack of mesoblastic differentiation. The uveal meshwork and the ciliary muscle were imperfectly formed. There was no canal of Schlemm. There were defects in the lens, the suspensory ligament and the ora serrata and a persistent hyaloid artery. The ring-shaped synechia tends to separate a small circular and central space from the peripheral annular anterior chamber around it.

4. Anterior staphyloma.

The iris may be so widely adherent to the cornea that the anterior chamber does not develop and a staphyloma appears (Reis, Swanzy, Bernheimer and others). An example is Meisner I with cyst-like distension of cornea and slight opacity at anterior pole of lens (Mohr's I was similar in appearance).

In a number of cases a cyst-like space lined by pigmented epithelium (Meisner I, Mohr I, Pinkus) or corneal epithelium (Peters and Wirths) is described. An even more complete arrest of development may produce another type of staphyloma in which the iris stroma is absent (*vide* Collins, 1909).

5. Microphthalmia.

This condition may result if, as a result of complete failure in the formation of Descemet's membrane, the lens and the fibrous tissue of the cornea unite so firmly that the ingrowth of the tissue that should form the iris is prevented (von Hippel's IV, Collins (1902), and Parsons). Though not examined anatomically it appears as if a patient described by Lawson (1905) had the following congenital defects of developmental origin: anterior staphyloma of one eye and corneal opacities and microphthalmia of the other eye.

If Descemet's membrane also fails to develop, the substantia propria of the cornea may be united to the iris stroma and even the pupillary membrane as in Mohr's case IV and Ballantyne's eight-month-old foetus. In this condition there is usually some corneal opacity and the iris and the cornea are adherent, so that hypertension and distension occur. The complete absence of Descemet's membrane and of the uveal meshwork in one globe suggested that in it ulceration was not the cause. It is more likely that the cause was a failure of mesoblastic differentiation or of the "loose postendothelial tissue" (Hagedoorn, 1937). In the extreme cases the tissue lying between the surface epiblast and the lens is converted into a vascularised mass of fibrous tissue instead of into Descemet's membrane and the anterior fibro-vascular sheath. This type was exemplified by the specimen of Marshall (1924). The very atrophic iris was almost completely adherent to the cornea and to an intercalary staphyloma. The anterior chamber was represented by a space 4·0 mm. wide. The lens rudiment was completely enclosed in a fibro-vascular capsule, to which was attached a persistent hyaloid artery. Marshall held that the connection between this sheath and the iris produced an iris bombé and glaucoma. Collins thought the iris had never completely separated from the cornea. Such a type of glaucoma must be due to a defect of earlier origin than that associated with persistent uveal meshwork. Collins stated that the presence of a fibrous congenital cataract and the persistent hyaloid artery implied a gap in the posterior capsule of the lens and therefore an early onset.

THE CAUSES OF CONGENITAL CORNEAL DEFECTS. *Anomaly or inflammation.* There has been much discussion regarding the probable origin of these varying degrees of ocular defect.

Collins, Peters and Meller considered that the majority of such cases were due to defective development. The following associations of staphyloma with other anomalies are of interest: persistent pupillary membrane, microphthalmia (Trattner, 1891), von Hippel's fourth case, dermoid (Bernheimer, Beal), coloboma (Mohr, Chauvel and others), embryotoxon (Peters). Peters considered that the following characteristics supported the developmental theory: the condition is symmetrical and bilateral, and it tends to affect several members of one sibship (Mohr, case IV); it may be associated with other defects in the eye and elsewhere in the body, but not with other diseases in the eye and the body of the child and the mother. He emphasised the absence of inflammatory phenomena in the cases in the literature. The following specimens were almost certainly developmental in origin: Meisner (3 cases), von Hippel (cases III and IV), Seefelder (1 case, 1920), Mohr (case IV, 1910), and Wirths' case.

Mussabeili (1934) held that there was a hypertrophy or giant growth in some of the cases with staphyloma that might obscure the picture.

Peters, Vossius and Seefelder assumed that the common "anlage" of the cornea and pupillary membrane had remained undifferentiated in these cases. Even von Hippel (1905) was inclined to forsake his idea of an "ulcus internum" and agree with this view, though he appears to have considered that both the developmental and the inflammatory explanations may be true.

The inflammatory theory. Nieden (1891) considered that the liquor amnii was the source of the infection, but the evidence in his case was not conclusive (Mohr). Seefelder held that the infection was endogenous. Leber (1898) and von Hippel stated that maternal endometritis could play a part in causing congenital ocular disease. Parsons (1904–5) emphasised the part that inflammation might play in arresting development. He stated that congenital anterior staphyloma was probably the most conclusive proof of the effects of intrauterine inflammation available. Coats (1910) was struck by the strong resemblance between the cases of congenital staphyloma and that which follows perforation in later life (Lawson and Coats, 1906). Coats suggested that in his specimen a corneal ulcer had perforated *in utero*, healed and formed a staphyloma before birth. Mayou agreed with Coats that these cases were due to a prenatal perforation. They held that in the case of congenital synechiae the state was quite different. They considered that in the latter the presence of a clear and not opaque cornea, of imperfect differentiation of the mesoblast of the anterior chamber and the absence of a staphyloma in any proper sense, were proof that the condition was purely developmental in origin and not due to a perforating corneal ulcer. Whilst Parsons expressed similar views he said that inflammation could not be positively excluded, for when it occurred early in intra-uterine life it might leave few or no traces, other than those of interference with normal developmental processes. On the other hand, when inflammation occurred so early as to leave no traces, it might be expected to have much more far-reaching effects than the comparatively slight and localised defects found. Clearing of the substantia propria, however, is not surprising at this period, for the young cornea clears with ease.

One must not apply knowledge of inflammation in adult tissues too rigidly in a consideration of intra-uterine inflammation for, probably, the reaction of embryonic tissues is different in many ways (Hoffman, 1931, 1932). The unvascularised state of these tissues makes actual bacterial invasion improbable, but toxins may reach them by the lymph stream. The avascularity of this area would facilitate their destructive work. There will be a greater tendency to destruction than to the formation of the usual reaction we call inflammation when the infection arises early. In other ways the response of foetal tissues to disease may differ from that commonly seen in the adult, *e.g.* variola (Mann, 1937).

The corneal opacities that are of inflammatory origin are almost always of the interstitial type and are often due to syphilis. There is some support for the view that they are due to exogenous infection from the amniotic fluid. Gonorrhoeal ophthalmia, panophthalmitis and even phthisis bulbi have been known to occur. Some protection is afforded by the fact that the lids are joined together from the third to the end of the sixth month of intra-uterine life. Meisner (1912) reported the association of purulent inflammation with corneal ulceration in two four-day-old guinea-pigs. Such direct evidence of exogenous infection must be very rare. Axenfeld thought that the internal ulcer was probably secondary to a cyclitis. Stock (1902) found corneal changes similar to those described by von Hippel in an eye that had had a typical interstitial keratitis. Gallenga's case (1903) was probably similar. Syphilis was present in cases reported by Reis (1924), von Hippel (1902) and Hosch (1901). Seefelder also described a case of parenchymatous keratitis in a 7-8-month foetus (1924).

Clausen (1922), however, concluded that his specimen of staphyloma had an inflammatory origin, because of the products of inflammation present. Even more definite evidence—the presence of thick infiltration of polymorphonuclear leucocytes—was present in both corneae of a new-born cat with partial staphyloma (Seefelder, 1930). Peters (1926) disagreed with the last two authors' interpretations, holding that the inflammatory processes may have been secondary. Peters considered that the freedom of the mother and the remainder of the litter from any sign of disease was against the inflammatory theory. If, as Seefelder suggested, the infection must have occurred at least fourteen days before birth surely micro-organisms would still have been present. None, however, was found. Neither were inflammatory signs found in the adherent iris, and the anterior corneal surface.

Very little evidence was seen in the shallow anterior chamber. Peters assumed that the ectoderm was unable to form a lens and it covered the centre of the cornea in a defective manner. The corneal tissue responded by granulation. He concluded "that neither in man nor in animals, until now, has a proof, free of pretext, been brought forwards to explain congenital staphyloma on the basis of a purulent or any other type of inflammation".

Even changes such as vascularisation, and a deep opacity with an ability to clear up, cannot be considered as certain proofs of an inflammatory origin, for they are now known to occur with developmental defects as well.

Embryology reveals the fact that if we wish to attribute the corneal opacity to some developmental defect (Peters) we must go back to the earliest stages of embryonic life to find its origin. The anomaly must predate the time for the normal separation of the lens and the cornea. The anterior pole of the lens separates from the posterior surface of the cornea early in the sixth month of intra-uterine life.

On the other hand, could an inflammatory process arising at this time, or even earlier, vanish completely by birth? Seefelder, for example, found no traces of inflammation in his specimen from a four-week-old dog (gestation period nine weeks). He wrote: "It would be unwise to regard a congenital corneal opacity as a developmental anomaly, simply because it became clearer and in the end vanished....I believe that the clearing up of a congenital corneal opacity points to an inflammatory origin" (1906). Mohr considered that the lesion arose in his four specimens after the iris had attained its full development—not earlier than the beginning of the fifth month. In his first specimen defects of the posterior corneal surface and of the iris endothelium were present in one eye. He considered that a synechia had separated as the result of growth and that the synechia present in the other eye would have separated if the child had lived longer.

The occurrence of a corneal opacity of one eye, or of microphthalmia, and a staphyloma of the other, and the association of the latter condition with persistent pupillary membrane, colobomata, etc., suggest that a staphyloma may be developmental in origin (France-schetti, 1930).

The process of corneal perforation. Light has been thrown on the effects of perforation by Elschnig, for in the Freiburg clinic special attention has been paid to the frequent perforation of Descemet's membrane in ulcus serpens, and other forms of purulent keratitis, prior to complete corneal perforation. This form is also accompanied by imbibition.

Elschnig pointed out that this perforation is usually overlooked because it is obscured by more obvious serious signs. It was due to leucocytic digestion and exfoliation. Similarly, when a rupture occurs at birth the other lesions that develop tend to prevent its recognition.

At times Elschnig detected the following signs of perforation: (1) A slight pain concurrent with the clouding of the cornea, (2) a slight stain of blood in the floor of the ulcer. As tension is lowered at the instant of perforation a minute haemorrhage from the iris may occur. As a rule within a few hours or days aqueous escapes because the cornea has perforated. Rarely, however, the corneal tissue in front of the perforation remains intact.

Elschnig held that the corneal imbibition which follows the rupture of Descemet's membrane might produce a clinical picture indistinguishable at the height of the clouding from that described by von Hippel as due to congenital corneal ulceration. Possibly the tendency of the former to clear up and of the latter to persist is an important guide.

Birth injuries. There is a group of corneal opacities that appear to be the result of injury during birth. Thomson and Buchanan (1903) referred to cases reported by Truc, Dujardin, Noyes and de Wecker. They described numerous forms of injury, including corneal opacities which show a definite tendency to clear up. They distinguished three types of opacity.

First, a comparatively frequent and temporary lesion which was probably oedematous in origin.

Secondly, a permanent opacity due to oedema with subsequent inflammatory changes. A variable degree of stripping of the posterior elastic lamina is found.

Thirdly, a rupture of the posterior layers of the cornea with the formation of cicatricial tissue. These authors considered that the rupture in some cases was due to direct pressure upon the eyeball. They were inclined to think these opacities were similar in origin to those that von Hippel classed as "ulcus corneae internum".

Summary. 1. We cannot yet be certain which congenital corneal opacities are due to endogenous infection and which are anomalies. It is very difficult to separate the effects of defective development from intra-uterine inflammation. In the absence of inflammatory signs, particularly if other anomalies, such as coloboma of the iris, are present, one is perhaps justified in excluding inflammation as a direct cause.

2. In this type defective development is not limited to the area round the angle, but its influence is found in the central area of the cornea and in the lens.

3. The insidious manner in which corneal perforation may occur is considered.

4. Injuries at birth may produce a corneal scar not unlike the congenital opacity under discussion.

5. The development of a normal anterior chamber is only possible if there is perfect balance between the varying regressive and constructive processes that concern the surrounding tissues.

CONGENITAL GLAUCOMA IN THE LOWER MAMMALS

In 1904 Lodata described the findings in a hydrophthalmic rabbit's eye. The iris and ciliary muscle were poorly developed, the angle of the anterior chamber was very wide, the trabecular tissue slightly thickened and Schlemm's canal was absent. Infiltration and pigmentation of the deeper corneal layers and particularly of Descemet's membrane were present. Rochon-Duvigneaud (1921, 1925) found signs of arrested development in the angle of a rabbit's hydrophthalmic eye. He considered that the apparent impermeability of the tissues at the angle was the result of arrested development.

In a hydrophthalmic eye of a pig described by Koby (1929) the ciliary body was completely absent and the iris was represented by three segments. One was attached to the cornea except for a small portion centrally, one occupied the periphery of the anterior chamber and the third occupied the normal position of the iris and consisted exclusively of a folded pigmented network. The canal of Schlemm was absent. The other eye of this animal was microphthalmic.

Reganati (1932) described the findings in the eye of a month-old rabbit, with congenital glaucoma. No trace of the canal of Schlemm could be found and even if it had been present its function would have been interfered with by the position of Descemet's membrane, which blocked its entrance. In the eye of a rabbit reported by Alajmo the base of the iris was attached to the cornea and the wide angle which was formed in this manner was full of pigmented tissue little differentiated from that of the iris. Neither uveal meshwork nor canal of Schlemm was found.

One is struck by the absence of reference to signs of inflammation in these reports and by the emphasis each author placed on development defects in the angle.

The following description is of interest. Beckh (1935) reported an adult rabbit which developed unilateral glaucoma with marked ocular distension. This followed 5½ months after a testicular injection which may have led to the development of yaws. Old peripheral anterior synechiae with complete obliteration of the angle and evidences of an old and healed chorio-retinitis were found.

EXPERIMENTAL EVIDENCE OF INTERFERENCE WITH FILTRATION

Leber and Bentzen (1895) by experiment showed that the rate of filtration was slower than normal in a hydrophthalmic eye.

Rochon-Duvigneaud (1921) injected a fluorescein solution into the vein of an ear of a rabbit with bilateral hydrophthalmia. The appearance of the dye in the anterior chamber was prolonged. The angle of the deep anterior chamber was expanded compared with that of a normal rabbit and the ciliary body was almost completely atrophied.

2. INFLAMMATION AS A CAUSE OF HYDROPHTHALMIA

INTRODUCTION

1. The significance of the signs of ocular inflammation.
2.   ,,   ,,   the state of the choroid.
3.   ,,   ,,   lowered resistance of the scleral coat.
4.   ,,   ,,   endophlebitis.
5.   ,,   ,,   the state of the vitreous.
6.   ,,   ,,   the association with general disorders.

The cause of any one congenital abnormality is difficult to ascertain. Parsons wrote: "The logical position to adopt is that of calling in the aid of inflammatory processes only when the conditions are such that simple arrest of development fails to account for them."

In considering inflammation in early embryonic life one must remember that such a process must be modified, firstly, because a fully developed vascular system is not present, and secondly, because it may arise from a placental, uterine, or other maternal focus, being transmitted by way of the blood stream.

We have already drawn attention to Parsons's view that there is conclusive evidence in favour of the intra-uterine inflammatory theory supplied by certain cases of congenital anterior staphyloma. They present the same features as do cases of the corresponding condition in the adult eye. "*A priori*, therefore we should be naturally inclined to attribute them to the same cause."

It appears, therefore, that intra-uterine inflammation is almost certainly the cause of at least some of the cases of congenital staphyloma. The probability of such a cause for one anomaly prepares the way for belief in a similar explanation for kindred conditions, such as the defects found round the angle of the anterior chamber, that concern us here.

THE SIGNIFICANCE OF THE SIGNS OF OCULAR INFLAMMATION

The following forms of inflammation have been held responsible: primary iritis (Venneman), cyclitis, choroiditis (Gallenga, May), and uveitis (Grahamer, Murray, Manz). A vascular sclerosis following choroiditis (Goldzieher) and chronic irido-choroiditis (Kalt) has been suggested, while other authors have deduced an obliteration of the angle following a primary cyclitis (Raab) and an intra-uterine irido-cyclitis producing aniridia (Pflüger). The presence of uveo-sclerotic adhesions has also been referred to (Schiess Gemuseus).

Great difficulty is experienced in interpreting the signs of inflammation that are found in eyes that are obviously hydrophthalmic. These signs may be secondary and in no way associated with the development of the initial disease. Take, for example, specimen IV of Seefelder's series (clinical case 39). The patient was eight years old and so ample time has passed for secondary processes to occur. Seefelder wrote: "Had the disease been unilateral I would have decided in favour of unusually severe inflammation in the anterior segment of the left eye as the primary cause of hydrophthalmia." The complete absence of any clinical evidence of inflammation in the right eye, also hydrophthalmic, made this an unlikely cause.

In many other cases one must discount the influence of inflammation because of previous operative interference with the eye. Seefelder's case VI (clinical case 16) for example had had two operations $6\frac{1}{2}$ years before enucleation.

In others some of the findings may be associated with the sudden death of the child after the anaesthetic.

E. von Hippel, Reis and Seefelder agreed that the absence of anatomically evident traces of inflammation in malformed eyes does not strictly disprove that the anomaly was due to foetal disease. Such traces in early life may be so scanty as to give a very poor idea of the severity of the inflammatory attack. Corneal opacities particularly show this ability to disappear. In one specimen with a congenital corneal opacity of undoubted inflammatory origin the only evidence that could be found of inflammation, nine months after the outbreak of the disease, was a clot of fibrin which extended from the ciliary processes along the posterior surface of the lens. Even this would soon have vanished and no sign then of the inflammatory process would have persisted.

In some cases, however, there appears to be a definite causal relationship. Seefelder's case VII (from Sattler's clinic) is of particular interest, but unfortunately no clinical notes are available. "There is here no doubt that a very severe inflammatory process in the centre of the cornea and the anterior uveal tract had led to the development of the disease", and this in very early life, because the cornea at the time of enucleation was described as being moderately clear even though extensive scars were present. There was a total peripheral anterior synechia, and the widespread pigment infiltration of the sclero-corneal network and of Schlemm's canal suggested that no block existed prior to the formation of the synechia.

The presence of pigment helps us in another way to understand the order of previous events. At times pigment granules are found included in the newly grown glass membrane that has proliferated to cover up a tear in Descemet's membrane. We can assume that the pigment, as is common with an anterior uveitis, adhered during the stage of inflammation to the cornea recently denuded of endothelium by rupture of Descemet's membrane. Such a finding proves rather the early occurrence of inflammation than its causal relationship. Seefelder found it in specimens V and VI (clinical cases 18 and 38). A similar deposit of pigment was found in specimen III and signs of an anterior uveitis were present. The latter, however, were of uncertain value, because an iridectomy had been performed six days before enucleation. Seefelder described an eye of an eight-month-old foetus with kerato-iritis that showed exactly similar signs of inflammation but without glaucoma. The anterior chamber was well formed and so hypertension had not and probably would not have appeared.

It is of interest that in the eyes of one very early case, viz. specimens II and III, aged seven days, Seefelder found no acute inflammatory phenomena but a very high albumen content of the aqueous and
vitreous and numerous polymorphs and traces of fibrin (Figs. 57 to 60).
He considered that simple tearing of Descemet's membrane could not
account for the following corneal changes: marked proliferation of
both the fixed and the wandering corneal cells, thickening of the
cornea, and the incomplete state of the endothelial layer. The changes
in this eye are of great interest, because it is the earliest specimen of
congenital glaucoma to be examined. The evidences of proliferation
in and close to Schlemm's canal in these cases were similar to those
described in this situation by Elschnig in interstitial keratitis (his
Figs. 6 and 8). Though the condition of the anterior chamber in Seefelder's cases was apparently normal a proliferating inflammation in
the region of Schlemm's canal was present. In Fig. 6 the chief lumen was
present but full of spindle cells and in Fig. 8 almost complete obliteration of the whole venous circle was seen. In Seefelder's case 39 tension
remained so low after an iridectomy with a cystoid scar that the
presence of a detachment was feared. After an attack of iridocyclitis
with fibrinous exudate the tension rose and remained high. It was
probably due to the albuminous aqueous and the effects that it had
on the channels of filtration.

Though in each of his seven specimens Seefelder found more or
less certain signs of inflammation he wrote that he was far from
recognising in it the main factor in the pathogenesis of hydrophthalmia.
He considered that both inflammatory processes, and any incident
such as teething that could promote hypersecretion by trigeminal
irritation, could excite hypertension if the usually efficient compensatory mechanism for the excretion of fluid was inadequate.

Lagrange wrote that hydrophthalmic eyes are chronically inflamed
but, as a rule, it is a cellular reaction or an aseptic inflammation
resulting from a developmental defect. "It is because the eye is not
congenitally provided with its excretory apparatus that the irido-
corneal region is irritated and that there are produced the infiltrating
and sclerosing processes which we have found in the ten eyes of which
we made an anatomical examination." He found peripheral anterior
synechia ("soudure de Knies") and signs of sclerosis at the angle,
corneal changes and the following changes in the ciliary body:
(a) invasion of the vascular sheaths with inflammatory cells, chiefly
mononuclear and plasmocytes, (b) dissociation of the muscles of

accommodation with numerous inflammatory elements in the inter-
vening spaces. "These are secondary phenomena due to the imperfect
functioning of an eye with a defective angle of filtration....If one
were present at the beginning of the disease and could make very
early histological examinations, there would be found a primitive
hypersecretion, like that in the essential, simple, true glaucoma which
always begins with a hypersecretion. On the subject of infantile
glaucoma, one might express this opinion, but one cannot prove the
fact, and it must be recognised that all the pathological anatomy is
dominated by the absence of the canal of Schlemm, sclerosis, and the
closing of the filtration angle. The inflammatory phenomena which
are found in such eyes probably result from this obliteration. They
are the consequence of the buphthalmia: they are not the cause"
(Lagrange, 1925).

Goldzieher (1890) upheld the inflammatory theory, and Christel
(1912) and Schlaefke (1913) from their studies considered that infection, probably intra-uterine in origin, produced the obliteration of
the filtration angle.

Magitot (1912) in two of his four specimens found inflammatory
foci in the region of the equator of the globe and an obliterating endophlebitis of the optico-ciliary vessels. It certainly seems that cases
such as those described by Magitot may have been inflammatory in
origin. He considered that the lesions of the posterior ciliary and the
vorticose veins, which he found in young subjects, produced hypertension by venous obstruction (Arlt). Syphilis may have been the
initial cause, for it is prone to attack vessels at an early stage.

von Muralt held that the irido-choroiditis was not primary, for
foetal irido-choroiditis is always associated with synechiae which
lead to pupillary occlusion and visual loss. Lagrange considered
that hypertension would not last so long as it usually does in hydrophthalmia if the underlying cause was irido-choroiditis for "hypotension is the outcome of chronic irido-choroiditis at all ages".

Inflammation appears to have been the primary lesion in Böhm's
first specimen (1914). The ocular defect was noticed the day after
birth. On examination 5½ years later foetal closing of the pupil and
extensive peripheral anterior and posterior synechiae were found.
A severe cyclitis had apparently led to extensive changes. The following
changes were found in Böhm's third case and certainly suggested
the early presence of inflammation: Extensive peripheral anterior
synechia, adhesions of the ciliary processes and the presence of con-

nective tissue. The persistence of part of the hyaloid artery and incomplete development of Descemet's membrane and its endothelium suggested a developmental origin. These corneal changes and the incomplete formation of the anterior chamber made the condition resemble that described by von Hippel as "ulcus corneae internum". Even though incomplete differentiation of the cornea from the iris and the lens would account for the condition, Böhm considered that the inflammatory changes predominated and probably an intrauterine inflammation was primary.

In Böhm's second specimen there were a defective anterior chamber and total peripheral anterior synechiae. He held that if inflammation were the initial influence posterior synechiae would also be present. Peters and Seefelder agreed that one or more anterior synechia may exist as a result of failure of differentiation of the mesoderm. As hypertension and distension develop, the original congenital changes tend to become obscured. This type of hydrophthalmia can easily be distinguished from the other forms by the complete or partial absence of the anterior chamber. If the defect were developmental, it is strange that the lens should have escaped.

In his third specimen posterior as well as anterior synechiae were present and he considered inflammation to be the initial influence.

Takashima (1913) reported the findings in five specimens and the angle was open in only one. In three anterior synechiae and signs of chronic iritis were present and in two of these the canal was obliterated. In a fourth case scarring of the root of the iris and iris atrophy with complete closing of the angle were found. The entire region where the canal usually lies was infiltrated with small cells and pigment in two of these cases. In the remaining case in which the angle was free the canal persisted only as a narrow lumen. In the wide open angle flakes of coagulated albumen and fibrin were found. This region of the canal showed no infiltration but was displaced backwards with the scleral spur—a finding noticed by Seefelder and others. The iris showed signs of a mild chronic inflammation. From these cases it was doubtful whether the peripheral synechiae were due to inflammation of the anterior uveal tract and so the primary cause of the hydrophthalmia, as Raab, Grahamer, May and others held, or due to secondary changes as Reis and others thought. Michelson-Rabinowitsch, Cabannes, Seefelder, Stimmel and Rotter, Takashima, Lagrange and others held that inflammatory changes were secondary.

As a rule when inflammatory changes are evident they are more marked in the posterior than in the anterior uveal tract. Some writers, who considered that inflammation is the main cause of congenital glaucoma, held that if no signs of anterior inflammation were present the meshwork of the pectinate ligament and Schlemm's canal had been damaged and later closed by a sclerosis as a result of inflammatory products carried forwards.

Eleonskaia (1935) removed a blind painful eye from a child aged $3\frac{1}{2}$ years and concluded that an intra-uterine uveitis with secondary changes in the angle had produced the congenital glaucoma.

As is well known glaucoma may be a late result of corneal perforation, particularly if peripheral anterior synechia develops. Obstruction at the angle or hypersecretion of fluid due to dragging on the ciliary region may account for the hypertension. Occasionally it may be trauma that has not produced obvious injury. Worms and Pesme (1925) reported the development of hydrophthalmia as the result of a non-perforating corneal burn. After the burn healed iridocyclitis appeared and the eyeball distended as the tension rose.

Sédan (1925) reported an interesting example of hydrophthalmia developing in a child's eye which was perforated at the age of $3\frac{1}{2}$ years. The iris prolapse was removed immediately, but as iridocyclitis and glaucoma developed a simple sclerotomy was performed nine months later. This operation was effective for sixteen months. At the age of five as the eye had distended and become painful another sclerotomy was done which led to reduction of tension. It was remarkable that the corneal diameter did not increase though the eyeball distended. At the age of six years there were from 4 to 8 D. of myopia present, at $6\frac{1}{4}$ years 12 D., at $6\frac{1}{2}$ years 16 D., and at $7\frac{1}{2}$ years 25 D. Sypkens (1924) described an injured eye that developed an anterior staphyloma and became greatly enlarged. The iris and the cornea formed the staphyloma and the ciliary body was so extended centrally that it appeared like a second iris.

THE SIGNIFICANCE OF THE STATE OF THE CHOROID

Congestion of the choroid. Dürr and Schlegtendal (1889) held the view that pressure of the oblique muscles on the venae vorticosae might produce choroidal congestion and a consequent rise of ocular tension. They also held that endo- and perivascular changes might develop in these veins. Cross, Reis, Seefelder and others failed to find supporting evidence for this theory. Only in Seefelder's case 47 did the exit of the upper vorticose vein and the insertion of the superior oblique muscle appear adjacent. As the other vorticose veins did not show similar relations to the other muscles, and as experimental investigations showed that compression of all the vorticose veins could not produce permanent hypertension, and as the anastomoses with neighbouring veins is so rich, no notice should be taken of such a finding.

Choroidal inflammation and atrophy. Goldzieher (1890) brought forward a theory that choroidal inflammation and its subsequent atrophy was the most frequent cause of hydrophthalmia. There is little support for such a view, for it has been shown that in the early stages the choroid is usually normal but in the late stages atrophy is the usual finding.

Cross, Reis, Seefelder and others failed to find any evidence, even when widespread atrophy was present, that hydrophthalmia could be attributed to such causes. In Seefelder's specimen IV signs of a chronic inflammation of the whole uveal tract were present. The changes were most marked in the anterior part of the tract and the choroid showed little sign of inflammation. Seefelder considered that this was the reverse of what one would find if the choroidal changes were primary. The thinning of the choroid in some cases is not due to atrophy but to the marked distension at an early age.

THE SIGNIFICANCE OF LOWERED RESISTANCE OF THE SCLERAL COAT

Dufour many years ago suggested that a weakness of the zonule of Zinn and of the sclero-corneal ring might permit over-distension of a globe even in the presence of normal tension. The manner in which this occurs is little understood, but syphilis, rickets and scurvy can probably act in this way. It is possible that any maternal infection may influence the developing eye during foetal life. This applies particularly to syphilis partly because of its presence throughout the whole nine months of gestation.

Is it unreasonable to assume that malnutrition, inflammation or even some little understood but inherited defect may so weaken the structure of the sclera and the cornea that they will distend abnormally during early life even though the intra-ocular tension remains normal? Such a conception has been included in the attempts to explain myopia, megalocornea and keratoconus. There is, however, more likelihood of such a diminished resistance playing a part in these diseases than in hydrophthalmia, for, after all, raised tension is at least an essential early feature of this condition. A globe uniformly distended in early life and devoid of signs of hypertension would be a myopic rather than a hydrophthalmic eye. Further examination would reveal the fundus findings associated with high degrees of myopia.

If it be true that an innate scleral weakness exists, a similar defect must exist in the cornea, for in certain early specimens of hydrophthalmia the cornea alone appeared to be distended. "Megalocornea" has been described as the first stage in the development of congenital glaucoma.

The conception of a weak sclera has been supported by evidence of the influence that endocrine disorders may have on the scleral coat. Theoretically one may hold that "the sclero-corneal coat is the skull of the eye and it must suffer under the influence of thyroid or pituitary disorders for the same reasons as the bones do", but clinical evidence of this is very scanty. Occasionally thymus, thyroid or pituitary extracts have been claimed as valuable in the treatment of hydrophthalmia, keratoconus, etc., but one can hope for little from this direction.

If such an explanation is ever applicable it might hold in the specimens of Cabannes and Kalt. In the former the eye was very distended, though the angle was open and the canal of Schlemm clearly visible, and so diminished excretion was a less likely explanation than usual. Kalt's specimen was an example of advanced hydrophthalmia. He considered that hypersecretion and diminished scleral resistance were the causes of distension. Atrophy of the uveal tract and enlarged excretory channels were the main findings.

Congenital glaucoma does not appear to be common in any series of cases of rickets, lymphatism or other deficiency disorders. One doubtful case was reported by Carlotti (1906). The condition according to Lagrange was not one of glaucoma but of ocular rachitis.

One may conclude that if a diminished scleral resistance is a factor in the production of the picture known as hydrophthalmia it can only play a small contributory part.

THE SIGNIFICANCE OF ENDOPHLEBITIS

Magitot held that the lesions found in early hydrophthalmic eyes enabled one to divide the causes of the condition into two groups.

(1) In one group there are at most only slight signs of inflammation. When such signs are present they are in the form of an obliterating endophlebitis of the scleral emissary and the anterior ciliary veins.

If no evidence of inflammation is present one always finds aplasia of the venous system at the angle and absence of Schlemm's canal. These congenital defects, he held, were probably due to an infection or a placental irritation transmitted from the mother. Magitot stated that such anomalous eyes may be associated with extra-ocular disorders such as neurofibromatosis, naevi and the hepatic insufficiency that explains the occasional deaths under anaesthetics that have been reported.

(2) In a larger group there are evidences of inflammation that vary greatly in severity. When slight in severity and extent they are found in the venous system at the angle and the scleral emissary veins. More frequently they affect the retro-ciliary and the choroidal areas. The whole of the uveal tract and the vorticose veins are included in the more advanced cases. The lesions may even be found in the central retinal and the posterior ciliary veins.

In all these cases the lesions are venous and not arterial. Therefore Magitot has the same conception for congenital glaucoma as for the simple senile form. "En un mot, c'est la jeunesse des tissus qui cree l'entite clinique du glaucome infantile."

Magitot considered the following explanations of hypertension inadequate: inflammation of the ciliary nerves leading to increased transudation (de Lapersonne, Abadie and Angelucci and the Italian school), passive hypersecretion of the vorticose veins (Stellwag, Sattler and others) and a secretion from the "ciliary glands".

Remembering that Bartels (1905) showed by experiments that hypertension could result from suppression of either the anterior veins only or the vorticose veins only, Magitot stated that the venous inflammation and consequent obstruction raised the arterial pressure and particularly that in the ciliary arterioles. The effect would be similar to that occurring when hypersecretion of urine follows a rise in renal arterial pressure. "The transudation of fluid, which normally is very slight, is considerably increased. As from the choroid plexus in meningitis, and the renal parenchyma in nephritis, a hyper-production occurs." Guyon has characterised this phenomenon by saying, "a cell secretes the more as the end of its life approaches". "Therefore", wrote Magitot, "it is unnecessary to blame a blockage of the aqueous outflow. Electrolysis of the angle (Erdmann, Parisotti) and cauterisation of the limbus must act simply by destroying venous channels and provoking inflammation. The injection of irritating substances into the anterior chamber may directly diminish the activity of the ciliary cells, and while indeed granular particles, such as Indian ink, etc., collect at the angle this may be due to their density and the centrifuging action of the ocular movements on the anterior segment."

Magitot considered that the initial inflammation must be less severe than in the majority of cases of iridocyclitis, which affects arteries as well as veins and leads to destruction of the ciliary cells and a consequent fall in tension. In congenital glaucoma the inflammation is essentially very chronic and so the production of fluid may continue for a long time. The hypertension is due to increased transudation through the anterior epithelial cells and sometimes an obstruction of one or more of the vorticose veins as well. Magitot supported his belief that the ciliary cells are not destroyed by stating that in hydrophthalmic eyes they appear as if they were living and so capable of secretion.

If then the inflammatory phenomena are not the direct cause of hypertension as Fuchs and Goldzieher held they appear to be at least the provocative cause (Magitot).

Birnbacher and Elschnig examined different eyes of a patient who had died very soon after the first attack of hypertension. Now, Elschnig found Schlemm's canal to be infiltrated with pigment, fusiform and round cells, while Birnbacher described the condition as normal. Bartels observed that it was a matter of interpretation, and that Elschnig must have taken the very slight lesions of the vorticose veins to be artefacts.

Magitot quoted many references to lesions of the vorticose veins in cases of senile glaucoma. He wrote: "As in hydrophthalmia the endo- and periphlebitis seems very rarely to exist without pronounced choroidal inflammation. Here again the lesions appear to be graduated from before backwards."

THE SIGNIFICANCE OF THE STATE
OF THE VITREOUS

Hydrogen ion concentration. From gonioscopy one learns that there is no direct relationship between the extent of peripheral synechiae and the height of the intra-ocular pressure in simple glaucoma. The angle may be open even in absolute glaucoma.

Troncoso found an angle open in 25 % of cases of congestive glaucoma whether acute or chronic and a great tendency for the angle to become closed in the chronic form. The angle was open in 55·8 % of eyes with simple glaucoma but partly or completely closed in six that had had a subacute exacerbation. In 61 % of cases with secondary glaucoma the angle was fully open. It was open in the early cases. Werner found the angle closed or almost so in a small series of congestive glaucoma and open in 73·3 % of eyes with simple glaucoma. Thorburn's findings in a small series agreed closely with the above.

The direct cause of hypertension in chronic adult glaucoma therefore is not the presence of a partial or total peripheral synechia. These are secondary changes, and according to Troncoso show that the disease is progressing and that the oedematous ciliary processes have pushed forward the root of the iris. The canal of Schlemm is fortunately not the only way of escape for fluid; the veins of the iris also play a part. Such a conclusion enables one to accept with greater readiness the experimental findings of Duke-Elder, Friedenwald and others as support for the conceptions of an increased capillary permeability, or an oedema of the vitreous due to an increase in the protein content of ocular fluids, as the local conditions underlying glaucoma.

Duke-Elder, however, stated that the perilental space is filled with a vitreous-like substance. If this undergoes a change similar to that apparently undergone by the vitreous in glaucoma, free transmission of fluid to the anterior chamber may be further restricted.

It is uncertain whether swelling of the turgescible part of the vitreous may play a part in the production of glaucoma. In the first place the necessary alteration in pH is hardly compatible with life, and in the second place the part that swells is simply 0·1 % of the whole vitreous (Cohen, Newell and Killian).

Duke-Elder measured the degree of turgescence of the total protein at various hydrogen ion concentrations. The turgescence reached its maximum at pH 3·5 and there were smaller secondary maximal turgescences near pH 8·0 and pH 9·5. Similar though less marked changes were observed when the vitreous humour was studied in sodium chloride solutions. A slight increase in volume was noticed from pH 6·0 to pH 8·0, which is the range for the normal and the pathological vitreous. Unless some compensatory adjustment occurs in the eye a slight increase in volume could greatly raise the ocular tension (Duke-Elder, 1930).

Little is known concerning the pH value of the vitreous humour at different ages. Nordenson (1921) studied the bovine foetus and found the pH of the vitreous to be low and constant until after birth, when it increased. Salit (1930), using the quinhydrone method, found that the pH of bovine vitreous humour showed the following increase with age: 3 months, pH 7·29; 8 months, pH 7·40; 18 months, pH 7·43; 24 months, pH 7·50.

The question may be asked, could some alteration in the rate at which the pH normally increases produce a swelling of the vitreous that might be the first stage in raising the intra-ocular pressure in hydrophthalmic eyes?

The increase in tension in adult primary glaucoma is probably the result of a fluid retention due to increased capillary permeability or of an increase in the protein content of the ocular fluids.

THE SIGNIFICANCE OF THE ASSOCIATION WITH GENERAL DISORDERS

If we consider Seefelder's cases we find that many of the patients are sickly children who come from families in which various diseases caused a high mortality, and that they belonged to a community in which unsatisfactory hygienic conditions prevailed.

There are probably two ways in which a disease may so affect the eye that its distension is possible:

(1) The first way is by producing a weakness of the cornea and the sclera so that distension is possible even in the absence of hypertension. This has already been considered.

(2) Excessive formation of intra-ocular fluid or some interference with its escape from the eye may also be the result of a general disorder. A vasomotor or sympathetic upset may be one of the ways by which the eye is affected (Fage, 1915).

The influence of syphilis. Syphilis is the best understood and the most common general disease to be associated with congenital glaucoma. While one remembers its far-reaching influence one must be on one's guard against calling all lesions in an affected patient "syphilitic". The relationship may be purely fortuitous, for the incidence of syphilis is high in the communities in which congenital glaucoma is found.

On many occasions in cases unconnected with syphilis the initial photophobia, the steamy and clouded cornea surrounded by a varying degree of injection, has led to the diagnosis of interstitial keratitis. Arnold observed one case for five months and Seefelder watched one for a similar period before other signs of hydrophthalmia were exhibited. Magitot's first case was originally diagnosed as interstitial keratitis. Gros, Haab and Jaensch also referred to this difficulty in diagnosis. As a rule the first sign of corneal involvement is observed later in life in interstitial keratitis than in the case of hydrophthalmia.

Interstitial keratitis as a cause of hydrophthalmia. Collins (1887) wrote regarding interstitial keratitis: "In rare cases where the whole circumference of the cornea is affected and becomes vascular the central portion of it may break down and ulcerate.... The infiltration of the cornea leads to softening and the normal intra-ocular tension may give rise to a local ectasia.... Yielding of the cornea may be so great as to produce a staphyloma" (Collins, 1912). Cross thought that a circumcorneal inflammation such as interstitial keratitis might seal Schlemm's canal and the spaces of Fontana and so prevent filtration at the angle. Schieck (1931) in his series of 707 cases of interstitial keratitis found that 164 were between six and ten years, 173 between eleven and fifteen years, 150 between sixteen and twenty years, and no mention is made of those under five.

Elschnig's work (1906) on an eye with cyclitis due to hereditary syphilis is of interest He found in one eye young connective tissue cells with round or spindle-shaped nuclei, amongst mono- and polymorphonuclear leucocytes in the wall of Schlemm's canal In the other eye the canal was partially filled with spindle-shaped cells and the venous spaces were almost destroyed. Schieck (1931) wrote that in rare cases as the result of hypertension and lowering of the corneal resistance a condition is produced the clinical picture of which is identical with "buphthalmos". Igersheimer reported raised tension in 22 % of cases with interstitial keratitis. Langendorff (1922) reviewed 165 cases of interstitial keratitis in Virchow's clinic from 1907 to 1921 and found 3·6 % with glaucoma. Intercalary staphylomata and keratectasia have been reported as sequelae (Schieck). Ch. Abadie and Morax (1920) preferred antisyphilitic treatment to operation for hydrophthalmia and Terson (1920) stated that syphilis was frequently associated with hydrophthalmia. Abadie held the view that specific chorio-retinitis was always the cause of congenital glaucoma (quoted by Elliot). Zentmayer (1913, 1914) considered that the prevalence of congenital syphilis amongst negro children explained their tendency to hydrophthalmia. The failure of the cornea to clear after operation and its subsequent vascularisation are suggestive signs. Lagrange considered that syphilis was a much more common factor in the development of juvenile and senile glaucoma than of the congenital form of this disease.

Lagrange wrote: "This disease acts on the sympathetic nerves and perhaps provokes hypersecretion by hypersympathicotonia, but most often the specific infection acts by disturbing the formation of the uveal tract, and in particular the angle of filtration. The resulting maldevelopment is initiated by an inflammatory infectious disorder, the chief result of which is an upset of the development of the excretory channels. It is this last fact which dominates all the pathological phenomena which characterise infantile glaucoma.

"We do not think that syphilis is the primary cause of the affection as often as might be believed. Three of our last patients gave an absolutely negative Bordet-Wassermann, and showed no sign of hereditary syphilis. Lieto Vollaro thinks that the aetiology must be looked for sometimes in syphilis, sometimes in tuberculosis, and Louis Dor has written to us that tuberculosis seems to him to have a far greater place in the aetiology than syphilis. Nothing proves that his opinion is not correct. Darier considered tubercle to be the cause of a sclerosing form of interstitial keratitis in a patient who developed hydrophthalmia in one eye."

Ginestous reported a patient with congenital glaucoma, whose father had active tuberculosis. Fracassi (1929) found that the sire of two albino rabbits with hydrophthalmia and coloboma had testicular tuberculosis. That interstitial keratitis may lead to this great ocular distension is shown by Seefelder's cases 42 and 44. Syphilis may have been a factor also in his cases 2 and 21. His case 9 was probably of the same nature, for the corneal opacity was of an inflammatory nature and was associated with an iris which resisted atropine. There was no improvement in the cornea after iridectomy and the disease progressed to complete blindness in both eyes. The history was that of hereditary syphilis and no antisyphilitic treatment was adopted. Gama Pinto's case XI, Scalinci's case I, one of W. Pyle's and two of Angelucci's cases, amongst others in the literature, were probably of the same nature. Mayou (1910, 1918, 1915), Zorab (1920), S. Stephenson (1905), Planchu and Gautier (1910) and Horton Brown (1913) are amongst those who have found inherited syphilis in their cases.

Harlan (1919) reported a case of hydrophthalmia following interstitial keratitis. He performed a cilio-optical neurotomy. Cousin (1920) described a patient aged fifteen years who during an attack of meningitis developed attacks of glaucoma which led to the appearance of bilateral hydrophthalmia. He had obvious signs of inherited syphilis. Bonnet and Paufique (1934) described a patient who when aged seven years had interstitial keratitis and when examined by them twenty years later showed the typical picture of "keratoglobus". Old corneal vessels were present and the Wassermann and Kahn tests were positive. Fuchs stated that the vertical diameter of the cornea may become greater than the horizontal in congenital syphilis. von Hippel (quoted by Seefelder) reported a boy with inherited syphilis who was treated for severe interstitial keratitis and uveitis and a year later, at the age of fourteen years, developed hydrophthalmia.

Goldenberg (1920) reported the history of a child who had had ophthalmia neonatorum and who at the age of six weeks showed corneal bulging. At the age of one year a bilateral leucoma adherens and nystagmus were present. Each globe was greatly enlarged, the tension was raised and the anterior chambers obliterated. An iridotasis was attempted but simply an iridectomy resulted. Such a condition is better described as a staphyloma, for its pathology is entirely different from that of the cases being considered. Perforation played an essential part in the production of the secondary glaucoma.

Early incidence of interstitial keratitis. Igersheimer wrote that interstitial keratitis was rare in the first few years of life. Collins stated that interstitial keratitis might arise as early as $2\frac{1}{2}$ years. Cunningham (1922) analysed a series of 336 cases of interstitial keratitis of which the ages of onset were known. The earliest was two years and eight months and only 3·5 % developed under five years. In Hutchinson's series (1863) one year was given as the age of onset in case 19. Of 231 children with congenital syphilis observed for a period of five years in Leningrad, only one developed interstitial keratitis. The corneal changes appeared at six weeks and the child died soon afterwards (Cherkovsky and Rautenshteyn, 1936). Seefelder (1906), Reis (1907), von Hippel (1908), Meisner (1912) amongst others have reported instances of foetal keratitis. See also section on Central Corneal Defects in Chapter v. In Sydney Stephenson's analysis (1907) the commonest age of onset was between five and ten years. Cunningham (1922) in his combined series of 581 cases found 59 % to be females. This is in marked contrast to the sex incidence in hydrophthalmia.

Parsons described congenital corneal opacities which after birth cleared up from the periphery towards the centre. Though it was not always possible to establish a syphilitic history he thought they were probably examples of interstitial keratitis. The changes were deep-seated, involving the part of the cornea that is related to the uvea.

In inherited syphilis corneal involvement, in contrast with chorioretinitis, appears to be rare in the first few years of life. This may be due partly to the fact that some of the cases are diagnosed simply as hydrophthalmia. In the questionnaire two cases were excluded on the ground that they were almost certainly infantile or congenital interstitial keratitis.

In interstitial keratitis the signs of inflammation may be so widespread that the corneal changes have been considered to be always secondary to a uveitis (Leber and his school) and sometimes so by von Michel and others. von Hippel found in one globe such extensive changes that he regarded the condition as a slight chronic panophthalmitis.

As a rule the corneal infiltration is densest in the deep layers and at times close to the angle of the anterior chamber. This may extend into the meshwork and the iris and the ciliary body.

The endothelium may be normal, thickened or so affected that deep staining with fluorescein may be produced (von Hippel, 1902; Benson, 1902 and others).

To illustrate the manner in which congenital interstitial keratitis can simulate hydrophthalmia due to other causes the following notes are of interest. They relate to two sisters C.P. and M.P. who were aged four and ten months respectively at the first examination. The corneae of each child were quite opaque at birth and no view of the pupil was possible until seven months. No congestion of the eyes was observed by the parents but the pupils of the elder child were small and atropine was used. On examination each cornea was almost opaque, though showing signs of clearing peripherally. The elder child after having mercurial inunctions at intervals for three years, developed some acute cerebral disturbance. Intense headaches, that made her bang her head on the floor, vomiting and diarrhoea appear to have been the most striking symptoms. She lost her ability to walk for eight months and her balance became upset. Pyuria and haematuria were present. The child's teeth became loose. The parents considered that the cause of the condition was mercurial poisoning; while one physician considered the condition was encephalitis lethargica. Another diagnosed meningitis. Now that the child is ten she is very deficient mentally and is quite indifferent to her family and quite incapable of learning. "She is in almost constant motion but no sign of either pyramidal or extra-pyramidal disturbance could be made out, and judging by the grace of her movements her proprioceptive system must be in good order" (Leonard Cox, 1937).

Both children had negative spinal serological tests at the ages of four and ten months. They had previously been given anti-syphilitic treatment. The parents had positive Wassermann reactions at this time, which became negative after treatment with neo-salvarsan. Prior to the birth of these children the mother had had a baby that lived for half an hour and a miscarriage at three and a half months.

The younger child was treated with neo-salvarsan, administered rectally, and iodides. She was not given any mercury. She had no mental upset and though she is handicapped by defective vision is making excellent progress in her education by correspondence.

It has not been possible to measure the corneae of the elder child, but they are exceedingly large and show dense central opacities and so much central apical bulging that they are almost conical. The horizontal diameter of each cornea of the younger child is 15·0 mm. and the vertical diameter is slightly greater. A few faint vessels are seen near the periphery of the cornea. It is difficult at present to estimate their depth. During the six years of observation by the author the corneae, particularly of the younger child, have cleared up greatly. One anticipates that in a few years the recognition of corneal opacities in this child will require a loupe. There is little room for doubt that the condition affecting these children was intra-uterine interstitial keratitis. The opacification at birth, the mode of clearing of the cornea, and the results of the serological tests of the patients and their parents make this highly probable. The difficulty in seeing vessels deep in the cornea suggests that they may clear away more completely when the keratitis arises before birth.

The following was probably a similar case. In a child reported by Marcus Gunn (1898) the corneae were described as "thick blue" at birth, at three weeks as hazy, and at 5½ years as appearing quite clear though careful focal illumination revealed a faint haze. The patient received only mercurial treatment and ung. flav. dil. cum atrop. locally. An eruption of the skin was present one week after birth. Rothan (1926) reported the development of high-grade hydrophthalmia after interstitial keratitis which appeared at the age of fourteen years.

Seefelder after reviewing forty-five cases of hydrophthalmia decided that congenital syphilis played little part in the pathogenesis of the disease. He (1906) examined the eyes of an eight months' foetus with recent kerato-iritis and of one that was seven months old and had keratitis. "Sure proof of foetal inflammation is also very important for the pathogenesis of hydrophthalmus congenitus. With the occurrence of inflammatory processes, filtration disturbances arise much more easily in foetal eyes than in later life, because the angle at this time is still partly or completely filled by the pectinate ligament." Of eleven patients with hydrophthalmia who had a Wassermann test made at the Wilmer Institute none had any stigmata of congenital syphilis. Only one had a positive reaction and even she showed no sign of congenital syphilis (Beckh, 1935).

Syphilis of the parents has often been found and many ophthalmologists have considered this to be the main cause of hydrophthalmia. Santonastaso (1936) reported a patient aged five years whose mother received specific treatment during lactation. Only one eye was affected and on histological examination Schlemm's canal was not found and slight infiltration of the iris and the ciliary body was found with marked endarteritis of all the vessels. de Lapersonne reported twins who were hydrophthalmic and they and their parents had positive Wassermann reactions.

A family reported by Rollet (1931) is of interest. The grandfather had syphilitic iritis and infected his wife. A daughter developed interstitial keratitis, periostitis of the right tibia and synovitis of the left knee. A granddaughter had hydrophthalmia. Santonastaso refers to a family reported by Cuenod and Nataf at a congress at Tunis in March 1934. Of four sons three had severe hydrophthalmia and the first two had positive reactions for syphilis. During the third pregnancy the mother underwent thorough treatment and the child was normal. Satisfied that the cure was complete she stopped all treatment and the fourth child had glaucoma.

Cattaneo's work (1924) on twelve foetuses with inherited syphilis is of interest. The ages varied from seven to nine months and in half he found cellular infiltration and lymphocytes, and in some spirochaetes in the ciliary body and the choroid. Santonastaso thought that the presence of these changes and the absence of alterations in the retina so resembled the state in both recent and old specimens with hydrophthalmia that this was further evidence of the importance of syphilis in producing glaucoma at birth. This author considered that two factors were present in congenital glaucoma. The first was uveal exudation with hypertension and the second was obliteration or arrested development of Schlemm's canal. Both, he thought, were due to a general infection, frequently syphilis, producing a local inflammation. Schlemm's canal and the ciliary vessels are damaged and so the reabsorption of the intra-ocular fluid is impeded.

In the questionnaire papers little reference was made to the influence of syphilis. The mother of one patient had a + + + Wassermann reaction. One other mother had had nine miscarriages.

Though syphilis cannot be considered of importance in the majority of cases with hydrophthalmia yet its importance is obvious in a certain proportion.

3. OTHER THEORIES OF ORIGIN: THE ASSOCIATION WITH NERVOUS AND ENDOCRINE DISORDERS

Hypersecretion as a cause. von Muralt suggested that as a result of irritation of the ciliary nerves hypersecretion appeared and glaucoma followed. Similar views were held, for a time at any rate, by Haab, Horner, Grahamer, Gallenga, Mayerhausen, Kalt and others.

This theory of hypersecretion "is *a priori* improbable on the same grounds which hold good for adult glaucoma" (Parsons).

Angelucci's theory. Angelucci considered that hydrophthalmia was due to an indefinite congenital trophoneurotic disease. He associated it with the following symptoms, which he thought were due to an abnormal vascular condition: tachycardia, irritability with melancholia, angina pectoris, enlarged vessels of face and head, sensations of heat, defective development of teeth and bones, etc.

In support of his theory Angelucci reported three hydrophthalmic brothers whose mother had Basedow's disease. In a child of six with bilateral hydrophthalmia, tachycardia was present—surely a not uncommon finding.

Gallenga, Lodato and several others agreed that all these conditions could be traced to the sympathetic system and that a disorder of this system produced hypersecretion and glaucoma. de Lapersonne (1902) supported these ideas, holding that the structural defects at the angle were secondary and that the origin of the hypertension was vascular or vasomotor.

Hardesky (1934) considered that one case of congenital glaucoma was associated with a hypertrophy of the thymus and that there was a suprarenal deficiency in another. Improvement was claimed after radiation of the thymus and the injection of ephedrine. It has been claimed that syphilis may be indirectly the cause of congenital glaucoma by its effects on one or more of the endocrine glands. Coronat (1913) reported a three year old patient with bilateral hydrophthalmia and severe congenital oedema of the lower limbs. von Imre junior (1922) considered that the tension of a young woman with hydrophthalmia was reduced by the use of ovarian extract. She was strongly sympatheticotonic and had signs of ovarian insufficiency.

Axenfeld, Seefelder, Heine and Reis stated that the above associations were quite inconstant. Schmidt-Rimpler considered that the above-mentioned disturbances might be the exciting factor producing attacks of glaucoma in a structurally defective eye. "The very detailed histories taken in respect of the cases investigated would allow the reader to arrive for himself at the conclusion that the pathogenesis of hydrophthalmia cannot be explained by Angelucci's theory" (Seefelder).

It is certain that irritating disturbances such as the cutting of teeth (Mayerhausen, Bergmeister and others) can lead to acute attacks of glaucoma in structurally defective eyes. These attacks are associated with corneal oedema and other signs of acute glaucoma.

The significance of endocrine disorders in this respect is not understood, but it is likely that they can produce a rise in tension particularly in an eye predisposed to glaucoma.

TWO MAIN TPYES OF HYDROPHTHALMIA

When we examine a series of sections from different specimens two main types of hydrophthalmic eyes appear. One type is characterised by a wide open angle, though frequently it is only apparently open, for closer study reveals the presence of persistent foetal tissue or the absence of Schlemm's canal. This is the type that in the past has been classed as developmental, and certainly its frequent association with other anomalies is further evidence of this origin. One must remember, however, that among the dystrophic influences that may have caused the defect of development inflammation and its effects may have been important.

The second type is characterised by a definitely closed angle. A more or less complete peripheral anterior synechia obstructs the angle. This is the "soudure de Knies" that fills so large a part in the writings of Lagrange and others. If this is a primary lesion it is almost certainly due to iridocyclitis of uterine origin.

It is not surprising that one finds widespread signs of inflammation in the older examples of all types of hydrophthalmia. Not only is such a defective distended organ a site where resistance is lowered and the development of infection facilitated, but the globe becomes so prominent that it is subjected to a lifelong series of injuries with the subsequent appearance of inflammatory signs. It is a surprise, however, when even in the earliest examples of the so-called developmental type we find traces of an almost vanished iridocyclitis. This was Seefelder's finding in specimens II and III, which were removed on the seventh day. These were typical in that the angles showed persistent meshwork (Figs. 57 to 60). Schlemm's canal was posteriorly situated and the iris, ciliary muscle and processes were foetal in type. In addition the following extra-ocular defects were present: cleft palate, enlarged palpebral veins, and micrognathia. Yet the pathologist found remains of an almost vanished iridocyclitis with secondary involvement of the inner corneal surface. Was this the actual cause of the anomalous state of the angle or an exciting cause of hypertension in a defective globe or merely the result of a superadded infection?

The problem of old specimens. A considerable number of reported specimens are too old and disorganised for one to learn anything of value regarding the initial cause. For this reason the following have been excluded—the specimen of Grahamer; Böhm V; Gallenga I, II, III; Dunphy; Jaensch IX; Lagrange V; Wheeler; unpublished specimen V; Zentmayer I, II; Pergens; Christel.

The interpretation of the older specimens is particularly difficult. Three of the main problems are:

1. The investigation of the closed angle in the presence of a peripheral synechia. As a rule no meshwork is found in these. Reis, however, in specimens V and VI described compressed trabeculae and their replacement by connective tissue (Figs. 68, 71).

2. The complete or partial obliteration of Schlemm's canal as a secondary change. In almost all the specimens with peripheral synechiae this canal is closed. In many with persistent uveal meshwork the canal is narrow and situated posteriorly.

3. The disappearance of Descemet's membrane in old specimens with extensive anterior synechiae. This makes it difficult to decide between a primary defect in the posterior layers of the cornea and a secondary degeneration.

The specimens II, III and V of Lagrange showed a thickening at the base of the iris—a chronic hyperplasia, which was without doubt due to secondary inflammation. In his specimen V not only the cornea but also the sclera was thickened. Similar changes were found by Cross in an eye that had been injured (1886, Fig. 13). Marked scleral thickening opposite the iris base is seen also in Fig. 779 (Parsons, *Pathology*, 3, pt. 1). Sclerosed connective tissue surrounded the base of the ciliary processes in another very late case. The probable cause was arrested development, and Lagrange's specimens have therefore been included with those showing persistent uveal meshwork.

In our analysis no reasonable cause for the glaucoma could be found in two specimens. They were:

1. Stimmel and Rotter II. Normal meshwork and canal of Schlemm. A good result was obtained in iridectomy because of the normal angle.

2. Cabannes. It was supposed that a subcutaneous angioma in the temporal region has led to hypertrophy because of hypernutrition. No other lesion was found.

There is little if any gain in clarity if we separate the cases of glaucoma with obvious causes from those that are less understood and call the former secondary and the latter primary. This division is artificial and not founded on fact. A rise in tension must have a cause. Are we justified in separating a very large group and classing them as primary? The immediate causes in them are more obscure than those associated with such conditions as hypoplasia of the iris and the posterior portion of the cornea or a congenital staphyloma. The latter are manifest on clinical examination, but their underlying pathological basis is no better understood than that of the hidden anomalies associated with so-called primary congenital glaucoma. When we consider adult glaucoma the secondary forms are better understood than that which is called primary. How ironical is our use of the term "simple glaucoma" for the latter group!

Therefore let us forsake such artificial divisions and let us consider all forms of congenital glaucoma (or hydrophthalmia) as secondary and equally so. The causes may be grouped as follows:

1. A lack of, or an imperfect development of, Schlemm's canal and its vascular connections.

2. An incomplete retrogression or aberrant development of the meshwork of the angle producing an obstruction to the entrance of this canal.

3. An imperfect development of the mesoblast that forms the iris stroma and the adjacent tissues of the cornea. Absence of crypts. Anterior pupillary synechia and even a staphyloma.

4. A perforation of the cornea with a prolapse of the iris that produces a staphyloma just before birth. It is uncertain whether such a condition ever occurs. It is difficult to draw a line between congenital glaucoma or hydrophthalmia and those staphylomatous eyes that are found to be glaucomatous and distended during the first few years of life. Apart from the central corneal defects and the iridic adhesions they usually show an anomalous state at the angle similar to that found in congenital glaucoma. Therefore these cases can be included in either group. One cannot include, however, those cases of distension that arise from a post-natal perforation even though striking distension occurs, and these cases constitute the great majority of staphylomata.

5. An intra-uterine keratitis or iridocyclitis that may either interfere with normal development or, by producing synechiae, obstruct the circulation of the aqueous, or, as a result of venous inflammation, block the channels of exit for this fluid. Interstitial keratitis arising soon after birth may produce distension with or without glaucoma. The clinical picture resembles congenital glaucoma, and strictly speaking this term is applicable, although the distension and the glaucoma are definitely post-natal.

6. Retinal gliomata and the well-known group of conditions that imitate them, including exudative retinitis or Coats' disease.

7. A variety of lesions such as dislocation of the lens that may be developmental or due to infantile injury. These constitute a very small group.

Fortunately examples of the last four groups are very rare and the value of classification is largely academic.

It is not necessary for the hypertension to have been present at birth for a diagnosis of congenital glaucoma to be made. It is sufficient if at birth there existed so defective a state that the onset of glaucoma was sufficiently early for ocular distension to occur.

The following figures are taken from the analysis at the end of this chapter, where an effort has been made to classify the specimens according to the probable cause of the glaucoma. Schlemm's canal was closed in the great majority. By including any one specimen in a certain group the author does not wish to infer that he considered that the characteristic lesions of the other groups were absent. This is not so and certain specimens, for example Mayou's specimen, could be included almost equally well under either of two groups.

Neither does the author wish to give the impression that signs of inflammation were absent in all these specimens, for they were present in many and particularly the older specimens, and doubtless in a certain proportion they represented the underlying basis of the whole condition.

	Not over 2½ years	Over 2½ and under 11 years	11 years and over	
Number of specimens:	28	39	45	
1. Compact trabeculae or persistent mesh-work	13	18	19	Developmental defects
2. Iris or iris-like tissue adherent to cornea	4	7	6	86 % 69 % 54 %
3. Congenital anterior synechiae	7	2	1	
4. Perforation with iris prolapse	1	0	0	
5. Iridocyclitis	1	0	1	Evidence of inflammation
6. Phlebitis	2	0	0	(probable) omitting
7. Uncertain	0	12	18	"Uncertain"
Peripheral synechiae	2	9	14	25 % 33 % 50 %
Proliferated endo-thelial or hyaline tissue	2	4	8	

The frequency with which the purely developmental lesions are found is less in the older specimens, because inflammatory and degenerative changes have developed and obscured the primary condition.

It is seen that peripheral synechiae appear to play an important part only in the late specimens. Therefore in the vast majority of cases they can be considered as a secondary and not a primary cause of congenital glaucoma. The presence of new connective tissue and hyaline material in a considerable proportion, viz. at least 18 % of specimens over eleven years, is of interest, for very little was found under this age.

If we combine the three series and omit the specimens marked "uncertain" we find that sixty-seven of eighty-two specimens, or 83 %, were associated with abnormal meshwork or an iris process or a united iris and cornea.

Ten of eighty-one specimens, or 12 %, were associated with central corneal synechiae.

If we include the uncertain specimens 25 of 112, or 22 %, were associated with peripheral synechiae and 12 of 112, or 10 %, showed signs of endothelial or hyaline proliferation.

The following specimens are omitted because the ages were not known: Lagrange IX and X (Mawas), Seefelder VII, Fischer (eight specimens). They may be analysed as follows:

Persistent uveal meshwork. Fischer (eight specimens), Lagrange X (possibly).

Peripheral synechiae. Lagrange IX.

Ulcus internum. Seefelder VII.

The following specimens were examined histologically, but either a detailed report was not available or the information in the literature is insufficient to justify their inclusion in the above analysis: Hippel III (forty-seven years). Gallenga IV and V, Schiess Gemuseus I and II, Raab, Haab, Brünhuber, Pflüger, Parkes Weber (1928–29), Hasse (1892), Eleonskaia (1935).

SUMMARY

1. In 86 % of twenty-eight specimens of early hydrophthalmia the cause of the condition was probably the foetal state or the abnormal development of the meshwork of the angle.

2. Failure in the differentiation of certain mesoblastic tissues or a persistence of their foetal form or even an aberration in growth is apparently largely responsible for the four types of lesion already discussed, viz. an absence of Schlemm's canal, persistent meshwork, peripheral synechiae, and congenital corneal opacities associated at times with adhesion to the iris and the lens.

3. Particular importance should be attached to the bundles of equatorial fibres which, by their appearance in man and in the late stages of embryonic life, produce so striking a change in the vicinity

of the angle. Their normal development means a well-developed scleral spur and an adequate canal of Schlemm. They may also determine the type of distension that occurs (see unpublished specimen V). A marked atrophy of the meshwork is essential if the entrance to this canal is to become patent.

4. The frequent association of other ocular anomalies and defects in development elsewhere is further evidence of the part played by errors in growth. It is of interest to note that in each of the eleven cases of neurofibromatosis associated with congenital glaucoma an "iris process" or persistent meshwork was found in the angle.

5. Inflammation as a cause of peripheral anterior synechiae is probably rarely a factor in producing congenital glaucoma. Though signs of inflammation and synechiae are frequently found in late specimens, they are rarely found if specimens are examined under the age of $3\frac{1}{2}$ years.

6. If inflammation is the cause of the developmental defects referred to above, few traces are found even in early specimens. It appears that if one relies on a study of early specimens, there is little evidence of inflammation as the predominant factor in the production of congenital glaucoma. Though little is known of the nature of pre-natal inflammatory processes, it is probable that the relative avascularity of many of the tissues at this time will limit the obvious signs of tissue reaction and that the normal regressive tendency of so many vessels in the anterior parts of the globe will remove some of the remnants of an inflammatory state. Therefore we need not be surprised if a defect in development persists as the only relic of such a state.

7. Inflammation of and around the ciliary veins appears to play an important rôle in rare cases. Its significance is not clearly understood.

8. The relationship between congenital and juvenile glaucoma is intimate and depends mainly on a varying degree of obstruction at the angle. If the whole circumference is not obstructed the onset may be delayed even beyond the time when the cornea and the sclera can respond to hypertension by distending.

SUMMARY OF SPECIMENS OF CONGENITAL GLAUCOMA

The following is an attempt to recognise the initial lesion in twenty-eight early and eighty-four older specimens.

(a) Compact Sclero-Corneal Trabeculae or Persistent Uveal Meshwork

Various types are included here. The condition may be apparently one of arrested development, or a thickening of the meshwork, or a process of iris-like tissue may be present, whilst in others one can merely say "aberrant growth". In all, however, interference with the entrance into Schlemm's canal is probable.

Early specimens:

Seefelder I, II (and III)	Kalt
Meller	Würdemann
Wagenmann ⎫ with neuro-	Spielberg
M. Rabinowitsch ⎬ fibromatosis	Pesme II
(Mayou) ⎭	Manz (?)
Jaensch I (and II)	Kalt (?)
Stimmel and Rotter I (Seefelder	
VIII)	13

Later specimens:

Seefelder IV, V, VI. Reis II, IV,	Cross I, II
VII	Stimmel and Rotter II, III
Unpublished specimen IV, VI	Jaensch III, IV, V, VI
Magitot IV	Dürr and Schlegtendal I, III
Sachsalber (neurofibromatosis)	Römer
Safar	Takashima II
Rumschewitsch	P. Smith I
Panico II, III	Gallenga II, III
Santonastaso	Collins
Lagrange I, II, III, VI, VIII	37

(b) Iris or Iris-like Tissue Adherent to Cornea Peripherally

Early specimens:

Unpublished specimen II (neuro-	Clapp
fibromatosis)	von Hippel II
Wiener	4

Later specimens:

Pesme I	Murakami ⎫
Reis III, V, VI	Schiess Gemuseus III ⎬ Neurofibro-
Dürr and Schlegtendal II (?)	Collins and Batten ⎬ matosis
Böhm I	Snell and Collins ⎬
Lamb	Knight ⎭
Marshall	13

(c) Congenital Anterior Synechiae.
"Ulcus Corneae Internum"

In this group also varied conditions are included. As a rule a central defect in the posterior layers of the cornea is present. This, however, was not so in Marshall's old specimen.

Early specimens:

Cosmettatos	Jones	
Mayou	Meisner I, II, III	
von Hippel I		7

Later specimens:

Schlaefke	Böhm II, III	3

(d) Congenital Corneal Perforation

Juler (?)   1

(e) Iridocyclitis and Peripheral Synechiae

Early specimen:

Cross, M.P.   1

Later specimen:

Byers   1

(f) Phlebitis

Magitot I (and II), III.   2

(g) Uncertain

Takashima I, III, IV, V	Dürr and Schlegtendal IV	
Zentmayer I, II	Lagrange IV, V and VII	
Pergens	Grahamer	
Böhm IV, V, VII	Jaensch VII, VIII, IX	
Unpublished specimen I, III, V	Christel	
Seeligsohn	Dunphy ⎫	
Seidel	Cabannes ⎬ (Naevus)	
Oguchi	Stoewer ⎪	
Wheeler (neurofibromatosis)	Love ⎭	30

$$\overline{112}$$

REFERENCES

Developmental Theory

Significance of Ocular Anomalies

1920 Terson, M. A. *Soc. d'Ophtal. de Paris,* Feb. 21.
1925 Terson, M. A. *Bull. et Mém. Soc. franç. d'Ophtal.* **38**, 220.
1934 Pesme, P. *Arch. d'Ophtal.* **51**, 524.

Significance of Persistent and Aberrant Mesoblastic Tissue

1876 Raab. *Klin. Monatsbl. f. Augenheilk.* **14.**
1889 Horner, P. *Gerhart's Handb. der Kinderkrankheiten.*
1905 Reis, W. *Arch. f. Ophthal.* **60,** 1, Figs. 3–7.
1910 Seefelder, R. *Ber. d. deutsch. Ophthal. Gesell. Heidelberg,* **26,** 308.

Significance of the Meshwork

1891 Cross, F. R. *Trans. Ophthal. Soc. U.K.* **11,** 231.
1893 Collins, E. T. *Trans. Ophthal. Soc. U.K.* **13,** 114.
1896 Cross, F. R. *Trans. Ophthal. Soc. U.K.* **16,** 340, Figs. 11–13.
1900 Hopf. Inaug. Dissert. Jena. Quoted by Seefelder.
1907 van Duyse. *Arch. d'Ophtal.* **27,** 1.
1908 Engelbrecht, K. *Arch. f. Augenheilk.* **61,** 390.
1909 Seefelder, R. *Arch. f. Ophthal.* **70,** 65.
1920 Axenfeld, Th. *Ber. d. deutsch. Ophthal. Gesell. Heidelberg,* **38,** 301.
1921 Clausen, W. *Versamml. Augenärzte Sachsen und Thüringen.* Abst. *Klin. Monatsbl. f. Augenheilk.* **67,** 116.
1921 Holm, E. *Klin. Monatsbl. f. Augenheilk.* **66,** 730.
1923 Velhagen, K. *Münchener Med. Wochenschr.* **70.**
1924 Vogt, A. *Klin. Monatsbl. f. Augenheilk.* **72,** 244.
1926 Mann, Ida. *Proc. Roy. Soc. Med.* Sect. on Ophthal. **3,** 51.
1934 Rieger, H. *Wien. Klin. Wochenschr.* **155.**

Significance of Iris Processes

1893 Collins, E. T. *Trans. Ophthal. Soc. U.K.* **13,** 128, Figs. 1 and 5, Plate V.
1901 Fisher, J. H. *Trans. Ophthal. Soc. U.K.* **21,** 166.
1911 Thomson, A. *The Ophthalmoscope,* **11,** 472.
1926 Mann, Ida. *Proc. Roy. Soc. Med.* Sect. on Ophthal. **3,** 51.

Significance of Peripheral Anterior Synechiae

1905 Parsons, J. H. *Pathology of the Eye,* **3,** 1, p. 791. *Graefe-Saemisch Handb.* pt. 11, chs. 7, 8, 9, Sect. VII.

The Significance of Congenital Pupillary Synechia and Corneal Defects

1891 Nieden, A. *Klin. Monatsbl. f. Augenheilk.* **29,** 353.
1891 Trattner, A. *Klin. Monatsbl. f. Augenheilk.* **29,** 331.
1894 Collins, E. T. *Lancet,* **2,** 1463.
1898 Leber, Th. *Arch. f. Ophthal.* **48,** 193.
1901 Hosch. *Arch. f. Ophthal.* **52,** 490.
1902 May, C. H. *Berliner Ophthal. Gesell.* May. Quoted by Reis.
1902 Stock, W. *Ber. d. deutsch. Ophthal. Gesell. Heidelberg,* **20.** Quoted by Reis.
1902 von Hippel, E. *Arch. f. Ophthal.* **54,** 509.
1902 Collins, E. T. *Trans. Ophthal. Soc. U.K.* **22,** 148.
1903 Thye, A. *Klin. Monatsbl. f. Augenheilk.* **41,** 374.
1903 Gallenga, R. *Arch. di Ophthal.* **2.** Quoted by Reis.
1903 Thomson and Buchanan. *Trans. Ophthal. Soc. U.K.* **23,** 299.

1904–5 PARSONS, J. H. *Pathology of the Eye*, 3, pt. I. London: Hodder and Stoughton.

1905 BALLANTYNE, A. J. *Trans. Ophthal. Soc. U.K.* 25, 319.

1905 LAWSON, A. *Trans. Ophthal. Soc. U.K.* 25, 314.

1905 VON HIPPEL, E. *Arch. f. Ophthal.* 60, 3, p. 444.

1906 LAWSON and COATS. *Trans. Ophthal. Soc. U.K.* 26, 36.

1906 SEEFELDER, R. *Arch. f. Ophthal.* 64, 231.

1907 COLLINS, E. T. *Trans. Ophthal. Soc. U.K.* 27, 203.

1907 TERRIEN, F. *Arch. d'Ophtal.* 22, 329.

1908 ENGELBRECHT, K. *Arch. f. Augenheilk.* 61, 390.

1909 COLLINS, E. T. *Trans. Ophthal. Soc. U.K.* 29, 169.

1910 MOHR, TH. *Klin. Monatsbl. f. Augenheilk.* 48, 157 and 338.

1910 MAYOU, M. S. *Trans. Ophthal. Soc. U.K.* 30, 128.

1910 COATS, G. *Trans. Ophthal. Soc. U.K.* 30, 128.

1912 MEISNER, M. *Arch. vergl. Ophthal.* 3, Nr. 9. Quoted by Seefelder, *Kurzes Handb. der Ophthal.* 1, 591.

1913 RÜBEL, E. *Klin. Monatsbl. f. Augenheilk.* 51, 1, p. 855.

1918 VON HIPPEL, E. *Arch. f. Ophthal.* 95, 2, p. 307.

1918 WIRTHS, M. *Klin. Monatsbl. f. Augenheilk.* 61, 625.

1920 SEEFELDER, R. *Klin. Monatsbl. f. Augenheilk.* 65, 539.

1920 AXENFELD, TH. *Ber. d. deutsch. Ophthal. Gesell. Heidelberg*, 38, 301.

1921 DOYNE, P. G. *Proc. Roy. Soc. Med.* Sect. on Ophthal. Nov. 11

1921 THIER, A. *Arch. f. Augenheilk.* 89, 137.

1922 CLAUSEN, W. *Arch. f. Augenheilk.* 91, 198. Quoted by Reis.

1922 GLOOR, A. *Klin. Monatsbl. f. Augenheilk.* 69, 126.

1922 KAYSER, B. *Klin. Monatsbl. f. Augenheilk.* 68, 82.

1923 MEISNER, M. *Arch. f. Ophthal.* 112, 3–4, p. 434.

1923 WAARDENBERG, P. J. *Amer. Jl. Ophthal.* 6, 142.

1923 LINDBERG, J. G. *Klin. Monatsbl. f. Augenheilk.* 70.

1924 MARSHALL, J. *Trans. Ophthal. Soc. U.K.* 44, 176.

1924 REIS, W. *Arch. f. Ophthal.* 113, 237.

1924 SEEFELDER, R. *Wien. Klin. Wochenschr.* 37, 39.

1925 FRANK-KAMENETZKI. *Klin. Monatsbl. f. Augenheilk.* 74, 133.

1926 PETERS, A. *Klin. Monatsbl. f. Augenheilk.* 76, 803.

1930 SEEFELDER, R. *Kurzes Handb. der Ophthal.* 1, 591.

1930 FRANCESCHETTI, A. *Kurzes Handb. der Ophthal.* 1, 733.

1931 HOFFMAN, R. *Arch. f. Augenheilk.* 105, 162. Abst. *Klin. Monatsbl. f. Augenheilk.* 1932, 88, 871.

1933 MANS, R. *Arch. f. Ophthal.* 129, 180.

1934 MUSSABEILI, U. *Klin. Monatsbl. f. Augenheilk.* 92, 827.

1935 RIEGER, H. *Arch. f. Ophthal.* 133, 608.

1937 HAGEDOORN, A. *Arch. of Ophthal.* 17, 223.

1937 MANN, IDA. *Developmental Abnormalities of the Eye.* Cambridge, p. 18.

CONGENITAL GLAUCOMA IN LOWER MAMMALS AND EXPERIMENTAL EVIDENCE OF INTERFERENCE WITH FILTRATION

1895 LEBER and BENTZEN. *Arch. f. Ophthal.* 41, 3.

1904 LODATA, G. *Arch. di Ottal.* 11. Quoted by Lagrange.

1921 ROCHON-DUVIGNEAUD, A. *Ann. d'Ocul.* 158, 401. Abst. *Ophthal. Lit.* 1922, p. 230.

1925 ROCHON-DUVIGNEAUD, A. *Bull. et Mém. Soc. franç. d'Ophtal.* **38**, 220.
1929 KOBY, F. *Ann. d'Ocul.* **165**, 200. Abst. *Klin. Monatsbl. f. Augenheilk.* **82**, 719.
1932 REGANATI, F. *Boll. d'Ocul.* **11**, 475.
1935 BECKH, W. *Amer. Jl. Ophthal.* **18**, 1141.

INFLAMMATORY THEORY

1889 DÜRR and SCHLEGTENDAL. *Arch. f. Ophthal.* **35**, 2, p. 88.
1890 GOLDZIEHER. "Hydrophthalmus", *Eulenburg's Realencyclopädie der ges. Heilkunde.* Vienna. Quoted by Schmidt-Rimpler, *Graefe-Saemisch Handb.*
1905 BARTELS, W. *Zeitschr. f. Augenheilk.* pp. 105 and 480.
1906 ELSCHNIG, A. *Arch. f. Ophthal.* **62**, 481.
1906 CARLOTTI, J. *Soc. d'Ophtal. de Paris*, Oct.
1912 CHRISTEL, P. *Arch. f. Augenheilk.* **71**, 247.
1913 SCHLAEFKE, W. *Arch. f. Ophthal.* **86**, 106.
1913 TAKASHIMA, S. *Klin. Monatsbl. f. Augenheilk.* **51**, 2, p. 187.
1914 BÖHM, K. *Klin. Monatsbl. f. Augenheilk.* **52**, 831.
1921 NORDENSON, J. W. *Upsala Lärkaref Förhandle.* **26**, 1. Ref. Krause, *Biochemistry of the Eye*. Baltimore: Johns Hopkins Press, 1934.
1924 SYPKENS. *Amer. Jl. Ophthal.* **7**, 957.
1925 SÉDAN, J. *Soc. d'Ophtal. de Paris*, p. 55.
1925 WORMS and PESME. *Soc. d'Ophtal. de Paris*, p. 81.
1925 LAGRANGE, F. *Bull. et Mém. Soc. franç. d'Ophtal.* **38**, 1.
1930 DUKE-ELDER, S. "The Nature of the Vitreous Body", *Brit. Jl. Ophthal.* Monograph Series, **4**.
1930 SALIT, P. W. *Biochemical Jl.* **24**, 596.
1935 ELEONSKAIA, B. *Sov. Viest. Ophthal.* **6**, 3, p. 330. Abst. *Amer. Jl. Ophthal.* **18**, 875.

THE SIGNIFICANCE OF THE ASSOCIATION
WITH GENERAL DISORDERS

1863 HUTCHINSON, J. *Syphilitic Diseases of the Eye and Ear*. London: Churchill.
1887 COLLINS, E. T. *Roy. Lond. Ophthal. Hosp. Reps.* **11**, 338.
1898 GUNN, M. *Trans. Ophthal. Soc. U.K.* **18**, 185.
1902 BENSON, A. H. *Ophthal. Review*, p. 121. Quoted by Schmidt-Rimpler.
1902 VON HIPPEL, E. *Arch. f. Ophthal.* **54**, 3.
1905 STEPHENSON, S. *Brit. Jl. of Children's Diseases.*
1906 SEEFELDER, R. *Arch. f. Ophthal.* **64**, 231.
1906 ELSCHNIG, A. *Arch. f. Ophthal.* **62**, 481.
1907 STEPHENSON, S. *Med. Press and Circ. Lond.* **84**, 648.
1907 REIS, W. *Arch. f. Ophthal.* **66**, 201.
1908 VON HIPPEL, E. *Arch. f. Ophthal.* **68**, 354.
1910 PLANCHU and GAUTIER. *Recueil d'Ophtal.* **32**, 220.
1910 MAYOU, M. S. *Trans. Ophthal. Soc. U.K.* **30**, 120.
1912 COLLINS, E. T. Pyle's *Internal System of Ophthal. Practice*, p. 419. Philadelphia: Blakiston.
1912 MEISNER, M. *Arch. vergl. Ophthal.* **3**, 11.

1913 HORTON BROWN. *Amer. Jl. Ophthal.* **30**, 20.

1913 ZENTMAYER, W. *Jl. Amer. Med. Ass.* Sect. on Ophthal. p. 140.

1914 ZENTMAYER, W. *Ophthal. Year Book*, **11**, 202, and *Ophthal. Record*, **22**, 25.

1915 MAYOU, M. S. *Proc. Roy. Soc. Med.* Sect. on Ophthal. April, **9**, 104.

1915 FAGE. *Arch. d'Ophtal.* **34**, 574.

1918 MAYOU, M. S. *Trans. Ophthal. Soc. U.K.* **38**, 146.

1919 HARLAN, H. *Amer. Jl. Ophthal.* **2**, 288.

1920 ABADIE and MORAX. *Arch. d'Ophtal.* May, p. 315.

1920 COUSIN, G. *Arch. d'Ophtal.* May, p. 313.

1920 GOLDENBERG, M. *Amer. Jl. Ophthal.* **3**, 140.

1920 TERSON, A. *Arch. d'Ophtal.* May, p. 315.

1920 ZORAB, A. *Trans. Ophthal. Soc. U.K.* **40**, 319.

1922 CUNNINGHAM, J. F. *Trans. Ophthal. Soc. U.K.* **42**, 44.

1922 LANGENDORFF, F. J. *Deutsch. Med. Wochenschr.* **48**, 490.

1924 CATTANEO, D. *Ann. d' Oftalm. e Clin. Ocul.* fas. VI. Quoted by Santonastaso.

1925 MORGAN, J. A. *Amer. Jl. Ophthal.* **8**, 813.

1926 ROTHAN. *Klin. Monatsbl. f. Augenheilk.* **77**, 237.

1929 FRACASSI, G. *XIII Cong. Internat. Ophthal. Amsterdam.* Quoted by Santonastaso.

1931 ROLLET. *Soc. d'Ophtal. de Lyon.* 13 gennaio. Quoted by Santonastaso.

1931 SCHIECK, F. *Kurzes Handb. der Ophthal.* **4**, 1, pp. 241, 302 and 314.

1934 BONNET and PAUFIQUE. *Bull. Soc. d'Ophtal. de Paris*, March, p. 232.

1935 BECKH, W. *Amer. Jl. Ophthal.* **18**, 1129.

1936 CHERKOVSKY, V. V. and RAUTENSHTEYN, E. I. *Sovet. Vestn. Oftal.* **7**, 289. Abst. *Arch. of Ophthal.* May, p. 932.

1936 SANTONASTASO, A. *Ann. di Ottal. e Clin. Ocul.* **64**, 405 and 437.

ASSOCIATION WITH NERVOUS AND ENDOCRINE DISORDERS

1902 DE LAPERSONNE, F. *Arch. d'Ophtal.* **22**, 565.

1913 CORONAT. *La Clin. Ophtal.* **19**, 85. Abst. *Klin. Monatsbl. f. Augenheilk.* **51**, 1, p. 545.

1922 VON IMRE, Jr. *Klin. Monatsbl. f. Augenheilk.* **68**, 652.

1934 HARDESKY, J. F. *Amer. Jl. Ophthal.* **17**, 689.

TWO MAIN TYPES OF HYDROPHTHALMIA

1892 HAASE. Inaug. Dissert. Strassburg. Quoted by Reis.

1929 WEBER, PARKES. *Proc. Roy. Soc. Med.* Neurol. Sect. **22**, 25.

1935 ELEONSKAIA, B. *Sovet. Vestn. Oftal.* Quoted by Santonastaso.

CHAPTER VI

TREATMENT

HISTORY OF TREATMENT

Soon after the first recognition of hydrophthalmia we find descriptions of the manner in which the early surgeons endeavoured to diminish the quantity of fluid in the eye. Boerhaave in 1749 advised, in addition to purgatives and mercurial hydragogues, a puncturing of the eye at the side of the lens from time to time until the eye recovered its normal size. Maitre-Jan (1740) proposed an anterior scleral incision in the external angle of the eye.

Pellier de Quengay (1789) wrote that if diuretics and hydrogogues failed one should not hesitate to puncture the eye. Amongst his good results one reads in his book of a certain "Ferrien of Cette, who after several punctures of the anterior chamber, the use of diuretics, and fondants and ophthalmic opiates, cured a buphthalmia so marked that the cornea was opaque and the globe of the eye so large that the lids could not cover it".

Though Gleize (1786) preferred local medication, finding operation difficult and insufficient, he reported the facts that Guerin and Woolhouse advised scleral puncture and that Mr Toubervil, an English oculist, also performed this operation and considered it capable of lessening the size of the eye and preventing cataract.

A thesis by Grellois (1836) summarised the treatment in use at the time. He reviews the advantage of anti-herpetic, anti-syphilitic and anti-scrophulous methods, recommending blisters to the forehead "sétons à la nuge", compresses of lead acetate, and the application to the globe of hot sachets of dry aromatic plants. He recalled the fact that the surgeons who compressed the globe were using a procedure already employed by Rhazes.

In *Annales d'oculistiques*, March 1841, we read: "M. O'Beirne, the clever Irish surgeon, who has published a work on the treatment of hydrophthalmia, thinks that in the majority of cases this disease may be cured without operation. According to him, the trouble is usually connected with a rheumatic diathesis, and may fortunately be dissipated with the aid of calomel, repeated until there is salivation. He reports a serious case which he cured in this way, and refers to

several others. Here is a new clinical history which supports this
assertion. A little girl, aged nine, cachetic, and suffering from measles;
during convalescence, she was exposed to cold; ophthalmia appeared
with chronic keratitis, and progressive hydrophthalmia. The two
eyes were no longer covered by the lids, the corneae were globular
in shape, the anterior chambers were three times their normal size.
Pupils, large, irregular, iris pushed backwards in an astonishing way.
Globes hard to the touch, immovable, myopic vision, but apparently
poor. Mercurial friction around orbit. Internally, sodium sulphate,
calomel and opium, blisters to the arm. Cured in the space of $1\frac{1}{2}$
months, vision clear and stronger, globes normal dimensions."

Rognetta (1844) enumerated the different surgical procedures advisable, in hydrophthalmia, after medical treatment: 1. Paracentesis,
agitating the canula if one wished to induce adhesive inflammation.
2. Injection of alcohol as into a hydrocele. 3. "Decreasing seton",
composed of several threads which are successively withdrawn.
4. A pad of wool left for several days on the eye. 5. Amputation of
the anterior hemisphere of the eye.

As an instance of dangerous treatment based on a faulty analogy
we find Chavanne (1855) stating that hydropsy of the eye was
comparable with a hydrocele and therefore injections of iodine were
indicated. The author described a good result obtained by Bonnet.
Five months after the treatment the eye was greatly diminished in
size, all traces of inflammation had disappeared and the globe
deprived of its substance and its vitality was nothing but "un informe
moignon" (Lagrange). What better example could one have of the
evils of therapy based on an attempt to interpret one morbid entity
by a study of an apparently analogous condition elsewhere? The
fact that the result was described as good also makes one cautious
in weighing the results of treatment from certain sources.

MEDICAL TREATMENT

As has been seen medical treatment was adopted in the earliest
days. More recently it was used with greater zest when men like
Abadie, Foulcher, Carlotti, Toulant and Worms stated that syphilis
was the main cause of the disease. Von Muralt Arnold, Schmidt-
Rimpler, Zentmayer, Casimatis and others held that this was not the
case, and Lagrange and many others adopted an intermediate attitude
and considered that it was apparently the main factor in a percentage
of patients.

In 1907 Abadie showed four patients who had been greatly improved by intravenous injection of arsenic and mercurial injections. One was a man who had had repeated sclerotomies and paracenteses without avail. In 1920 the same author reported another patient who possessed good vision eleven years after treatment.

Onfray and Plicque (1924) described a three-week-old child with strongly positive Wassermann and Hecht reactions. Spontaneous perforations of each eye developed on several occasions, but did not recur after novarsenobillon therapy.

Carlotti (1906), Roche and Fradkine (quoted by Lagrange) have claimed benefit from such treatment, and the last named used extracts of various endocrine glands in addition.

Lagrange wrote: "There is no doubt that specific treatment has its successes and when the syphilitic aetiology is obvious it should be employed; we even think it a good idea to use it when the aetiology is doubtful." He advised intravenous injections into a temporal branch of the epicranial veins in very young children when possible. Otherwise he advocated subcutaneous injections of sulfarsenal. In addition he used iodides and mercury in one of its various forms. He referred to the use of arseno-benzol suppositories in children under two years (see Lesné's report, 1924).

The other forms of medical treatment advocated depended on a desire to improve the general condition of the child and to treat the obvious disorders that are occasionally present, such as rickets or tuberculosis.

USE OF MIOTICS

When we remember the state of Schlemm's canal in the average specimen with hydrophthalmia we are not very hopeful of miotic treatment relieving the raised tension. Many oculists, however, have considered that the operative risks are so great and the results so poor that they have relied simply on miotics and medical treatment. Saemisch and Panas were amongst these. Wolff obtained gratifying results in five of nine patients by the use of miotics, but he considered that, owing to the transient nature of the improvement, miotics should be kept for patients who refused operation. Uhthoff after treating twenty-three patients, aged three to eleven years, without lasting success, arrived at the same conclusion. Seefelder wrote that after prolonged study of the use of miotics he and Sattler were convinced of their inadequacy, though a trial of them in addition to operation was worth while. Schmidt-Rimpler held the view that miotics were of value, and that in advanced bilateral cases it was wise to operate only on one eye and to rely on miotics for the treatment of its fellow. Jaensch concluded that purely medical treatment failed in hydrophthalmia. He injected adrenalin subconjunctivally in a three-year-old patient without success.

The majority of authors appear to have some faith in the value of eserine and pilocarpine. Naturally their belief varies with their conception of the underlying basis of the disorder. Those who hold that hypersecretion from "hypersympatheticotonia" is the main cause are more inclined to rely on miotics than those who consider that the great majority of cases are due to developmental defects. Lagrange held that even the latter could benefit from the use of miotics, as do old cases of chronic glaucoma with obstruction of the angle.

"Miotics are tension reducing; there is no doubt of it, and one should not fail to use this precious property against infantile glaucoma" (Lagrange).

There may still be uncertainty as to the exact manner in which miotics lower tension, but clinicians are satisfied that "the fall in tension coincides with the miosis and that the glaucomatous phenomena are accentuated when the pupil does not react to miotics".

The very interesting work of Asayama (1901), on the anatomy of the pectinate ligament, supports the ideas of Schnabel.

In the photographs of monkeys' eyes, taken by Heine to demonstrate the anatomical conditions in accommodation, the atropinised eye shows the meshwork in a collapsed condition, while in the eserinised eye they are wide open, giving easy access to the canal of Schlemm. This throws light on the related favourable action of efforts at accommodation in glaucoma, and helps to explain the effects of eserine. The traction of the ciliary muscle on the meshwork at the angle dilates the lacunae and the spaces it encloses. Fortin more recently has demonstrated the manner in which the ciliary muscle is found to have opened out the lumen of the canal of Schlemm in an eserinised eye rapidly fixed after excision.

These experimental facts seem indisputable, and favour the theory that eserine frees the angle. But may one affirm that this alone is sufficient to explain the action of miotics on ocular tension?

At the beginning of glaucoma, during the prodromal attacks, the lesions hindering excretion are not yet established, and mechanical freeing of the angle is perhaps not sufficient to explain the action of miotics. This is what many authors have thought, and, as we have seen above, they have called in an action of eserine on the intra-ocular vasomotor and secretory systems.

Recent work on the physio-pathology of the sympathetic system has thrown a little light on the indisputable vasomotor rôle of the vegetative system in the course of a glaucoma attack, and on the action of miotics.

Without giving a satisfactory explanation, they contain novel elements representing signposts on the road which will lead to the final solution of the question. According to these ideas, the sympathetic innervation of the eye is governed by two systems with antagonistic functions: the ortho-sympathetic and the para-sympathetic, if one adopts the terminology of Laignel-Lavastine. The action of mydriatics and miotics on these two systems is of great importance: pilocarpine excites the para-sympathetic and the vagal system, of which it is the homologue. Miotics by exciting the vagal system combat the sympatheticotonia which is at the base of intra-ocular hypersecretion. Lagrange wrote: "If we take the most recent work, such as that of Laignel-Lavastine for our guide, we are asked to admit that the mode of action of miotics and mydriatics, which are sometimes vaso-dilators and sometimes constrictors, is governed by the former condition of the patient." We will summarise the modes of action of miotics in infantile glaucoma in the following way:

1. By causing miosis, the angle may be freed.

2. The absorptive power of the iris is augmented by an increase in its surface.

3. By enlarging the diameter of the iris vessels, their capacity increases and so the ciliary vessels may discharge into them their superfluity of blood; this compensatory anaemia may reduce the secretion of aqueous.

4. Perhaps also the dilated vessels of the iris may compress the ciliary body and thus reduce the secretion.

If there are other actions they are still very much under discussion. Each fact is contradicted by another of equal importance. "We must wait till new proved facts can be added to those we have just discussed" (Lagrange).

Duke-Elder (1934) summarised the actions of eserine as follows:

1. It diminishes the blood supply to the anterior portion of the uveal tract by constricting the anterior ciliary arteries as they travel through the muscle belly.

2. It tends to open up the choroidal veins, and

3. It opens up the trabeculae of the angle and the canal of Schlemm by traction on the scleral spur.

If the last were its only action one would not expect any help in those cases of congenital glaucoma with an undifferentiated angle, but its other influences may enable eserine to be of value in these cases.

Results of miotic therapy. There are few oculists who would hold that one can safely rely solely on miotics, particularly in early cases. The majority value them as an aid to operative measures in restoring and maintaining normal tension. When they lower tension they have a very definite pre-operative value, and when tension persists after operation their use is certainly indicated.

Arnold (1891), Lodato (1904), de Lapersonne (1902), Lagrange and many others pointed out the danger of miotics when they lead to a postponement of operation. Gallemaerts's (1925) views were in accordance with these. He added that one should operate as soon as the diagnosis was established, whatever the age of the patient. There is little evidence to support the view that the use of miotics main-tained during the first three or four years of life would probably arrest the condition (Dufour, 1894).

Thiele (1930) stated that miotics could commonly keep tension normal and prevent further progress of the disease in early cases where glaucomatous changes, especially tears in Descemet's membrane and cupping, were absent.

Lagrange praised "the ophthalmic surgeon who, here as always, must be an attentive physician", and therefore made his diagnosis of the aetiology, instituted general treatment with mercury and other forms of therapy as indicated, and used miotics daily, remembering always, however, that while using them he was usually only preparing the way for surgical intervention. He gave the following example of pilocarpine-eserine treatment of hydrophthalmia.

An eight-year-old boy, with bilateral hydrophthalmia, glaucoma cups, and slight daily variation of tension in each eye. By using eserine and pilocarpine in drops and ointment, the tension was brought down to normal in the afternoon. Both drugs acted more strongly in the form of ointments. Since the tension always rose still higher overnight, 2 % pilocarpine ointment was applied twice during the seventh night. The tension sank below normal, as measure-ments carried out at the same time at night showed. It rose next day when no treatment was given. Pilocarpine ointment twice during the following night caused another rapid fall in tension. The nightly rise in pressure did not occur when pilocarpine drops were used three times daily, and pilocarpine ointment once at night. The treatment was continued in this way for many months. Then, as instructions had not been carried out sufficiently exactly, irregularities appeared in the pressure curve and a trephine was performed on both eyes. After observation for three years, there was no further increase in the cupping of the discs or further loss of function.

OPERATIVE TREATMENT

It is difficult to understand the exact manner in which the operations to be discussed give relief. In many cases there is little correspondence between the operator's plan and the state produced by the operation. In the following review a brief statement of the manner in which each operation is supposed to act will precede a summary of opinions expressed by various surgeons. We will refer to the gonioscopic studies of Troncoso and others, for they give valuable information regarding the *modus operandi* of various operations that meet with success in reducing raised intra-ocular tension.

One seeks in vain for a "best" operation in the treatment of hydrophthalmia. Apart from the difficulty any surgeon finds in doing equally well various operations on several series of similarly affected patients at the same age, which, after all, is the only way to find the best treatment, there is so much variation in the course that the disease may run in the two eyes of the same individual, or in two individuals in the same family, that a fair comparison is impossible. The so-called spontaneous cures discussed under "Prognosis" cause a further complication. Nevertheless, it is hoped that a perusal of the following paragraphs will be of value. The experience even of those who have operated on the largest numbers of hydrophthalmic patients is limited to thirty or forty individuals. The rarity of the condition is a major difficulty in studying the results of treatment.

IRIDECTOMY

It was natural that a re-opening of the angle of the anterior chamber was considered to be the means by which an iridectomy (von Graefe) reduced tension. This was Weber's idea in 1877. de Wecker disagreed, believing that a permeable scar or a communication with the veins rendered escape of fluid possible. Numerous other theories were put forward by different surgeons, including Fuchs, who stated that only a filtering scar could enable an iridectomy to restore normal tension in the presence of a permanently closed angle. Czermaki wrote that the most essential part of a coloboma was its peripheral part, for it may open up the obstruction to Schlemm's canal. Coccius, Leber, Bowman and Ulrich considered that improved communication between the anterior and posterior chambers was the result of value after iridectomy.

Gonin (1925) considered that the thin scleral wall facilitated the production of a fistula after iridectomy. He obtained a complete success following an iridectomy in 1911 and nine years later Morax considered that a sclerectomy had been done in addition because the fistulisation was so effective (see Schoen's and Picqué's cases below).

The following reports of eyes that have had an iridectomy performed on them are of interest: (1) Stimmel and Rotter (1912) examined a specimen of Seefelder's case I (clinical series). For almost nine years the tension had remained normal, then after a cataract extraction panophthalmitis led to enucleation. The conjunctiva had healed over the scleral wound but the lips of the latter were separated by iris and ciliary tissue, which produced a cystoid scar. (2) Spielberg (1911), after reporting histological findings of the eyes of a patient aged five months, stated that he agreed with Siegrist that an iridectomy of itself accomplished little in the cure of hydrophthalmia due to a primary or secondary absence of Schlemm's canal. He considered that the gain resulted from the incision in the sclera in the region of the angle and that this could be obtained far better by an anterior sclerotomy. He published an illustration of one of Siegrist's specimens that had been unsuccessfully treated by an iridectomy. From it we can see that the iris could only be excised in the iridectomy where it had not formed a synechia with the posterior wall of the cornea. Siegrist, Haab, Spielberg and Stölting all preferred an anterior sclerotomy to an iridectomy. The first-named sometimes combined a sclerotomy with an incision at the angle (de Vincentiis). (3) Michelson-Rabinowitsch's case was examined six months after an iridectomy. As the most peripheral portion of the iris had not been excised she considered that the lowering of tension was due to suprachoroidal filtration, as suggested by Fuchs and Axenfeld.

Treacher Collins wrote in 1896 that he had examined microscopically several eyes in which the operation of iridectomy had been unsuccessfully performed, and in all these he found the angle was closed by an adhesion of the root of the iris to the cornea, both in the region of the coloboma and elsewhere.

This finding emphasised the difficulty of obtaining good results by iridectomy.

Troncoso and Werner found on gonioscopic examination of adult glaucomatous patients, total scleral synechiae even in eyes that had been satisfactorily treated by iridectomy. The synechiae persisted unchanged after operation in some of these cases and no filtering scar was found. Troncoso considered that though the separation of such synechiae was beneficial it was not a condition *sine qua non* for the re-establishment of normal tension. He thought that an iridectomy might confer benefits in the following ways:

(1) By providing a large aperture between the chambers which allows the liquids of the eye to circulate freely and to equalise the pressure on both sides of the iris-lens diaphragm.

(2) By re-opening, in some cases, the normal outlets of the chamber blocked by anterior peripheral synechia.

(3) By relieving the pressure on the veins of the iris and ciliary processes and permitting the absorption of the aqueous in larger quantities.

(4) By opening a new, although small, outlet to excretion through the edges of the coloboma, which are never cicatrised.

Troncoso thought that a complete iridectomy should be made in adult glaucoma and that an attempt to tear the root of the iris frequently fails. Such an attempt is not indicated if gonioscopic examination shows the angle open at the site of operation. From clinical observation of non-inflammatory chronic glaucoma it has been established in Heidelberg that (1) if miotics do not reduce tension in spite of the onset of miosis, iridectomy is unlikely to produce a satisfactory result, and (2) iridectomy is only likely to reduce tension if miotics show a tendency to lessen it.

Until the introduction of corneo-scleral trephining, iridectomy appears to have had as many supporters as any other method of treatment for congenital glaucoma. A. von Graefe considered that though a policy of *noli me tangere* was wisest for most cases, yet if the damage due to hypertension were rapidly progressive, iridectomy might prove of value. Marc Dufour reported five not very good results. Gallenga (1885) reported four successes and ten improvements from iridectomy in a series of forty cases operated on by various methods. Gorecki (1897) and Stephenson (1908), Bergmeister (one case cured),

Mellinger (1887) and Besselin (1898) (each reported two good results), Gros (several good results) and others favoured iridectomy. Gros in his thesis referred to several successes obtained by Panas and Meyer. Hirschberg (1907) examined a child on whom he had performed an iridectomy on each side thirteen years before, and found the vision to be J. 2 and 1/1000 respectively. In 1907 Motais entered a protest against the view that iridectomy was usually useless and dangerous in congenital glaucoma. He stated that he had performed iridectomy in the first year of life in at least six cases and at least ten years later had found no advance in the condition. Schoenemann obtained good results in a series which were followed for from three to six years. He performed an iridectomy in eleven cases and combined it with paracentesis in five.

SCHOENEMANN: IRIDECTOMY, 1900

Age at operation	Operations	Severity	Period of observation	Vision	Tension
5 months	I	+	6 years	1/2	N
5 ,,	I	+	6 ,,	1/3	N
3½ ,,	I	+	6 ,,	Good	N
3½ ,,	I	+	6 ,,	Good	N
8 years	I	Early and mild	5 ,,	1/2	N
10 days	P, I, P, Xtn	Early and very marked	3 ,,	Fair	N
10 ,,	P, I, P	Very marked	3 ,,	Good	N
12 ,,	P, I, 2 P, Xtn	,,	4 ,,	Good	N
12 ,,	P, I, 2 P	,,	4 ,,	Good	N
5 years	I	+	3 ,,	1/2	N
5 ,,	I, 2 P, I	+	3 ,,	1/5	N

I = iridectomy; P = paracentesis; Xtn = extraction.

In addition one patient was reported who one year after an iridectomy had normal tension and apparently good vision. Schoenemann referred to a reduction in the size of the globe in six of his cases after operation.

Angelucci reported three successes in children, aged fourteen, sixteen and forty-one days respectively, and two failures. Schweigger considered that an early iridectomy was the means of avoiding blindness, but, and Schoenemann agreed with him, the incision must end in the centre angle of the limbus and not be peripheral. Dufour, Haab and others emphasised the need for deep narcosis. Gama Pinto recommended that the incision should be corneal and made with a Graefe knife. Lagrange considered that it was wise to excise the anterior lip of the scleral wound in addition to the iridectomy.

Seefelder's report shows that iridectomy can lead to most satisfactory results in early cases. In the great majority of the cases conditions were unfavourable, chiefly owing to the long duration of the disease. There were eleven successes among forty-three eyes. In seven an immediate arrest of the disease took place, but only four of these were followed for from two to seven years. In twenty-three cases the operation had no effect, and in seven cases the condition was aggravated. Operations on both eyes of case 7 had what was considered a unique result, for full vision and an almost emmetropic refraction were found five years after iridectomy.

Fleischer quotes Wolff's experience with forty-nine eyes. In this series tension was restored to normal in fourteen, no success was claimed in twenty-seven, and ten eyes were lost from the results of the operation. Schoenemann had no failures in a series of thirteen eyes of seven patients. Reber's results were poor. Uhthoff obtained good initial results in 77 % and lasting success in 63 %.

JAENSCH: IRIDECTOMY, 1927

Age at operation	Operation	Severity	Period of observation	Final vision	Final tension
4 months	{ 1 Scler.	+	6 years	Gradual	?
	{ 1	+	6 ,,	failure	?
6 ,,	1	+	9 ,,	O	+
10 ,,	1	+	6 ,,	H.M.	N
11 ,,	{ 1	?	6 ,,	5/24	N
	{ 1	?	6 ,,	5/60	N
1 year	{ 1	+	9 ,,	C.F.	−
	{ 1	+ +	9 ,,	Xcn	Xcn
2 years	{ 1	+ +	9 ,,	H.M.	N
	{ 1	+ +	9 ,,	Xcn	Xcn
2¾ ,,	{ 1 Scler.	+ +	4 ,,	C.F.	N
	{ 1	+ +	4 ,,	O	+
4 ,,	1	+ +	8 ,,	O	N
4 ,,	{ 1	+ +	6 ,,	O	+
	{ 1	+ +	6 ,,	6/24	+
5 ,,	1	+ +	8 ,,	H.M.	N
5 ,,	{ 1	+	6 ,,	1/10	−
	{ 1	+	6 ,,	1/12	N
7 ,,	1	+ +	8 ,,	H.M.	N
11 ,,	1	+ +	2 ,,	C.F.	O

	6/5–6/12	6/18–6/24	6/36–6/60	<6/60 Fair	H.M. Poor	P.L.	O	Xcn
20 eyes	0	1	2	2	9	0	4	2

In Jaensch's series of twenty eyes there were five good results. Sixteen had normal tension without visual improvement. Though his results with trephining were better, 48 % being classed as complete successes against 25 % after iridectomy, yet he considered iridectomy the *sine qua non*, preferring it because of the danger of infection by way of the filtering scar in trephining. Jaensch described as failures those cases where the steamy clouding of the cornea did not disappear permanently after the operation. According to the classification Jaensch made of the effects of the operation: I, complete success, the eye retaining a vision of 1/10 and better; II, partial success, the residue of vision being retained or only lost to a slight degree, the eye after operation uninjured, no fresh attacks; III, failure, the hypertension not reduced, the eye blinded and painful, and finally phthisic; he had complete success in 48 %, as far as could be judged in the children who were too young to have the vision tested, and 35 % of failures. It is worthy of remark that Jaensch found no late visual loss after Elliot trephines, though the period of observation extended in eight cases over 1–12 years.

Only four eyes described in the replies to the questionnaire were subjected to an iridectomy alone. Little can be learned by a study of the results. The operation was performed on one eye at the age of two months and the eye was removed three months later. Another was operated on at the age of one year and eight years later the vision was 5/36. The remaining two eyes were observed for short periods only.

Many favourable results have been reported by various surgeons, and it is impossible to tell what proportion of the whole they constitute. Unfortunately there is little tendency to publish a series of failures from any particular form of treatment. Amongst the untoward effects are retinal detachment leading to enucleation. Wray (1908), Streatfeild (1882), and Böhm (1915) reported four cases in which enucleation was necessary after iridectomy. At the Edinburgh Seventh International Congress, held in 1894, Dufour stated that he had used iridectomy in five cases without success, and neither de Lapersonne (1902) nor Weekers was in favour of iridectomy. Probably most of the dangers could be obviated by using this method in early cases only.

Possibly, of the above opinions, that of Seefelder's is most valuable, for in his clinic various operations were performed and carefully compared. His results from iridectomy were variable. It is of interest to notice that in several successful cases reported by various observers a filtering scar was not uncommonly found. For an example a case of Picqué's referred to Lagrange may be studied. At the age of two an iridectomy had been performed on each eye. When fourteen he discontinued the use of miotics and vision began to fail. A sclerotomy was performed on each eye and after the excision of the iris prolapse which appeared, a cystoid scar developed with an improvement in vision and a clearing of the cornea. Schoen's case (1905) is also of interest. An iridectomy was performed on each eye at the age of four years. Twenty-one years later it was found that the wound of the right eye had healed smoothly and that in the left was cystoid. The vision of the latter was partially retained, while the other had been blind for eleven years. These findings certainly add support to the view that "fistulisation is the best method of treatment".

One must remember that in performing an iridectomy one makes a larger incision than one does in any of the fistulising operations and so runs a greater risk of iris and vitreous prolapse and of dislocation of the lens. In addition, the probabilities of success appear to be greater in certain of the latter type of intervention, *e.g.* a trephine or Lagrange sclerectomy. Lagrange held that though some of the results of iridectomy may appear to be good, in his opinion they would have been even better if a sclerectomy had been performed as well.

The only safe time, according to various surgeons, for the performance of an iridectomy is in the very early stage before distension and its consequent degeneration is too great, but surely as there are fewer risks and a greater possibility of obtaining permanent drainage by an operation such as a trephining it is wisest to consider the iridectomy as part only of the main operation. Whether a complete iridectomy has any advantage over a peripheral one will be discussed later.

PARACENTESIS OF THE CORNEA

In the section dealing with the history of treatment of congenital glaucoma, this method has been referred to. In more recent years it has been used mainly as an adjuvant to other operations. At times the surgeon has been impressed with the prolonged fall in tension following its use.

Snellen (1894) reported the arrest of the progress of this disease in three cases following a puncture at the limbus every day and the use of miotics. Seefelder reported lasting benefit in three cases following repeated paracenteses.

In nine eyes in the questionnaire the operation of paracentesis was used. In all except two it was combined with other operations. These two are of importance, for the right eye received four paracenteses at and soon after the age of three months, and the left eye received seven at the same ages; two years later the tension was normal and the patient could "see everything". The outlook might have been considered good in one other case but the result was poor. A trephine was performed after a paracentesis and the vision became reduced to less than 6/60.

POSTERIOR SCLEROTOMY

Various forms of sclerotomy have been devised and tried with a considerable measure of success. The posterior operation has been the most popular. Horner was the first to propose its use and Mauthner later strongly supported him. This operation found favour chiefly amongst Swiss oculists; Haab, Arnold and Siegrist particularly writing in its support. One of its advantages has been the ease with which it can be repeated.

The various forms of sclerotomy could be included under fistulisation operations, for, though it was not always apparent to the older surgeons, when success was attained it was the result of a cystoid cicatrix. Now that means of fistulisation have been improved the chief field of sclerotomy is in the advanced cases where the very thin corneo-scleral coat makes vitreous loss or loss of the lens a serious risk from more extensive operations.

The treatment by this operation may cover a long period, e.g. Haab operated on fifty-eight eyes of children and performed 104 sclerotomies. The average duration in hospital was fifty-one days. In six of these eyes the operation was performed only once, in thirteen twice, in ten three times and in nine from four to seven times. He claimed twenty-nine successes, nine failures, and in his opinion the prognosis was always good with early cases.

Arnold (1891) reported the results of Haab's treatment of sixteen patients. They may be summarised as follows:

ARNOLD (SURGEON: HAAB) SCLEROTOMY, 1891

Age at operation	Operations	Severity	Latest observation	Vision	Tension
8 weeks	1	Earliest	7 years	1/3	N
8 ,,	2	,,	7 ,,	1/20	N
2 years	3	+	4 ,,	—	N
2 ,,	2	+	4 ,,	No P.L.	+2
8 months	3	−	5 ,,	—	N
8 ,,	3	+	5 ,,	—	N
7 years	2	+	5 ,,	Poor	N
7 ,,	3	+	5 ,,	Good	N
1 ,,	4	+	3 ,,	Good	N
7 months	3	−	3 ,,	Good	N
1 year	2	−	2 ,,	Good	N
1 ,,	2	−	2 ,,	Fair	N

In addition four patients were too old to justify expectations of good results, two patients died a few weeks after the operation and two other patients were followed for too short a time for the observations to be of value. The prospects in these at the end of six months were, however, not bright.

Haab wrote that sclerotomy was the only operation free from danger in hydrophthalmia. He strongly opposed the use of an iridectomy.

Kunzmann (1899) also reported results obtained in Zürich. In twenty-nine cases good results were obtained and in nine they were unsatisfactory. If the patients were omitted who were not followed for a year 65 % could still be classed as good results. Hirschberg (1906, 1907) published a series of satisfactory results obtained by sclerotomy. Stölting had ten good results among sixteen eyes and Gadowiski described three good results in Wagenmann's clinic.

Fage (1915) claimed that five in a series of fourteen patients regained normal tension and the globes ceased to distend after one or more sclerotomies comprising merely puncture and counter puncture without opening up the angle.

These surgeons were interested chiefly in comparing sclerotomy and iridectomy, for sclerotomy was as yet little known. Fage, however, wrote to Lagrange expressing the view that a sclerectomy, particularly a circular resection such as would follow trephining, might prove to be the best procedure. Lagrange wrote that it would suffice for his colleague to see only once a sclerectomy performed with the punch or the knife with the resection of a strip, to realise that it is a more rational procedure than trephining, and less prone to postoperative infection.

De Schweinitz, Baer and Holloway followed Haab's example and preferred repeated sclerotomies. Zentmayer (1919) held that except for the very earliest stage of the disease, this was the only justifiable treatment. Peter (1919) performed a posterior sclerotomy every second month until four had been done on each side. The patient was seventeen months old. Optical iridectomies improved central vision and it was claimed that they almost removed the nystagmus which was rapidly developing.

ANTERIOR SCLEROTOMY

Delord (1925) reported success after two sclerotomies at the ages of three and four months. This case was followed for fifteen months. It is of interest that this child's father when aged seven months had had a successfully performed sclerotomy by Galezowski. His method of making an anterior sclerotomy was that described by de Wecker at the Heidelberg Congress in 1869. Lagrange stated that Gueren and Mackenzie had previously made scleral incisions to lower ocular tension.

JAENSCH: SCLEROTOMY, 1927

Age at operation	Operations	Severity	Latest observation	Final vision	Final tension
2 years	1 S.	+	6 years	H.M.	+
11 ,,	1 S.	+	1 year		Excision
14 months	3 S., 1 T.	+	12 years	H.M.	N
	3 S., 1 T.	+	12 ,,	3/18	N
14 weeks		+	12 ,,	0	–
		+		0	–
3 years		+	11 ,,	0	N
		+	11 ,,	0	N

8 eyes:	6/5–6/24	6/36–6/60	6/60 Fair	C.F., H.M. Poor	P.L.	0	Excision
	0	1	0	2	0	4	1

It is important to consider the varying effects that may follow the use of different instruments and slight differences in technique.

Quaglino, Galezowski and Snellen used a large lance capable of retaining the iris at the moment of withdrawal. de Wecker used a narrow inflexible knife and his description of his own operation is as follows: "An incision is made with a narrow Graefe knife at a distance of 1 mm. from the corneal margin. The knife is advanced very slowly, parallel with the iris, and the counter puncture is made at the point exactly opposite the puncture. In pushing the knife forward, a scleral incision is made so that the uncut bridge is equal in extent to the cut parts lying on each side. These two lateral incisions may be made by simple propulsion of the knife, or when the eye is not too much distended, by faint sawing movements, made very slowly and without displacing the iris against which the surface of the knife is lying. The method of withdrawing the knife deserves the greatest attention. At the moment of withdrawal the iris is retained in position with the flat of the blade during the escape of aqueous, then while withdrawing the knife from the anterior chamber, the handle is lowered so as to incise with the point, the arches of the 'rigole de Fontana', leaving nothing of the bridge, which measures one-third of the incision, but the external layers of the sclera'' (Lagrange).

Rochon-Duvigneaud described a "reduced" sclerotomy in which a narrow knife was used and simply a puncture and a counter puncture were made without attempting to enlarge the openings. It was recommended for use in young restless children as the risk of iris prolapse was small. In addition to the puncture there is in de Wecker's operation an attempt to open up the spaces of the meshwork. When a permanent cure followed these operations most probably a filtering scar had been obtained even though the surgeon was not always conscious of its presence or its value.

Weill and Bartels wrote in support of anterior sclerotomy. One very interesting patient was reported by Bartels (1931); hydrophthalmia developed during the first month and six months later an anterior sclerotomy was performed on each eye. The corneae cleared immediately but soon clouded over again. After two more anterior sclerotomies, one paracentesis, and one trephine during the next five months, the tension of the left eye became normal. Six years later the eye could count fingers. The right eye fared worse, and surely no other eye has received such operative attention during a period of seven months. The measures adopted were a second sclerotomy, six trephines, one paracentesis, one iridectomy and one cyclodialysis. Five years later the tension was normal and the cornea clear, but a cataract was present and the eye was blind. A very marked degree of myopia developed in the left eye. 10 dioptres of myopia were found at the end of the fourth year and two years later, even though the tension was normal, the myopia doubled. There was a striking absence of myopic degeneration.

One of the numerous operations devised by Herbert (1907, 1911, 1913, 1914, 1920, 1921) has been advised by several surgeons, including Whiting (1935) and Laws (1920). Laws reported a child that was operated on during the first year. In only one eye was a basal inclusion of the iris obtained. For nine years the tension was normal in both, and then it rose in the eye without an iris inclusion. As the disc was cupped the operation was repeated. The other eye remained in a satisfactory state.

Whiting in a personal communication described his experience with a patient over thirty years: "I did a corneo-scleral trephine on one eye, but with permanent reduction of pressure. I then did a Herbert's sclerotomy on the other eye. The pressure went down and has remained down ever since. I then did a Herbert's sclerotomy on the first eye, again with satisfactory results. Since then Herbert's sclerotomy is the only operation which I have employed for this condition. It is unusual for one sclerotomy to be sufficient and I have done as many as three, but the operation is not a severe one, and it is not at all difficult to do a second or third—as would be the case if the trephine had to be repeated. Unfortunately, I have not been able to collect the results, which date back to about 1921, but so far as my memory serves, I have only had failures in four eyes—all of which were nearly blind and in a hopeless condition before the operation. In the other cases, where a reasonable degree of vision was still present, I have obtained uniformly satisfactory results and some of these eyes have now been under observation for as long as eight or nine years."

"The technique of the operation is exactly that originally described by Herbert. The instruments used are a straight or angled broad needle and Herbert's secondary knife. No conjunctival flap is raised but the broad needle is entered about 4 millimetres from the limbus and is pushed into the anterior chamber, gradually deepening the section so that the point enters at the angle and just in front of the iris. The needle is pushed on until the incision is of uniform breadth throughout, and is then withdrawn. The secondary knife is then inserted into the incision on the flat, and when the point is well into the anterior chamber the cutting edge is turned directly forwards; short to and fro movements of the knife cut through the sclera up to, or nearly up to, the limbus, but not through the conjunctiva. These secondary cuts are made at each side of the original incision. The operation is now complete unless there is any tendency for the iris to prolapse. This is unusual, but if it does occur an iridectomy must be done. The operation is not really difficult. The points that require care are:

1. The original section must not go deeply at the beginning, or there is liable to be a localised ciliary staphyloma.

2. The section should enter exactly in the angle. Owing to the abnormal structure at the angle of the anterior chamber, I have in one or two cases found that the knife pierced the root of the iris. Where this occurred it did not appear to affect the success of the operation.

3. While the sclera must be cut through sufficiently to isolate the scleral wedge, the conjunctiva overlying it must be left intact."

Whiting added: "My object is to indicate my view that Herbert's sclerotomy is by far the best operation for this condition."

Lagrange concluded that the necessity to intervene several times in almost all cases was the most serious disadvantage to sclerotomy.

He considered that the operation of sclerotomy was useful very early in the disease and also very late when the eye is greatly distended, the vitreous is fluid, and the zonule stretched. He, however, preferred sclerectomy in the early stage—for it is then free from danger. Sclerotomy may also have the advantage of preparing an eye for a fistulising operation by reducing tension.

Anterior sclerotomy was resorted to in sixteen out of ninety-six cases in the questionnaire, i.e. was used only as a preliminary or supplementary method of treatment. Little can therefore be learned of its intrinsic value. Both eyes of one patient aged eight months had an anterior sclerotomy, a trephine and then two more anterior sclerotomies, and eight and a half years later the vision was 5/25 and 5/5. The condition was apparently advanced when first observed, the corneal diameters being 14·6 and 14·4 mm.

Professor J. B. Coppez, of Brussels, showed in 1901 at a meeting of the Société Belge d'Ophtalmologie, a young man with hydrophthalmia who had had a sclerotomy many years before. This sclerotomy had led to the formation of a cystoid scar as large as a pea, yellowish in colour, rather like a lipoma. Here the filtration had been what one looks for and such as is obtained by sclerectomy. By sclerotomy this filtering scar is invisible to the naked eye. This is the result sought for and often obtained by de Vincentiis and his pupils by the operation known as "debridement" of the angle.

INCISION OF THE ANGLE: THE OPERATION
OF DE VINCENTIIS (1893–95)

Since this operation was described by de Vincentiis (1893–95), numerous Italian surgeons and Valude and Duclos and others in France have made use of it.

The operation is an attempt to incise the tissue at the angle, particularly peripheral synechiae if present, and to open the meshwork in the region of Schlemm's canal. One of the extremities of the horizontal diameter of the cornea is pierced with the needle of de Vincentiis, 1·5 mm. from the limbus. The needle is directed across the anterior chamber to the opposite side till the point is engaged. At this moment the instrument should be lightly turned so that its cutting edge is turned towards the sclera. A semi-circle is now described using the point of entry as a pivot. The point is moved slowly beneath the limbus cutting open the angle as the needle is withdrawn. When the blade, which is still in the angle, approaches the point of entry the handle is raised again and the instrument is withdrawn.

Bocchi (1896) reported two satisfactory results, though neither case was followed for long. In one of these iridectomy and a simple sclerotomy had failed. Sgrosso (1895) reported a good result after six months' observation.

Valude and Duclos (1898) in three cases found that the incision went through Descemet's membrane a little behind the corneal margin and did not touch the sclero-corneal meshwork, the canal of Schlemm or the scleral veins. In another three cases the needle had opened "the lymphatic and venous sinus of the limbus", probably Schlemm's canal, and cut the tendon of the ciliary muscle. They therefore modified the needle of de Vincentiis and in experiments were then able to reach the apex and walls of the true angle. They operated on four eyes with the Graefe knife, performing the anterior sclerotomy described by de Wecker, and they obtained results identical with those in the experiments. These two operations evidently act in the same manner and good results may be obtained. It is likely, however, that the results may not be permanent, but they may prevent hypertension until it is too late for distension to occur.

Scalinci (1900) described the results obtained by de Vincentiis after thirteen operations on nine patients. They may be summarised as follows:

SCALINCI (SURGEON: DE VINCENTIIS), 1900

Age at operation	Operations	Severity	Latest observation	Vision	Tension
2½ years	1	–	4 years	"Good result"	"Good result"
2½ ,,	1	–	4 ,,	,,	,,
2 months	1	Early	2 ,,	,,	,,
2 ,,	1	,,	2 ,,	,,	,,
1 year	1	– –	4 ,,	1/9	sl. –
15 months	1	– –	3 ,,	Improved	N
15 ,,	1	– –	3 ,,	,,	N

In addition five patients followed for 2 months, few days, 14 months, 5 days, 3 months respectively, were reported. In the majority of these an arrest of the condition could be anticipated.

Of seven cases followed for periods of at least two years good results were claimed in all. In only one was there an elevation of tension at the latest examination, and this patient had vision of 1/8 four years after the operation. It is of interest to observe that a single operation only was performed on each eye.

Scalinci concluded that this operation always reduced the tension immediately, and that in the majority of cases this reduction persisted with disappearance of the corneal oedema and improved vision: results which are the more to be appreciated since they are obtained without risk even when marked ocular distension is present. The small haemorrhage produced in the anterior chamber is not serious, and a small iris prolapse at the side of the puncture occurs only if the child is very restless. Such a prolapse does not seem in any way regrettable. "The operator has only to excise as large a piece as possible of the prolapsed iris to transform the operation into a sclero-iridectomy, which many authors (Terson senior) rightly consider to be a very useful operation." Lagrange, de Vincentiis and de Wecker each once, however, experienced profuse intra-ocular haemorrhage.

Lagrange held that in spite of the good results described in the Naples school this operation does not appear preferable to the anterior sclerotomy of de Wecker. The former does not free the angle as much as the latter can, and as rapid cicatrisation is apt to follow the incision of the meshwork of the angle it has the disadvantage of sclerotomy, viz. the need for frequent repetition. Lagrange held that an anterior sclerotomy was more certain in its results than the operation of de Vincentiis.

One wonders how this operation can lead to permanent success, as after all the angle is already open in many cases (47 % Polya) and in others the canal of Schlemm so poor that a new passage to it means little gain. If, however, the primary cause was an arrested development of the uveal meshwork this operation might, in early cases, have a special indication.

It is difficult to foresee what possibilities Barkan's (1936–1938) "intra-ocular microsurgery" may have for the treatment of congenital glaucoma. The frequent corneal opacities would limit the use of a contact lens. His operation of goniotomy or incision of Schlemm's canal may prove of value in certain chosen cases.

Many other operations have been used in the treatment of hydrophthalmia. They all, with one exception, depend on the establishment of a scleral fistula to facilitate the escape of aqueous. The exception is Heine's cyclodialysis, and in it an attempt is made to make a fistula into the subchoroidal space. A consideration of the merits of these operations will be introduced by the following paragraph dealing with the rationale of fistulisation.

THE THEORY OF FISTULISATION

It would be difficult to find a better instance of the value of a filtering cicatrix than that described by Terrien and Goulfier (1924). It concerned a girl of thirteen years who had bilateral hydrophthalmia which arose in infancy. An almost total aniridia was present on each side. The left eye was grossly distended and the sclera ectatic in the upper part and the disc cupped. The tension was 45·0 mm. (Schiötz). The tension of the right eye was normal. The globe was of normal size and the disc of normal appearance. The explanation of this was a large distended sub-conjunctival cicatrix, which was due to a spontaneous scleral rupture and had led to a cure of the hydrophthalmia. Treacher Collins in 1913 stated that he had examined microscopically several eyes with filtering scars following the operation of iridectomy and that he had found a fold of iris tissue in the wound preventing it from closing completely. He doubted whether a filtration scar could be formed without such entanglement of iris until Colonel Herbert demonstrated that such was possible. In 1914 he wrote that the establishment of a permanent gap in the corneal endothelium was the most essential feature in the operation of corneo-scleral trephining. The cleanly cut circular opening appears to be ideal in this respect. He referred to two other essentials for permanent fistulisation, viz. (1) the bathing of the substantia propria by aqueous humour. This and freedom from sepsis would prevent granulation; (2) prevention of a down-growth of epithelium into the wound by having a large flap which would keep the conjunctival and the corneo-scleral wound remote.

Holth believed that the permanence of fistulisation was dependent on the walls of the wound being lined with uveal pigment (Verhoeff, 1915). Elliot's investigations have shown the difference between a clinically and an anatomically iris-free scar. "The latter must be very rarely met with, the former can be attained very frequently by the adoption of a correct technique" (Elliot). The anatomical investigation of these surgeons confirmed the existence of the clinically iris-free scar that functions as a filter. For further discussion on this topic it is wise to refer to the writings of Holth, Elliot, Lagrange and Herbert (see Fig. 113).

It is sufficient here to mention Elliot's contention, that an iris impaction may be rather an event that one would expect to occur in a scar that was filtering freely, than the actual cause of this filtering. He admitted with Holth that suitably performed iris-inclusion operations might promote adequate filtration but they differed in their aims. Elliot considered that iris inclusion might occur but should not be sought after, but Holth held, originally at least, that filtration depended on the presence of a lining of uveal pigment. Both agreed, however, on this point, that a fistula was the object to obtain.

Fistulisation or the attempt to produce a "filtering scar" goes back to the days of von Graefe and de Wecker. The latter surgeon in 1867, realising that iridectomy was not the ideal treatment for chronic glaucoma, searched for a means of producing a "cicatrice à filtration" and one that was free from incarcerated iris. He proposed the operation of sclerotomy, which proved itself of great value, though its frequent repetition was often necessary.

During the following forty years many modifications were suggested. The majority of these were of little value. They were neither simplifications of technique nor means to more lasting and more frequent cures. These should surely be the requisites before a surgeon recommends any departure from an established operation of proven merit. The dissatisfaction of many imitators is due much more to the imperfection of their imitation than the operation itself, which in the hands of a von Graefe, de Wecker, Elliot or Gonin had led to such desirable results.

JAENSCH: TREPHINE, 1927

Age at operation	Operations	Severity	Latest observation	Vision	Tension
3½ months	⎰ 2 T ⎱ 1	+ +	3 years 3 ,,	P.L. 5/20	+ N
10 ,,	⎰ 1 ⎱ 1	+ +	12 ,, 12 ,,	1/4 1/10	N N
2 years	1	+	1¼ ,,	H.M.	N
2½ ,,	⎰ 1 ⎱ 1	+ + +	10 ,, 10 ,,	1/12 1/10	N N
5 ,,	3 T	+ +	1 year	O	–

8 cases: 6/5–6/12. 6/18–6/24. 6/36–6/60. <6/60 Fair. H.M., C.F. Poor. P.L. O Xcn
        0   2   2   1   1   1   1   0

(Other cases followed for less than 1 year.)

Jaensch found connective tissue and degenerated ciliary processes in the trephine wounds of his specimens I and II (aged ten months). He stressed the need for careful iris replacement and absolute asepsis. He considered that the dangers of trephining were as formidable as those of iridectomy. Even though he split the cornea the ciliary tissue has been caught by his trephine. The vitreous, which is fluid, is ready to escape on the slightest undue pressure. Deep narcosis lessens this risk but the mortality under anaesthesia is high. He compared the results from iridectomy with those of trephine as follows:

Iridectomy, 20 eyes: 25 % good results, 35 % satisfactory, 40 % bad results.
Trephine, 23 eyes: 48 %   ,,   ,,   17 %   ,,   35 %   ,,   ,,

Iridectomy appeared preferable to him because of the danger of late infection and of ciliary prolapse after trephining.

Various modifications were of value and will be referred to later. They include Herbert's several forms of sclerotomy (1903 to 1910), Heine's cyclodialysis (1905), Holth's iridencleisis (1907 to 1909).

In 1906 Lagrange described his "epoch-making operation" under the title of "sclerecto-iridectomy". His aim was that of de Wecker, the production of an iris-free filtering scar.

Then followed amongst others Brooksbank James's sclerectomy (1909), Bettremieux's simple anterior sclerectomy (1907 and 1908), and Fergus's scleral trephining with cyclodialysis (1909).

It was in 1909 and 1910 that Robert H. Elliot introduced to other oculists his invaluable operation of corneo-scleral trephining. It has been the fate of few widely practised operations to be so roundly condemned and so warmly praised as Elliot's operation. One explanation of the disappointed is their failure to follow the steps of the operation as outlined by the originator.

It is quite likely that some of the modifications of Elliot's and Lagrange's operations are due to surgeons getting away from the main object—an iris-free filtering scar—and concentrating on some less important part of the operations. It is rarely wise for a surgeon to introduce a modification of an operation of proven value until he has mastered the technique of its deviser. The failures at the hands of imitators are so often due to errors in technique and not to intrinsic defects in the operation itself. If we are to obtain results comparable with those claimed by a master we must perfect our imitation of his technique. Take, for example, the criticism of trephining that it predisposes to late infection (see later).

A discussion of the operations of Lagrange and Elliot will be given first, as this raises most of the problems of importance.

Lagrange studied the anatomy of the limbus to ascertain the average distance between the lower limit of the detachable conjunctiva and the ciliary tendon. At "12 o'clock" this was found to be 1·75 mm., at "6 o'clock" 1·45 mm., and "3 and 9 o'clock" 1·0 mm. As Rochon-Duvigneaud and Ducamp measured from the corneo-conjunctival border to the tendon of the ciliary muscle their measurements are slightly greater. These three observers and Le Magourou (1914) agreed that the corneal wedge overlapping the sclera is of constant dimensions, viz. 1·0 mm. above and 0·80 mm. below, and that the scleral zone or the zone of filtration averages 0·75 mm. above and 0·65 mm. below.

It is wise to keep these measurements in mind when fistulising an eye for glaucoma. In the child of course the dimensions are less, but in hydrophthalmia they will vary according to the degree of distension, to the state of the eye and to the state of development of the structures at the angle.

Trantas's early method of gonioscopy and the later method of Troncoso, as well as biomicroscopy with the slit-lamp, may help one to judge the variation from normal in hydrophthalmia in suitable patients. It is probably wise before deciding to trephine to attempt by these methods to exclude two variations that may jeopardise the result. They are the absence of conjunctiva that can be dissected off over the angle of filtration and the presence of ciliary processes on the posterior surface of the iris.

Lagrange said that the two dangers that made him avoid trephining for adult glaucoma may not exist when operating in this way for hydrophthalmia. They were (1) wounding the ciliary body when the trephine opening is entirely subconjunctival and (2) cutting the flap when trying to avoid the ciliary body. He added, however, that at the very time when one should operate for hydrophthalmia, that is, when distension is just beginning, a trephine is not only contra-indicated, but a very dangerous procedure, because of the risk of wounding the ciliary body. The scleral zone at this stage is never larger, and may even be smaller, than a trephine of 1·5 mm.

In the later stages Lagrange considered that an elongated opening was more inclined to gape and so prove more effective than the circular aperture left by a trephine. The former is more apt to re-open the spaces of Fontana and free them from debris than is the circular aperture left by a trephine. Lagrange's aim was to restore over as great a distance as possible the blocked spaces of Fontana and to construct over as great a distance as possible an artificial subconjunctival canal of Schlemm.

de Lapersonne wrote that it was prudent to resort to the use of a trephine if one had not learned how to do a sclerectomy according to the methods of Holth, Lieto-Vollaro or Lagrange.

Lagrange's sclerecto-iridectomy. Fistulisation in the treatment of chronic glaucoma was the finest advance in ophthalmology in the first twenty years of this century. Just as Gonin's name is associated with the second period of twenty years for his work on retinal detachment, so should the names of Lagrange and Elliot be associated with the first for their work on glaucoma.

Before considering the use of Lagrange's operation in congenital glaucoma it is of interest to recall his summary (1922) of the results obtained in the treatment of chronic glaucoma. In 240 cases not a single instance occurred of infection, vitreous loss, ciliary involvement, expulsive haemorrhage or traumatic cataract. Of the last forty-nine cases, if we include those who developed senile cataract, 82·5 % gave good visual results and 80 % normal tension. Lagrange was dissatisfied with the occasional case that developed a tension below 15 (Schiötz).

Lagrange emphasised several points in connection with sclerecto-iridectomy that are worth recalling: (1) The value of this operation is beyond dispute, but, he says, "we would jeopardise the future of this treatment if we said that it was applicable to all buphthalmic eyes". The critical moment for its use is when general treatment and miotics can no longer control the disease. These must not be persisted in unless they are obviously of avail, for it is desirable to operate on tissues as normal as possible and while vision is good. (2) If tension is high a retro-bulbar injection may be of value. (3) Even though anatomical studies prove that the point of election is above it may be wise to operate below the cornea because of the tendency for upward rotation of the eye under a general anaesthetic. Forcible rotation downwards is apt to promote the escape of vitreous.

Lagrange considered that owing to the greater tendency for the wound to gape even a simple sclerotomy might permit sufficient filtration if tension were high. He recommended a sclerectomy if tension were normal or slightly raised and a sclerecto-iridectomy if the tension were very high. The amount of sclera removed should vary inversely with the height of the tension.

As the scleral filtration zone averages only 0·75 mm. above, even the narrowest trephine will include not only this area but in addition encroach more or less on either the ciliary body or the cornea. Lagrange held that excision of corneal tissue encouraged its proliferation and a tendency for the aperture to close. A further disadvantage of trephining too close to the cornea is the poor protection that the emaciated conjunctiva gives when the limit of the detachable zone of conjunctiva is passed. Lagrange also emphasised the danger of trephining too far back and so injuring the ciliary body or producing its incarceration in the aperture. In Lagrange's sclerectomy the filtration angle and it alone is opened into longitudinally and extensively and a thick mucous membrane covering is provided for pro-

LAGRANGE (SURGEON: LAGRANGE), 1925

Age at operation	Operations	Severity	Latest observation	Vision	Tension
5 years	L	+	16 months	0	N
5 ,,	L	+	16 ,,	Poor	N
18 months	L	+⎫	Only followed	Volume	T = N
18 ,,	L	+⎬	13 months	reduced	
28 ,,	L	+⎫	Cyclitis, cataract	Atrophy of globe	
16 ,,	L	+⎭	3⅔ years	Poor	N
16 ,,	L	+	3⅔ ,,	Poor	+
11 ,,	L	+	7 months	Poor	Full
2½ years	L	+	15 ,,	Poor	N
2½ ,,	S, L	+	3 ,,	Poor	N

tection and for the escape of aqueous. Lagrange described his operation in detail in his monograph (1922) and in a paper (1914 and 1922). He emphasised the necessity of making the resection several millimetres long and a little less than 1·0 mm. broad, and restricting it to the scleral band in the anterior wall of the angle. He preferred to use Holth's punch to scissors.

Only four of these globes were re-examined after periods of more than three years after operation, and in three the vision was poor, in one it was nil, in three the tension was normal and in one it was still raised. It is of interest to find frequent reference to the operative reduction in the size of the globe and also the not uncommon finding of an oedematous cicatrix.

In the questionnaire reports only one patient was treated by sclerectomy alone. Van Lint operated on both eyes of a patient at the age of seven years. Seven years later the vision was C.F. and P.L. In one of these eyes the vision had been 1/8 at the time of operation. The condition was evidently advanced when first observed as each disc was atrophic.

Morax performed sclerectomy on the eyes of two children who succumbed to chloroform anaesthesia, and whose eyes were studied by Magitot. Lagrange, however, classed another of Morax's cases as a complete success. Nine years after a sclerecto-iridectomy the vision was 2/10 with glasses, tension was below 20·0 mm. and the fields were normal.

Satisfactory results were claimed by Lawson (1909), Adams (1912) and Allport (1910) each in one case, but the periods of observation were not longer than eighteen months.

Van Lint advised sclerectomy; Holth sometimes used this operation and at other times iridencleises with meridional iridotomy. Lacroix (1925) advises sclerecto-iridectomy. In his opinion the iris rarely presents if one does a trephine, owing to the very frequent peripheral synechiae. He considers that one can only expect good results in recent or not very advanced cases. In an acute attack he suggested doing an iridectomy first and later a sclerectomy in the scar, "une oulectomie".

It is at times necessary to repeat a sclerectomy several times, and fortunately this can be done with impunity. A patient reported by Valois and Lemoine (1925) had an ineffectual iridectomy on his only eye at eighteen. Two years later a sclerectomy was performed, and during the next two years two sclerotomies, one trephine and six sclerectomies after Lagrange were performed. At the end of the patient's twenty-fourth year the vision was 0·3 and the tension was 30·0 mm. (Bailliart). Coppez operated successfully on several cases of congenital glaucoma (1911). He summarised his method of making a sclerectomy as follows: "I begin by cutting a conjunctival flap, measuring about a centimetre wide by a centimetre high, adhering to the superior part of the corneal limbus. In order to dissect this better, I spread it out by holding one angle with the forceps, while the assistant does the same with the second angle. Arriving at the level of the limbus, I cut the conjunctiva as far as possible using blunt-pointed scissors. The extension of the conjunctiva helps to avoid making a gash, which is unfavourable from the point of view of the formation of the fistula. I then free the sclerotic from all episcleral tissue; I lay much emphasis on this practice which Gama Pinto recommended a long time ago. The proliferation of the episcleral tissue is sometimes one cause of the obliteration of the fistula. I then introduce the probe, perform an iridectomy, resect the anterior lip of the scleral fold with the punch, and retract the conjunctival flap."

Many surgeons have been struck by the thinness of the conjunctiva of young subjects affected by hydrophthalmia. It has to be dissected with great caution. "It is no longer a question of Prof. Lagrange's flap of velvet, it is scarcely a flap of cotton. One must be careful to insert the probe very far back. One must at all costs prevent the escape of vitreous which endangers the final result. Concerning the performance of iridectomy on infants, I perform it only if the iris presents of its own accord in the fold, but I do not systematically look for the iris in the anterior chamber, a practice that I consider very dangerous, as it gives rise particularly to haemorrhages. Finally, I advise sclerectomy and eventually, if the circumstances are suitable, sclerectomy-iridectomy."

"The results are certainly less favourable than with adults. The chief risks in operating, as I have just said, are tearing the conjunctiva, allowing the vitreous to escape from a distended globe, and haemorrhage. Fistulation is equally risky: the young tissues proliferate easily. It is also sometimes necessary to perform two and even three sclerectomies, before obtaining a satisfactory result.

"We need not hide from ourselves the fact that we are in the presence of one of the most delicate of ocular surgical operations, but such as it is, it represents an enormous progress on the old methods" (Coppez, 1925).

Gonin wrote that he usually performed an iridectomy for congenital glaucoma, but that in about one-third of the cases a sclerectomy was necessary in addition.

Lawford obtained several good results from repeated sclerotomies. In one patient a sclerectomy had given an excellent result for one eye and had failed for the other eye.

de Lapersonne also advised sclerectomy but without an iridectomy, which in his opinion was dangerous because of the distension at the limbus, and the degeneration of the ciliary body.

Sourdille considered that an early sclerectomy was the best operation. In the late stages he preferred a sclero-iridotomy.

Dehouges (1926) operated successfully, by Lagrange's method, on both eyes of a patient with hydrophthalmia and cataracts.

Holth's sclerectomy. This surgeon described his method in 1907 and various modifications up to 1921. A translation of his original description is found in *The Ophthalmoscope*, 1909. His object was to lessen the risks of escape of the lens and of expulsive haemorrhage. In 1911 he stated that in congenital glaucoma he always used the obtuse-angled flap and usually operated below the cornea. The pupil should be strongly contracted before operation and he used deep anaesthesia. After the keratome incision he did not attempt to empty the enormous anterior chamber, which might promote haemorrhage. He made a sclerectomy ($3 \cdot 0 \times 1 \cdot 5$ mm.) in the anterior lip and as quickly as possible a peripheral iridotomy. As a rule little aqueous was lost. He then tied the previously inserted conjunctival suture which was reindeer tendon No. 000.

Lagrange held that this operation was more complicated and required more special instruments than his own sclerectomy. Later Holth preferred iridencleisis, which operation is discussed in another place.

Lieto Vollaro's modification, 1923. This surgeon dissected a conjunctival flap with a keratome or small Graefe knife after the method of van Lint for cataract and Dupuys-Dutemps for glaucoma. He emphasised the necessity of directing the point of the keratome towards the periphery of the iris and, once the anterior chamber is entered, of lowering the handle so that the instrument is parallel with the plane of the iris. If the keratome is introduced at a tangent to the plane of the iris the sclera will be cut obliquely, which prevents a complete and sufficient scleral resection. The resection is made with a cataract knife after the method of Kalt. A peripheral iridectomy is performed and the flap sutured in position by two sutures.

Corneo-scleral trephining. Elliot considered that the following were some of the advantages of his operation: (1) The conjunctiva in congenital glaucoma can be very easily detached, and so the trephine can be placed sufficiently far forwards. (2) The anterior chamber is so deep that the trephine may be manipulated with confidence. (3) The tissues are so thin that it is easy to perforate them with the trephine and to obtain an opening that will remain open.

Owing to the disproportion existing between the dimensions of the globe and those of the orbital opening it may be difficult to commence the conjunctival wound far enough back. Hamilton held that the tissues, being very thin, offered little resistance to the trephine and so made the operation difficult.

Fleischer in 1918 was able to collect the following good results from trephining: Zeeman (in six of eleven eyes), Grunert (in four), Dubois (in three) and Clegg (in one). In Zeeman's series (1918) three eyes were lost from escape of vitreous, late retinal detachment (in an eight-year-old boy), and infection eighteen months after the operation. In two the operations made no difference. To avoid retinal detachment Zeeman forbade trephining in old cases. Iridectomy was a desirable addition to a trephine or a sclerotomy.

In Fleischer's series (1918) from Tübingen no ill effects were observed though vitreous was lost once. He considered that good results were obtained in all. Only two required a second operation. If we exclude those patients that were not observed for a period of at least one year after operation, and those that were operated on late, there remain eleven eyes of seven patients operated on during the first year of life. They were followed for periods of from two to six years. In all these cases the tension was "permanently" reduced to normal, the cornea became clear, and the eye free from signs of irritation. He was impressed by the general improvement in the children after operation. They became less restless and irritable and free from photophobia. Fleischer's other conclusions were: that it is probably wiser to do a complete iridectomy, that atropine is only required if signs of inflammation are present, that pilocarpine may be needed for some years, that it is wise to wait for some months before deciding that any given operation was inadequate (for in one of his patients, case VII, tension returned to normal after six months), and that a second operation will probably be required if after three months hypertension and corneal opacities have persisted. Fleischer obtained arrest of the disease in two patients aged twenty and twenty-four and in the former he claimed an actual improvement in vision. In contrast with the flat scar that develops in children's eyes a cystoid cicatrix appeared in this patient.

Whilst Fleischer claimed that an early trephine with complete iridectomy was the operation of choice, he was at a loss to explain the nature of its effect. He observed that Seefelder and Schoenemann had admirable results from iridectomy, and that he had to repeat the operation when he performed a peripheral iridectomy. He also noticed that trephining without iridectomy may at times lead to a cure, and yet the rapid and complete blockage of the trephine aperture by scar tissue appeared to prevent the formation of a fistula.

Fleischer concluded that trephining under the age of one year put an end to the hypertension in hydrophthalmia. After the age of one, damage to the optic nerve would interfere with the visual result. He considered that the flat scar, which developed in all the patients but one aged twenty, lessened the risk of late infection.

In 1925, when Blake collected notes of 472 cases from 178 ophthalmologists, he found that 156 operations had been done, including 78 iridectomies, 50 trephines, 15 anterior sclerotomies, 10 Lagrange operations and 3 iridotases. His conclusions were that trephining was the operation of choice and that this should be done during the first year. In the same year Patton (1925) found from his American questionnaire that 45 % of oculists in that country were advising no treatment but enucleation when indicated by pain. He concluded that early operation was advisable and that one of the filtering operations held out most hope of success. Lagrange held that such operations in extreme hydrophthalmia with badly diseased tissues were dangerous.

Some surgeons found the incidence of late infections to be 10 or even 20 %, but Elliot (1922) and Kirkpatrick, each with over 1000 trephines for glaucoma to their credit, had no experience of it. "As we approach the limbus we should work down to the sclera, and should expose the latter bare in the last two-thirds of the wound" (Elliot). If surgeons in general had followed this instruction more carefully they would have avoided many late infections. Admittedly in some eyes the cutting of a thick flap is difficult, but in these a measure such as that adopted by Wright of Madras, who cuts a second flap consisting of episcleral tissue, will be efficacious. To avoid the danger of a late infection he thought that one should follow Staub's example and make a small scleral flap after the conjunctival flap so as to give safer though more limited drainage. He prepared a thick conjunctival flap to within 1·5 mm. of the corneal margin and then dissected a thin scleral flap until the corneal tissues shone through. The flat oedematous scar and not the raised vesicular one must be sought. One must also remember that a late infection may follow any intra-ocular operation. When one remembers the sudden popularity and the widespread adoption of corneo-scleral trephining it is not surprising that many surgeons failed to take proper precautions, and that a large number of late infections occurred. "The danger of vitreous prolapse makes it wise", Wright held, "to cut through the sclera with Taylor's knife and not with the trephine." In this way he made a larger subconjunctival sclerotomy.

To lessen the risk of late infection which has been stressed by Meller and others, Bentzen (1927) advised the following modification of Elliot's procedure: a conjunctival dissection extending 2·0 mm. beyond each end of the horizontal diameter of the cornea, a scraping with a cataract knife of the epithelium of the superficial layer of the cornea over an area 2·0 mm. beyond the site chosen for the trephine and the insertion of two sutures.

Thiele (1930) wrote that though Elliot's operation is becoming increasingly popular the risk of secondary infection must not be treated lightly. "In the great majority of operated cases a fistula scar does not seem to be formed, as the wound tends to close quickly with scar tissue as a result of the altered conditions at the limbus. This, however, need not prevent the success of the operation."

Dettmering (1932) found no infection in a series of thirty-six trephined eyes. Of these nineteen healed flat and seven showed pad formation. Of those in which the trephine only was used six were classed as complete cures according to Jaensch's standard, four as partial cures and thirteen as failures. Dettmering considered that his findings did not demonstrate the superiority of trephining over other operations. Spital considered that this tendency to the formation of a flat scar was a disadvantage. In twelve eyes he obtained normal tension in only one case. In one eye he repeated the operation five times, in one eye three times, on two eyes twice and on the remainder once only. Goerlitz (1923) reported the restoration of normal tension in four eyes that were trephined.

Poulard and Lavat (1925) performed Elliot's operation sixteen times and Holth's operation twice in eighteen eyes (eleven patients). They reported permanent reduction of tension to 28·0 mm. (Schiötz) or less in two-thirds and apparent preservation of good vision in six patients who were operated on in the first year of life. One patient twelve years after operation had vision equal to 1/4 in each eye. This patient's eyes were only slightly enlarged then and each had had a filtering scar. These authors concluded that if one operated during the first few months of life the patient had every chance of retaining useful vision in at least one eye.

Their results may be summarised as follows:

POULARD AND LAVAT (SURGEON: POULARD): TREPHINE, 1925

Age at operation	Operations	Severity	Observation period	Final vision	Final tension
6 months	T	+	12 years	1/4	–
6 ,,	H	+	12 ,,	1/4	–
6½ years	T, 2 P	+ +	12 ,,	C.F. ½ m.	N
6½ ,,	T	+ +	12 ,,	P.L.	N
8 months	T, H, P	+	6 ,,	1/50 After needling	N
5 ,,	T, H	+	4 ,,	C.F. ½ m.	+ +
5 ,,	H	+	4 ,,	1/10 After needling	N
9 ,,	T	+	3½ ,,	H.M.	? full
9 ,,	T	+	3½ ,,	1/10	? full
7 ,,	T	+	3½ ,,	1/10	? full
16 ,,	T, P	+	3 ,,	Poor	+1
16 ,,	T, P	+	3 ,,	Poor	+1
4 ,,	T	+	2½ ,,	Fair	N
4 ,,	T	+	2½ ,,	Fair	? full
4 ,,	T	+	2 ,,	P.L.	+2
4 ,,	T +	+	2 ,,	Fair	+
7 years	T	+ +	2 ,,	C.F. 1/3 M.	N
10 ,,	T +	+ +	1½ ,,	H.M.	+ +

T = Trephine; H = Holth's sclerectomy; P = Paracentesis.

Summary:

Final vision	6/5–0/6	6/9–0/12	0/18–0/24	6/36–6/60	<6/60 Hm.		P.L.
					Fair	Poor	
Number	0	0	2	3	4	7	2

Of these eight globes were operated on before the end of the second year and followed for periods of over three years. The vision was 1/4 in two, 1/10 in three, 1/50 in one, C.F. in one, H.M. in one. The tension was reduced to normal in four, ? full in three and + + in one.

The sclerectomy was made with only a trephine in four of these eyes, in two others with a punch and in two the latter instrument was used to enlarge the trephine opening. It is of interest that in the whole series of eighteen globes a single operation was sufficient to restore the tension to normal (not more than 28·0 mm. Hg pressure) in eleven.

Sattler reduced tension in twelve of sixteen eyes which he observed for many years, and in two others after repetition of the operation. Jaensch reported sixteen successes in a series of twenty eyes. Eight of these were followed for one to twelve years. He claimed 48 % complete successes, *i.e.* vision of 1/10 or better regardless of tension. In the absence of further hypertension and operative damage and the maintenance of a remnant of vision a partial success was claimed. Blindness, pain, phthisis bulbi or persistent hypertension led to the declaration of failure. Goerlitz's (1924) results and opinions were similar to those of Fleischer. In four affected eyes useful vision was retained, high tension relieved and cloudy corneae cleared and no cupping of the discs was found. No fistulising scar developed, but he believed that trephining was technically relatively simple and easier than iridectomy to perform and more likely to lead to lasting benefit. In one of these two paracenteses were necessary later. Two globes developed a cataract, and after surgical treatment the vision was 1/10 and 1/50.

Though the tension was not reduced below 36·0 mm. (Schiötz), in a patient reported by Spratt (1930) the ability to count fingers remained for seventeen years after trephining.

Hymes (1934) reported the apparent arrest of glaucoma as a result of trephining in two sisters. The younger child was nine months old at the time of her operations. Five and a half years later her vision was 6/6 and 6/12.

Weeks (1920) considered that trephining was the most suitable procedure and on account of the thinness of the sclera he used a small trephine, 1·5 mm. In very young infants he thought that paracenteses were of great temporary benefit. He held the view that the wound was apt to gape and to be inadequately covered by the conjunctival flap after Lagrange's operation.

"Green, Lancaster, Peter Robertson, Beddell, Ellett and Feingold were encouraged by their results of trephining." Gifford (1934) and Elliot (1922) referred to good results obtained by Dubois, Calhoun, Wessely, Zentmayer, Hamilton and Lebensohn. Elliot stated that Hallet obtained a good final result in a child of seven years after three trephine operations.

Zeeman lost three eyes from vitreous loss, retinal detachment, and late infection. The first catastrophe appears to be a much greater danger than the last mentioned. H. Gifford (1916) reported two cases in which trephining failed because the scar healed so firmly that no filtration occurred. He held the view that the trephine should enter the anterior chamber as peripherally as possible to gain the advantage of the looser conjunctiva. He referred to Quackenboss having had to abandon an attempt to trephine because of the extreme thinness of the sclera. Axenfeld emphasised the danger of late infection and Lundsgaard considered that the bleb might be injured by the trauma to which children are subject. Snellen thought it wisest to make several openings with a small trephine. He was disinclined to operate in advanced cases.

Bentzen (1927), when describing his results with the trephine operation and inverted flap, included six cases of hydrophthalmia. The three which he was able to follow showed bad results. Kerasek (1934) reported a partial prolapse of the retina into the anterior chamber after trephining the eye of a seven-year-old girl. Morlet (1937) obtained good results by suturing the lids of both eyes after trephining. The eyes are dressed on the fifth and eighth days after operation.

Dettmering summarised the results of operation on forty-five of a total series of fifty-five hydrophthalmic eyes. In an attempt to analyse the results it is wise to exclude five for the following reasons: Case 16 was operated on at the age of fifty-two. Case 15 was previously reported, cases 20 and 21 (left eye) were not followed after operation and the nature of the operation performed on the left eye of case 26 was not known.

The remaining 40 eyes may be classified as follows:

A. One method of operation, 26 eyes   Reference
   1. Iridectomised, 3 eyes   16 R.E., 31 R.E. and L.E.
   2. Sclerotomised, 3 eyes   3 L.E., 2 R., 14 R.
   3. Trephined, 21 eyes   5 R., 8 L., 9 R. and L., 10 L., 11 R. and L., 19 R. and L., 19 R. and L., 21 R., 23 L., 26 R., 27 R., 28 L., 29 R. and L., 30 L.
   4. Cyclodialysis   28 R.
B. Several operative methods, 14 eyes
   I. Sclerotomy as final operation   6 R. and L., 7 R. and L.
   II. Trephine as final operation   12 R. and L., 13 L., 14 L.
   III. Cyclodialysis as final operation   2 L., 4 R. and L., 23 R.
   IV. Not known which was final operation   25 R. and L.

If Jaensch's (1927) classification is adopted the following results are obtained:

Group:	I	II	III
Operated in the first year of life	5	6	10
,, after ,, ,,	7	4	8
Total	12	10	18
Trephined as only or final operation	6	4	13
Sclerotomy as ,, ,,	1	3	3

Jaensch did not specify the state of intra-ocular tension but in this table two cases with vision of 1/10 have been excluded because of raised tension.

The great advantage of trephining over iridectomy, according to Fleischer and Dettmering, lies in the fact that its technique is simpler and less dangerous, particularly in small children, and that it is associated with fewer complications.

Meller emphasised the view that there was a tendency to get either solid cicatrisation with raised tension or a cystic scar with the risk of infection.

Further indications of the results to be expected from trephining are given by the following summaries of replies to the questionnaire issued by us in 1935–6 and of Colonel Wright's reported cases.

QUESTIONNAIRE: TREPHINE, 1936

Nineteen eyes were trephined before the age of two years and received no other operative treatment than one or two preliminary paracenteses. The three eyes which received such preliminary treatment were unrelieved for seventeen years later, two being blind and painful were excised and the third $9\frac{1}{2}$ years after operation saw $< 6/60$.

Of four cases who had the trephine opening enlarged with a punch all were reported to be satisfactory two and three years later.

The visual results may be classified as follows:

6/6	6/12	6/18	6/60	Satisfactory	Poor	Blind
1	4	1	1	6	1	5

Three patients became blind four, seven and eight years after the operation in three cases. Six eyes received a series of operations of which a trephine was either the first or the last and the final vision was:

6/8	6/18	6/24	C.F.	Blind
1	1	2	1	1

Eleven eyes were operated on after the age of two, and the results were:

6/9	6/12	6/36	1/60	C.F.	Fair	Blind
1	1	1	1	1	1	4 ? 5

Ten eyes in this series were excised as a result of injury. In only two was the loss of vitreous reported, but no direct question related to this, and so probably many surgeons omitted reference to it.

WRIGHT: TREPHINE, 1936

Age at operation	Operations	Severity	Observation periods	Final vision	Initial vision	Final tension
2 years	T	++	5 years	1/60	?	N
26 ,,	T	Mild	4 ,,	6/60	6/36	N
15 ,,	T	,,	3 ,,	6/5	6/5	N
23 ,,	T	+	3 ,,	H.M.	C.F.	+
13 ,,	T, L	+	2 ,,	H.M.	H.M.	+
19 ,,	T	+	2 ,,	6/12	6/18	N
19 ,,	T	+	2 ,,	6/36	6/36	N

In this series of seven globes observed for at least two years after operation the final vision was practically the same as when first estimated in five cases, worse in one and probably worse in another case. The tension remained raised in two cases. It is difficult to compare these results with those in other series because of the high average age, viz. seventeen years, none of the patients being under two years.

It is of interest to compare these results with those found in four cases which were treated with miotics or not at all. Probably in two cases the vision became worse and in only one was the tension maintained within normal limits.

WRIGHT: NO OPERATION, 1936

Age when treated	Severity	Observation periods	Final vision	Initial vision	Final tension
2 years	Mild	5 years	6/9	?	N
26 ,,	,,	4 ,,	No P.L.	6/24	+
15 ,,	,,	3 ,,	6/5	6/5	+
23 ,,	+	3 ,,	P.L.	H.M.	+

Holth's Iridencleisis. By iridencleisis one attempts to produce a fistula, the walls of which are covered with iris epithelium, so that the opening does not close with non-filtering cicatricial tissue, as is a frequent occurrence after scleral trephining (Meller). Werner from gonioscopic investigation concluded that the presence of extensive peripheral synechiae did not interfere with the action of this operation in reducing ocular tension. As with trephining, he found the angle closed after operation in eyes in which it was open prior to operation. The borders of the coloboma were incarcerated in the scar, usually in front of or in Schlemm's canal itself. Holth (1907–09) considered that this operation was indicated for hydrophthalmia, though he gave no results.

Gifford (1934) considered that the risks of trephining were so great that he preferred iridencleisis. He operated on five eyes (three cases) and considered that the results were very satisfactory in three. The time of observation was too short in another to justify a conclusion, and the fifth maintained vision for only two years, though the tension was normal. He encountered no complications. He followed Holth's technique, except that he made a horizontal incision just in front of the insertion of the superior rectus and that he used a "water-tight" suture in the conjunctiva. One patient was aged fourteen and the corneal diameter was 12·0 mm. in diameter at the time of operation. In the absence of reference to increased size of the eyes, one cannot dismiss the possibility of juvenile glaucoma being the disease present. Five years later one eye read 20/15 and the tension was normal. The other eye could perceive hand movements and at times the tension rose. The second patient was undoubtedly hydrophthalmic. The corneae measured 13·5 mm.; they were hazy and tension was very high. One disc was pale but not excavated and the other was difficult to see. An iridencleisis was performed on one eye, and an iridectomy on the other at the age of three months. It was necessary to repeat the iridectomy on this eye. Two years later the tension was normal and the corneae clear and the child appeared to have excellent vision. The third patient had large and cloudy corneae. Each eye was operated on at the age of ten months and a second operation was necessary on one eye two months later. Six months later tension was normal and the corneae clear and vision appeared to be good. These successes represent the good results obtained from thirteen treated by H. and S. R. Gifford and Patton, with the exception of one good result from sclerotomy and trephining.

Fowler (1934) reported two advanced cases treated by iridencleisis but without success.

Gjessing (1931) reduced the tension in the blind eye of a child aged eight years by this operation.

Blaickner (1930 and 1935) considered that iridencleisis was contra-indicated in "juvenile glaucoma in which the danger of forming ectatic scars or even staphylomata" seemed to be too great. Another contraindication was the presence of iridodonesis, owing to the danger of vitreous loss. In these cases Blaickner preferred cyclodialysis. Blaickner (1935) wrote: "I do not think iridectomy is of much value and the greatly stretched globe is not suitable for iris-inclusion. For congenital hydrophthalmia I mostly use Elliot's trephine with peripheral iridectomy. Only when one or other of the trephine holes has closed do I think iridencleisis worth considering. When the globe is not stretched I prefer cyclodialysis as the first operation." Wessely (1914) obtained from iridencleisis one success, and Vaeger claimed to have arrested the condition in two of five cases operated on by a modification, viz. Schloffer's operation (Elliot).

Lagrange considered that it was unwise to attempt to produce a fistula by iris-inclusion and without sclerectomy.

Seven eyes in the questionnaire were treated by iridencleisis. It was always combined with at least one other kind of operation. In three cases it was one of two operations and in the others two, three, five and seven other operations were performed. There is not sufficient data to make sure that all these were average cases, but it is interesting to observe that in all hypertension persisted.

Iridotasis. Borthen (1910) claimed that he had obtained satisfactory results in each one of fifty patients with simple or absolute glaucoma by using the operation he described as iridotasis.

Verhoeff (1926) employed a modified iridotasis for chronic glaucoma and hydrophthalmia. "A button-hole is made in the iris midway between the pupil and the limbus, the iris is grasped at the upper margin of the hole and pulled out beneath the conjunctival flap. In this way the sphincter is allowed to remain within the eye, so that the pupil is displaced slightly if at all."

Heine's Cyclodialysis. Heine's conception of the rationale of cyclo-dialysis was based on the assumption that a choroidal detachment, if produced, would result in reduction of tension, just as occurred after iridectomy for glaucoma and extraction. Fuchs had already pointed out that this accident was associated with a reduction in tension which was probably due to the escape of aqueous into the suprachoroidal space through tears in the "ligamentum pectinatum."

Meller considered, however, that such a detachment did not develop. He wrote (1923): "The occasional success is accomplished by the undermining of the angle of the anterior chamber. Cyclodialysis should be regarded as an operation to free the angle." Elschnig, after histological examination of an eye that had been satisfactorily treated by cyclodialysis fourteen years previously, stated that the formation of the cleft between the anterior chamber and the supra-choroidal space was the chief means in reducing hypertension. He considered that the freeing of the angle would not help because the "pectinate ligament" was too sclerosed and compressed to render fil-tration possible (Elschnig, 1932). Barkan (1936), who also examined an eye successfully operated on by this method, found evidence of drainage into the suprachoroidal space.

Barkan and others (1936) after gonioscopy concluded that Elschnig was correct in his view. After one hundred cases of glaucoma, de Grosz (1932) concluded that the effects were transient, and that the operation should be repeated. Of three hundred cases of glaucoma, 62 % were satisfactory at the end of one year and 50 % after five years.

When this operation was introduced by Heine, he considered that its relative freedom from danger might render it a suitable operation for hydrophthalmia. Instead of opening drainage channels as by iridectomy, or of establishing a scleral fistula by trephining, one endeavours by this operation to open up a communication between the anterior chamber and the suprachoroidal lymph spaces. Zeeman reported three complete successes in his series of eleven operations on five children. The first was a success, but even though the operation was repeated in the second and third cases the results were unsatis-factory; in the fourth child cyclodialysis led to improvement in one eye, in the other a trephining was necessary. In the fifth patient a trephining led to an excellent result in one eye, and two trephining operations failed and normal tension was restored after a cyclodialysis in the other. Jaensch found cyclodialysis of some value as a secondary operation. At the age of three months one patient with marked hydrophthalmia had two cyclodialyses and soon after, two trephines. Four months later he was blind and had raised tension. Another patient had two cyclodialyses at the age of two years and six months but later had only perception of light and hypertension.

In the questionnaire reports seven eyes received a cyclodialysis as the only operative treatment. Two of the patients died and the remainder were followed for a short period only. One eye was apparently mildly affected, for at the age of twelve years the vision was still 6/8. One year after cyclodialysis the vision was 6/12. Five other eyes received cyclodialysis, but from two to nine other operations as well. When first observed the outlook for four of the twelve eyes on which cyclodialysis was performed could have been considered good, but only one good result was obtained, and on this the cyclodialysis was the last of four operations, the first being performed at six months; of the three other eyes the tension was reduced, but late observations were not made in two, and the third case died from an abdominal tumour soon afterwards. The outlook for the remaining eight eyes might have been thought poor, and yet two good results were obtained. For one eye the cyclodialysis was the last of three operations starting at the age of ten, and for the other it was the last of four operations starting at six years. These were evidently mild cases, for the vision was 5/15 at ten years and 20/36 at six before operation.

OTHER OPERATIONS

Extraction of the lens. As an endeavour to arrest the development of myopia Fukala advised the removal of the lens. This operation has not been widely adopted because of the late risk of retinal detachment and of its failure to arrest the progress of shortsightedness. Lagrange considered, however, that this operation had not taken the place it deserved in ophthalmology.

Gallenga (1922) advised this operation in the treatment of congenital glaucoma. He was interested to find, when other measures including an iridectomy and several paracenteses had failed to relieve the tension in a glaucomatous eye of an eighteen-month-old child, that removal of the opaque lens at the age of three years led to a distinct reduction in the size of the globe. After a series of paracenteses a large discission was made and, with Daviel's curette, a large part of the lens was extracted. Six years later the cornea was clear, the globe was smaller and indistinct vision was present. He then treated two other globes in the same manner with similar results. He held that the undue stretching of the zonule of Zinn was relieved by extraction and that as less aqueous was produced tension was lowered. The ocular membranes could then shrink, reducing the size of the globe. Truc (1895) showed that removal of the lens led to a reduction of about 0·6 mm. in the antero-posterior axis of the globe and of 0·13 c.c. in volume. It is possible that in the eye of a child these results might be greater and might even ameliorate the state of the globe with hydrophthalmia.

Extraction of a cataract did not retard the progress of hydrophthalmia in Jaensch's case XVII. The operation was performed at eight years of age, and six years later both eyes were blind. The risks from retinal detachment infection and an expulsive haemorrhage are extreme in such an interference.

For results of extraction of cataract in hydrophthalmia see "Treatment of Complications", p. 341.

Resection of the cervical sympathetic ganglion has been recommended for glaucoma at all ages. Few can claim more than transient reduction in tension from this measure. Grunert (1900) had one good result among four, but it was observed only for two months. Wolff (1910) reported four satisfactory results from this operation when performed on a series of five children with glaucoma. Elschnig's paper (1912), however, according to Elliot, dealt this operation its *coup de grâce*— "a procedure which had outstayed all too long its scanty welcome at the hands of ophthalmologists".

Instead of removing a blind hydrophthalmic eye Desmarres and Lagrange recommended ablation or a partial excision. This operation consists of detaching the recti muscles, putting a purse-string suture in the conjunctiva and excising the anterior portion of the globe by rapidly cutting behind the ciliary body. The recti muscles are then tied together and the purse-string drawn tight. A considerable part of the vitreous is thus retained and a moveable stump obtained.

THE RELATIVE MERITS OF VARIOUS OPERATIONS

Zentmayer (1913) analysed the replies from a number of surgeons on the subject of the best operation to perform in the case of hydrophthalmia. According to him, iridectomy gave good results in 42 % of the cases, and bad results in 58 %; with sclerotomy 28 % were favourable and 72 % bad; with sclerectomy the results were satisfactory in 40 %, encouraging in 20 %, and bad in 40 %. It must be remembered that the operation of trephining was not in general use at this time.

The following is a summary of the results found in the questionnaire and the series of Seefelder, Stölting, Dettmering and Fleischer (see overleaf):

	1st op., 1 year and under		1st op., over 1 year	
	6/24 and better	<6/60	6/24 and better	<6/60
Herbert's sclerotomy (2 cases)	100 % out of 2	0 %	—	—
Anterior sclerotomy (as 1st or only op.)	50 % ,, 16	38 %	0 % out of 15	94 %
Trephine (as 1st or only op.)	33 % ,, 40	50 %	13 % ,, 55	63 %
Sclerectomy (as 1st or only op.)	25 % ,, 4	25 %	0 % ,, 14	86 %
Iridencleisis (as only op.) (3 cases)	0 % ,, 1	0 %	50 % ,, 2	50 %
Cyclodialysis (as 1st or only op.)	— ,, 0	—	8 % ,, 13	92 %
Iridectomy (as only op.)	0 % ,, 10	60 %	0 % ,, 17	80 %
Paracentesis (as only op.)	0 % ,, 6	67 %	0 % ,, 8	90 %
Cyclodialysis (as final op.)	25 % ,, 4	25 %	50 % ,, 4	25 %
Trephine (as final op.)	20 % ,, 7	30 %	0 % ,, 3	100 %

It must be pointed out, regarding anterior sclerotomy (operation at one year and under), that 75 % of the patients were from one clinic, and a big percentage were mild, whereas of the trephines not more than 30 % were from any one clinic. One would therefore expect a lower percentage of good results.

Trephining is a more complicated operation, has greater risks and the data concerning it are from many more sources than that for anterior sclerotomy.

Anterior sclerotomy and Herbert's sclerotomy (two cases only) gave the best results of operations done under one year. Paracentesis and iridectomy gave the worst results of operations done under one year.

The only good results from operations done over one year were from trephinings, cyclodialyses and iridencleises. When other operations had failed a cyclodialysis and trephining were the only operations to produce good results.

Therefore one may conclude that Elliot's operation is the most useful, but in early cases one or a series of sclerotomies, or a Lagrange's operation, may occasionally produce satisfactory results.

MULTIPLE OPERATIONS

There has been a tendency for surgeons to carry out an operative campaign somewhat regardless perhaps of the influence of such on the patient. Take, for example, the following instances: on the left eye three sclerotomies, one paracentesis, one iridectomy and one cyclodialysis. The result was normal tension but blindness.

Valois and Lemoine refer to a patient who had the following operations performed on one eye: an iridectomy, two sclerotomies, one trephine and six sclerectomies (Lagrange). The age at the first operation was eighteen years and the final vision was 0·3 and the tension = 30 (Bailliart). One admires the confidence of the patient even more than the courage of the surgeon in such a case.

In the series reported by Dettmering and Stölting and the questionnaire, including the cases of Zeeman, the following eyes received at least four operations excluding paracenteses.

Reference	No. of operations	Nature of operation	Age at first operation	Cornea	Final vision	Final tension	Optic Disc
Q. 14 R.	9	2 AS, T, (P), 3 T, I, C, T	7 months	15 mm.	O	+	Cup
Q. 47 L.	8	AS, T, Ik, T, AS, 2 D + T, G + T	2 years	.	.	Stony hard	.
Q. 44 L.	6	AS, T, T, Ik, AS, T	10 months	.	.	+	.
St. 9 R.	5	3 AS, 2 I	3 ,,	11–12 mm.	Xcn	?	Cup
Dett. 8 L.	5	5 T	7 ,,	?	{ P.L. Cat.	+	?
Dett. 6 L.	4	T, AS, T, AS	4 ,,	?	C.F.	+ +	Cup
Zeem. 6 L.	4	C, 3 T	3 years	15 mm.	O	.	?
Zeem. 8 L.	4	4 T	6 months	Large	Xcn	N	N
Q. 13 R.	4	3 AS, (P), T	8 ,,	14·6 mm.	5/25	+ +	N
Q. 13 L.	4	3 AS, T	8 ,,	14·4 mm.	5/15	+ +	N
Q. 14 L.	4	3 AS, T	7 ,.	15 mm.	C.F.	+	Cup
Q. 30 R.	4	AS, 3 T	3 ,,	?	6/24	?	N
Q. 32 L.	4	3 T, C	5 ,,	14 mm.	6/8	N	N
Q. 40 L.	4	T, C, T, C	6 years	14 mm.	6/9	+	Cup
Q. 42 R.	4	T, AS, 2 T	4 months	.	.	30	.
Q. 47 R.	4	AS, T, Ik, T	2 years	.	.	−	.

AS = Anterior Sclerotomy; T = Trephine; I = Iridectomy; C = Cyclodialysis;
D = Diathermy; G = Galvano-cautery; Ik = Iridencleisis.

It is rather remarkable that of the twelve cases whose vision was recorded some years later two had 6/9 or better, and three others had from 5/15 to 5/25. All had the operation performed before the age of nine months except one who was six years old before the operation was done. The corneal diameter was 14·0 mm. and a cup was present, and yet nine years later the vision was 6/9. The possibility of this being an example of very mild hydrophthalmia must be considered. The vision of the remaining seven cases was:

2 count fingers.	2 blind.
1 perception of light.	2 excised.

Of the sixteen cases the operation of trephining was the last performed in eleven and the first in six.

THE QUESTION OF OPERATION

Before deciding on an operation for any patient with congenital glaucoma, the following points should be considered: What is the outlook without operation? What are the prospects of arresting the condition by operation? Has the general condition of the patient been studied and adequate treatment supplied? What are the risks in operating? One must certainly remember the relatively frequent reports of deaths under anaesthetics of these children. One must recall the all too common bad results and the excisions following operation, not forgetting the worse results from lack of treatment. One must also bear in mind the possibility of enabling a patient to retain sufficient vision to earn his living anyway for a time and so to store his mind with knowledge that if blindness does ensue he may put to use his education and possibly even earn his living. Such an example is H. McK., who at the age of one year was operated on by the late Percy Webster of Melbourne even though the general opinion at the time was that the condition was hopeless. Twenty-five years later the patient was earning his living as a dispatch clerk. When six years later, as a result of a detachment of the retina, he was forced to give up this work he had learned sufficient of business methods and of life in general to be able to prove himself a most valuable social worker amongst the blind.

THE TIME FOR OPERATION

As a rule one may advise operation as soon as the disease is recognised provided that steps have been taken to improve general health and an attempt made to restore normal tension with miotics. In the very early stage before tears in Descemet's membrane and cupping have developed, as well as in the late stages, when secondary degenerative changes are advanced, one may hesitate to operate for very different reasons. A certain proportion of those found in the earlier stage will remain unchanged throughout life—the abortive type already discussed. These obviously will require no operation, but after all there is no way of recognising the fortunate few and any operation is accompanied with fewer dangers when performed at this stage than later. One is justified in treating an early case with miotics provided one makes careful and repeated searches for cloudiness of the cornea, for loss of function or for early cupping or for a failure to maintain normal tension. If these signs are found, or if in the eye, when first observed, one or more of these signs are present, operation, preferably sclerectomy, is indicated.

Not only are the risks less but also the results are better if operation is performed at an early stage. There is little prospect of regaining vision once it is lost, unless the loss is due to oedema and imbibition opacities of the cornea. The characteristic changes in hydrophthalmia that create difficulties are the stretching of the globe and particularly of the corneo-scleral junction, and the fluid nature of the vitreous. These are only slight if one operates early. Seefelder wrote: "All the successes so far known, practically without exception have been obtained in the early stages." Gallemaerts (1925) held that one should operate as soon as the diagnosis was made, whatever the age of the patient.

In the later stages, when the limbus is very stretched, the cornea shows numerous scars, the iris is atrophic, the transparency of the lens impaired and the disc deeply and widely cupped; a mental picture of the end result if no operation is performed will encourage one to operate even as a last resort. Some remarkably interesting results have followed late operations.

An attempt to make a fistula at this stage is dangerous because of the tendency to vitreous prolapse, dislocation of the lens and retinal detachment. Probably repeated paracenteses or sclerotomies hold out most hope of retaining the little vision that is left When these fail and vision has gone, pain and discomfort will probably lead to partial or complete removal of the eye.

If the eye is greatly distended and a little sight remains even though the tension is raised, any operative measures may have the effect of destroying the remnant of vision. If miotics failed to reduce tension in such cases Seefelder performed repeated sclerotomies and finally cyclodialysis. He claimed that repeated punctures of the anterior chamber were successful in three of thirteen eyes, though in one instance (case 22) the disease appeared to be at a standstill before operation.

Coppez wrote: "Operate as early as possible before disorganisation occurs." He reported the case of a six-year-old girl on whom he performed a double iridectomy in 1905. Twenty years later her vision had not failed further and her studies had been completed.

Sourdille held that one should operate as soon as the diagnosis is made. He never found a case of true infantile glaucoma to be cured by miotics and mercury.

TENSION AFTER OPERATION

Considerable importance should be attached to the question: can hydrophthalmia be considered to be cured if a state of normal tension is not attained? On our opinion of this matter depends our answer to a further question: should one operate if raised tension is the only manifest sign of hydrophthalmia?

In Dettmering's series six cases (19 L., 23 R. and L., 30 L., 31 R. and L.) were observed for a long time, and though normal tension had not been restored by operation yet vision remained unchanged. Can such eyes, it may be asked, have a high-normal tension? If so, we would expect no subsequent cupping of the optic disc. The length of observation and the state of the discs in these cases were 11 years, normal disc; 13 years, cup; 1 year, normal; $2\frac{1}{2}$ years, normal; 5 years, cupped; 5 years, cupped. These cases therefore suggest that the raised tension may be physiological for the eyes concerned. In an analysis of forty operated eyes, Dettmering showed that of fourteen with useful vision that had been observed for some years after operation, six showed normal tension and five of these had normal discs. Of the seven with raised tension only two were free from cupping. Of the unoperated eyes in this series six retained useful vision for a long time and the state of the disc varied with the tension in these cases. There was no instance of a normal disc with raised tension. Therefore only two in this series support the contention that a high-normal tension is possible.

If one finds a hydrophthalmic eye with useful vision, clear cornea, and only physiological cupping, one is probably wise to adopt conservative measures in treatment even though the tension is slightly above normal. If the patient cannot remain under constant supervision an operation is indicated. Operation is also indicated as soon as cupping appears or tension rises or the cornea becomes steamy.

If one could be sure of establishing normal tension by a single operation less importance would be attached to these considerations. Twice (4 R. and L.) in Dettmering's series three operations were necessary to produce normal tension, and thrice (6 R., 9 L. and 25 L.) two operations were necessary. In only two eyes (1 R. and 5 L.) was one operation enough. In five of these cases only did the cornea become clear and remain so after a single operation. In one eye, 1 R., the cornea was clear before the operation. Therefore the later operations in four cases were performed purely to obtain normal tension.

TREATMENT OF COMPLICATIONS

Cataract. It is not surprising that lens opacities are frequently found in late cases of hydrophthalmia. As they appear to be most common in those eyes that have been operated on, there is a possibility that the operation may have hastened the development of cataract.

Dettmering found cataract in seven of thirty-seven operated cases and in only one or two of eight unoperated cases in his series. No lens opacities were found in his cases for varying periods after operation, *e.g.* 2, 16, 16, 16, 24, 28 months, whilst 24, 18, 18, 33, 54, 54 months later lens opacities were found.

If the cause of the opacities was a rupture of the capsule by reduction of the tension, one would expect an earlier onset for these opacities. In this respect it is of interest to recall the fact that Meissner (1920) found a zonule defect and a lens coloboma in the region of the iris coloboma in the eyes of two children aged seven years upon whom iridectomies were performed at the ages of two and nine months respectively.

There is probably undue strain on the stretched suspensory ligament and probably also on the capsule prior to operation.

Dislocation of the lens may lead to hypertension and marked ocular distension. Marlow (1903) reported this state in a patient aged four years. The luxation was congenital. Brown (1937) and others have reported similar cases.

Seefelder held that primary linear extraction was a more suitable operation for these cataracts than simple discission. The already reduced filtration channels would scarcely be able to cope with the extra demands made after the latter operation. Seefelder extracted the cataract from his cases 5, 13, 15, 16, in two without any loss of sight, in two, which were very advanced, with slight vitreous loss, and in one with a late retinal detachment and subsequent shrinkage of the globe. Twice he found the anterior lens capsule thickened and it had to be removed with Mathieu's forceps. His attempt at discission was a failure because a complete posterior synechia formed.

McCaw (1919) extracted a cataract from a hydrophthalmic eye in an elderly man. The incomplete history prevents a definite exclusion of megalocornea as the disease present.

In the questionnaire only two instances occur of attempted extraction. They were both in the same patient, who was $3\frac{1}{2}$ years at the time. Nystagmus was present and the lenses dislocated forwards. In the right eye after a keratome incision vitreous loss occurred, but nineteen months later after a similar incision the lens escaped through a vectis back into the vitreous. The cataract was removed from the other eye with a scoop, but $5\frac{1}{2}$ years later the eye was excised after an injury. There was no perception of light in this eye, but hand movements in the other at the first examination.

Detachment of the retina. Though no reference has been found to the treatment of such a complication in an arrested case of hydrophthalmia there is no reason why such should not be attempted.

SUMMARY

1. Little can be expected from medical treatment, though it is wise to improve the patient's general condition and treat any bodily disorders.

2. In certain cases miotics appear to be beneficial and are therefore worthy of trial. The result is determined by the actual pathological state.

3. The operative measures attempt either to open up the channels for the escape of fluid at the angle or to establish a fistula into the subconjunctival or the subchoroidal spaces. The former are of value in early cases and while the latter have not produced such high percentage of successes under the first year they constitute the only hope for those over this age.

4. The superiority of Elliot's operation is possibly masked by the fact that it is in more general use and therefore performed by more inexpert operators.

5. Much can be hoped from the operation described by Barkan as "goniotomy" for this gives the surgeon a reasonable chance of esta-

blishing a channel of escape through obstructive tissue at the angle, by making an incision under direct and magnified vision.

6. Regarding the time of operation one may say that any hope for success almost vanishes after the first year. The exceptions are probably mild cases or those that are arrested spontaneously.

REFERENCES

MEDICAL TREATMENT

1906 CARLOTTI, J. *Soc. d'Ophtal. Paris*, Oct.
1924 LESNÉ. *Presse Médicale*, Oct.
1924 ONFRAY and PLICQUE. *La Clinique Ophtal.* 28, 681.

USE OF MIOTICS

1901 ASAYAMA, J. *Arch. f. Ophthal.* 53, 113.
1934 DUKE-ELDER, S. *Recent Advances in Ophthal.* 2nd ed. p. 128.

RESULTS OF MIOTIC THERAPY

1891 ARNOLD, TH. *Beitr. z. Augenheilk.* 3, 16.
1894 DUFOUR, M. *Trans. VII Internat. Congress*, Edinburgh.
1902 DE LAPERSONNE, F. *Arch. d'Ophtal.* 22, 565.
1904 LODATO, G. *Arch. di Ottal.* 11, 220.
1925 GALLEMAERTS, E. *Bull. et Mém. Soc. franç. d'Ophtal.* 38, 201.
1930 THIELE, R. *Kurzes Handb. der Ophthal.* 4, 828.

IRIDECTOMY

1882 STREATFEILD, J. F. *Lancet*, 1, 263.
1885 GALLENGA, R. *Ann. di Ottal.* 14, 322.
1887 MELLINGER. *Klin. Monatsbl. f. Augenheilk.* 5, 25.
1896 COLLINS, E. T. *Researches into the Anatomy and Pathology of the Eye*, p. 105. London: Lewis.
1897 GORECKI. Quoted by Lagrange.
1898 BESSELIN. *Münch. Med. Wochenschr.* No. 25. Quoted by Lagrange.
1900 SCHOENEMANN, C. *Arch. f. Augenheilk.* 42, 175.
1902 DE LAPERSONNE, F. *Arch. d'Ophtal.* 22, 565.
1905 SCHOEN, W. *Zentralbl. f. prakt. Augenheilk.* 29, 289.
1907 MOTAIS. *Bull. et Mém. Soc. franç. d'Ophtal.* 24, 379.
1907 HIRSCHBERG, J. *Zentralbl. f. prakt. Augenheilk.* 31.
1908 WRAY, C. *Trans. Ophthal. Soc. U.K.* 28, 100.
1908 STEPHENSON, S. *Trans. Ophthal. Soc. U.K.* 28, 100.
1911 SPIELBERG, C. *Klin. Monatsbl. f. Augenheilk.* 49, 314.
1912 STIMMEL and ROTTER. *Zeitschr. f. Augenheilk.* 28, 114; Abst. *Klin. Monatsbl. f. Augenheilk.* 61, 544 (1913).
1913 SEEFELDER, R. *Zeitschr. f. Augenheilk.* 26, 2 and 3. Abst. *Klin. Monatsbl. f. Augenheilk.* 51, 544.
1915 BÖHM, K. *Klin. Monatsbl. f. Augenheilk.* 55, 556.
1925 GONIN, J. *Bull. et Mém. Soc. franç. d'Ophtal.* 38, 220.
1927 JAENSCH, P. A. *Arch. f. Ophthal.* 118, 1, p. 27.

Paracentesis of the Cornea

1894 Snellen. *Soc. néerland. d'Ophtal. Leyden*, May. Quoted by Lagrange.

Posterior Sclerotomy

1891 Arnold, Th. *Beitr. z. Augenheilk.* **3**, 16.
1899 Kunzmann. Inaug. Dissert. Zürich. Quoted by Lagrange.
1906, 1907 Hirschberg, J. *Zentralbl. f. prakt. Augenheilk.* July, vol. 30, 1906; June, vol. 31, 1907.
1915 Fage. *Arch. d'Ophtal.* **34**, 574.
1919 Zentmayer, W. *Amer. Jl. of Ophthal.* **2**, 696.
1919 Peter, L. C. *Amer. Jl. of Ophthal.* **2**, 695.

Anterior Sclerotomy

1907, 1911, 1913, 1914, 1920, 1921 Herbert, H. *The Ophthalmoscope*, **5**, 292; **9**, 76; **11**, 398; **12**, 2; *Brit. Jl. of Ophthal.* **4**, 550; **5**, 183.
1920 Laws, W. G. *Trans. Ophthal. Soc. U.K.* **40**, 376.
1925 Delord, E. *Bull. et Mém. Soc. franç. d'Ophtal.* **38**, 227.
1927 Jaensch, P. A. *Arch. f. Ophthal.* **118**, 1, p. 28.
1931 Bartels, M. *Zeitschr. f. Augenheilk.* **75**, 17.
1935 Whiting, M. Personal Communication.

Incision of the Angle—The operation of de Vincentiis

1893 de Vincentiis. *Ann. di Ottal.* p. 540. Also *Ann. di Ottal.* 1895, p. 582. Quoted by Lagrange.
1895 Sgrosso. *Lav. di Clin. Ocul. Napoli*, **4**, 235. Quoted by Lagrange.
1896 Bocchi. *Arch. di Ottal.* **4**, 3–4, p. 130.
1898 Valude and Duclos. *Ann. d'Ocul.* **119**, 28 and 241.
1900 Scalinci, N. *Ann. di Ottal.* p. 324.
1936 Barkan, O. *Amer. Jl. Ophthal.* **19**, 966.
1938 Barkan, O. *Amer. Jl. Ophthal.* **21**, 1099.

The Theory of Fistulisation

1905 Heine. *Ber. der deutsch. Ophthal. Gesell. Heidelberg*, **24**. Quoted by Elliot.
1907–8 Bettremieux. *La Clin. Ophtal.* Quoted by Elliot.
1907 Holth, S. *Bull. et Mém. Soc. franç. d'Ophtal.* **26** 326.
1909 Brooksbank James, G. *Trans. Ophthal. Soc. U.K.* **29**, 266.
1909 Elliot, R. H. *The Ophthalmoscope*, Dec. 7.
1909 Fergus, F. *Brit. Med. Jl.* **2**, 983.
1909 Lawson, A. *Trans. Ophthal. Soc. U.K.* **29**, 263.
1910 Allport, W. *Brit. Med. Jl.* **1**, 563; *Rev. gén. d'Ophtal.* p. 41.
1910 Elliot, R. H. *The Ophthalmoscope*, **8**, 482.
1911 Coppez, H. *Arch. d'Ophtal.* **31**, 443.
1912 Adams, P. H. *The Ophthalmoscope*, **10**, 261.
1914 Le Magourou. *Arch. d'Ophtal.* **34**, 85.
1914 Collins, E. T. *The Ophthalmoscope*, **12**, 589.
1914 Lagrange, F. *Arch. d'Ophtal.* **34**, 71.
1915 Verhoeff, F. H. *Arch. of Ophthal. N.Y.* **44**, 129; *The Ophthalmoscope*, **13**, 352.

1922 LAGRANGE, F. *Glaucoma and Hypertony.* Paris: Doin.
1924 TERRIEN and GOULFIER. *Soc. d'Ophtal. Paris,* **41,** 516.
1925 LAGRANGE, F. *Bull. et Mém. Soc. franç. d'Ophtal.* **38,** 143.
1925 LACROIX. Communication to Lagrange.
1925 VALOIS and LEMOINE. Quoted by Lagrange.
1925 COPPEZ, H. *Bull. et Mém. Soc. franç. d'Ophtal.* **38,** 221.
1926 DEHOUGES, J. L. *Arch. de Oftal. Hisp.-Amer.* **26,** 29. Abst. *Ophthal. Lit.*
          1927, p. 118.
1927 JAENSCH, P. A. *Arch. f. Ophthal.* **118,** 1, 27.

HOLTH'S SCLERECTOMY

1907 HOLTH, S. *Ann. d'Ocul.* **6,** 137, May.
1909 HOLTH, S. *Bull. et Mém. Soc. franç. d'Ophtal.* **26,** 326.
1911 HOLTH, S. *The Opthalmoscope,* **9,** 487.
1921 HOLTH, S. *Brit. Jl. Ophthal.* **5,** 544.
1923 LIETO VOLLARO. *Arch. d'Ophtal.* **40,** 344.

CORNEO-SCLERAL TREPHINING

1916 GIFFORD, H. *Ophthal. Record,* **25,** 462.
1918 FLEISCHER, B. *Klin. Monatsbl. f. Augenheilk.* **61,** 152.
1918 ZEEMAN, W. P. C. *Klin. Monatsbl. f. Augenheilk.* **60,** 400.
1920 WEEKS, J. E. *Arch. of Ophthal.* **49,** 316.
1922 ELLIOT, R. H. *A Treatise on Glaucoma.* 2nd ed. p. 598. London:
          Frowde.
1923 GOERLITZ. *Klin. Monatsbl. f. Augenheilk.* **72,** 778.
1924 GOERLITZ. *Klin. Monatsbl. f. Augenheilk.* **73,** 778.
1925 BLAKE, E. M. *Arch. of Ophthal.* **54,** 1.
1925 PATTON, J. M. *Trans. Amer. Acad. Ophthal.* **30,** 38.
1925 POULARD and LAVAT. *Ann. d'Ocul.* **162,** 496; *Bull. et Mém. Soc. franç.*
          d'Ophtal. **38,** 212.
1927 BENTZEN, C. F. *Trans. Ophthal. Soc. U.K.* **47,** 275.
1927 JAENSCH, P. A. *Arch. f. Ophthal.* **118,** 1, p. 27.
1930 SPRATT, C. N. *Arch. of Ophthal.* **4,** 338.
1930 THIELE, R. *Kurzes Handb. der Ophthal.* **4,** 828.
1932 DETTMERING, M. Inaug. Dissert. Göttingen.
1934 GIFFORD, S. R. *Arch. of Ophthal.* **11,** 751.
1934 KERASEK, O. *Klin. Monatsbl. f. Augenheilk.* **92,** 389.
1934 HYMES, C. *Amer. Jl. Ophthal.* **17,** 132.
1936 WRIGHT, R. E. Personal Communication.
1937 MORLET, C. Personal Communication.

HOLTH'S IRIDENCLEISIS

1914 WESSELY, K. *Ophthal. Year Book,* p. 204.
1930 BLAICKNER, J. *Zeitschr. f. Augenheilk.* **72,** 265.
1931 GJESSING, H. *Arch. of Ophthal.* **6,** 489.
1934 FOWLER, J. G. *Amer. Jl. Ophthal.* **17,** 252.
1934 GIFFORD, S. R. *Arch. of Ophthal.* **11,** 751.
1935 BLAICKNER, J. Personal Communication.

Iridotasis

1910 Borthen, J. *Arch. f. Augenheilk.* **65**, 42. Quoted by Lagrange.
1926 Verhoeff, F. H. *Arch. of Ophthal.* **56**, 386.

Heine's Cyclodialysis

1923 Meller, J. *Ophthal. Surgery*, p. 269. Philadelphia: Blakiston, Son and Co.
1932 Elschnig, A. *Ber. der deutsch. Ophthal. Gesell. Heidelberg*, **50**, 277.
1932 de Grosz, E. *Arch. d'Ophtal.* **49**, 625.
1936 Barkan, O. *Amer. Jl. Ophthal.* **19**, 21 and 957.

Other Operations

1895 Truc, H. *Bull. et Mém. Soc. franç. d'Ophtal.* p. 316.
1900 Grunert, K. *Ber. der deutsch. Ophthal. Gesell. Heidelberg*, **19**, 15.
1910 Wolff. Inaug. Dissert. Tübingen. Quoted by Lagrange.
1912 Elschnig, H. H. *Klin. Monatsbl. f. Augenheilk.* **50**, 598.
1922 Gallenga, R. *Boll. d'Ocul.* **1**, 477.

The Relative Merits of various Operations

1913 Zentmayer, W. *Jl. Amer. Med. Assoc.* **61**, 1110.

The Time for Operation

1925 Gallemaerts, E. *Bull. et Mém. Soc. franç. d'Ophtal.* **38**, 201.

The Treatment of Complications

1903 Marlow, F. W. *Arch. of Ophthal.* **32**, 470.
1919 McCaw, J. A. *Amer. Jl. Ophthal.* **2**, 528.
1920 Meissner, W. *Arch. f. Augenheilk.* **85**, 222. Abst. *Klin. Monatsbl. f. Augenheilk.* **64**, 722.
1937 Brown, Edgar. Personal Communications.

CHAPTER VII

PROGNOSIS

THE FINAL PICTURE

Few diseases lead to such visual loss, discomfort and disfigurement. Lagrange referred to the final stage of a hydrophthalmic eye as completely "désorganisé, disgracieux et douloureux".

A visit to a Blind Asylum and a search of its records afford ample evidence of this statement.

With head hung, watery eyes and every effort made to avoid light the victim seeks refuge in the dark. Relief may follow only bilateral enucleation.

One finds enormous eyes, infected and bleary, with lids that give very incomplete protection. The bluish sclera may be staphylomatous and the cornea so opaque that the iris is obscured. From the presence of retinal detachment and vitreous shrinkage there may be a greyish yellow reflex. The tension may be low from ciliary atrophy and phthisis bulbi or raised from an intra-ocular haemorrhage due to rupture of a branch of a long posterior ciliary artery.

A permanent cure. When one remembers the deep-seated cause of hypertension in the majority of cases of congenital glaucoma it is not surprising that complete and permanent cures are very rarely known. Even if the operation is performed in the earliest stages there is little chance of such a cure. However, since Seefelder's day the methods of treatment have improved so much that his views may be considered as unduly pessimistic. He wrote: "I intentionally do not use the term 'permanent cure', since I know of no case of operated hydrophthalmia where undiminished sight has been retained till later life. In my opinion there can be no definite point of time at which we can decide that a hydrophthalmia is permanently cured. Such observations as that of our case 20 must be highly disconcerting. Here, ten years after dismissal from the clinic, there was vision of 6/30 corrected with normal tension—definitely a gratifying result—while four years later the vision had inexplicably sunk to 6/100 and could not be improved by any correction."

The oldest person with congenital glaucoma in Jaensch's own experience was a man aged forty-four years. He had been able to see until he was twelve when a detachment appeared in one eye. The other failed when he was thirty-six and both eyes developed phthisis bulbi. In his summary Jaensch wrote: "Thus hydrophthalmia is prognostically very unfavourable and therapeutically very difficult to influence."

When more than one member of a family is affected there is as a rule little similarity between either the initial finding or the response to operation in the several affected members of the family. For examples of this, reference may be made to Dettmering's cases 2, 20, 21 and 23.

It is universally recognised that the treatment of hydrophthalmia is almost hopeless. Seefelder wrote: "There is apparently no other field of operation in ophthalmology which offers the surgeon so many failures and disappointments." One naturally wonders whether any treatment is worth while. One asks what will happen to the eye if no operation is performed? is a spontaneous arrest of the disease possible?

I. THE SPONTANEOUS ARREST OF CONGENITAL GLAUCOMA: MILD CASES

For long it has been recognised that the course of hydrophthalmia in certain eyes appears to be self-limited. It is supposed that, as a result of distension, obstructive tissue in the angle of filtration may become stretched and torn and an adequate channel formed for the escape of fluid.

Collins in 1896 recognised this when he described the eye of a four-year-old child in which such a cure had occurred, though pain, following a blow, later led to enucleation. The iris was much displaced backwards and the angle was open, but delicate fibrils extended from the sclero-corneal meshwork to the root of the iris. The appearances suggested that the congenital adhesions had stretched as the eye distended and that as some of them gave way, filtration became possible and ultimately normal tension was established.

The following history is that of a patient who probably had congenital glaucoma which was spontaneously arrested in very early life (Figs. 114, 115, 116). On examination, at the age of forty-two years, this woman showed slightly prominent eyes with blue sclerae and corneae larger than normal (horizontal diameter R. 13·0 mm., L. 12·6 mm.). Her vision had always been defective and her refraction was R. − 16·0 D.S. and − 2·0 D.Cyl. 90° = H.M. L. − 12·0 D.S. and − 3·0 D.Cyl.

= 6/12 partly. The tension of the right eye was full and that of the left eye normal. The anterior chambers were deep. Each optic disc showed a shallow but wide cup with a sharp edge. Neither tears in Descemet's membrane nor new vessels in the cornea could be seen. The Wassermann reaction was negative. The right nasal field to a 20·0 mm. white object at 1/3 metre was lost and a small central scotoma was present. The left nasal field was almost completely lost to a 5·0 mm. object and showed a very enlarged blind spot. Probably at a very early age this patient developed glaucoma which produced the enlarged corneae, blue sclerae, the cupped discs and the field loss. This condition, for some unknown reason, was arrested spontaneously.

Snellen (1919) emphasised the impossibility of foretelling a spontaneous cure. To confirm this view Zeeman (1918) described two children with signs suggestive that the disease would take a grave course, and in whom nevertheless it became arrested.

Axenfeld (1924) described an "abortive" case of hydrophthalmia. At the age of fifteen years the condition spontaneously came to a standstill with full vision and normal disc but slightly raised tension. "Glaucoma simplex juvenile" developed later and at the age of twenty-five years the patient was blind. Frequent tonometry and perimetry are essential when watching such a patient. Elschnig stated that he had seen even almost porcelain-white corneal opacities clear up spontaneously. They certainly do not of necessity mean a bad prognosis. Much depends on their actual cause, for if due to corneal imbibition they may vanish.

It must be remembered that certain authors have regarded cases of megalocornea as arrested hydrophthalmia. In 1916 Seefelder wrote: "I have supported this idea for a number of years, but have lately changed my opinion." Therefore it is possible that some of reports made before this may have been examples of megalocornea. An exaggerated impression of the frequency of good results without operation may thus have been obtained.

As a rule the presence of tears in Descemet's membrane or of obvious signs of glaucoma in the other eye decide the issue. Mulock Houwer (1932) described a child with typical megalocornea in the right eye and a similar condition of the left eye with typical tears in addition. The horizontal diameter of the latter cornea was 15·0 mm., that is 1·0 mm. greater than that of the former. The explanation of this association is difficult. Could the tears be due to a birth injury of an eye already prominent because of megalocornea? Against this view is the following finding: the tears were horizontal and as a rule after such injuries they tend to be vertical. Mulock Houwer was inclined to class these eyes and similar ones reported by Seefelder, and in fact all cases of megalocornea, as examples of hydrophthalmia with a special tendency to recovery and a different type of heredity. If hypertension were the cause of the condition in his case its effects vanished to a remarkable degree, for it must have been marked at one stage to produce such corneal distension.

A survey of the various series that have been published, and of the questionnaire, lends support to the view that occasionally a spontaneous arrest of the disease occurs.

Let us consider first the reports of patients who were not operated on and who retained relatively good vision for at least six years after the first examination.

In this discussion we will exclude the eyes in which hypertension disappeared but not before serious visual loss had occurred. In two of Fleischer's (1918) cases (12 R. and L.), for example, the tension became low, 12·0 mm. Hg, by the age of twenty-four years, but one eye was blind and the other could only detect hand movements. It is doubtful whether two of the eyes described by Dettmering (1932) can be included, because the only positive sign of hydrophthalmia appears to have been single readings of hypertension. In 13 R. the tension was 30·0 to 40·0 mm. Hg at 6/12 and on three subsequent occasions 26·0 mm. or under. In 30 R. at the end of the first month the tension was 48·0 mm., six months later it was 35·0 mm. In neither of these cases were any other signs of hydrophthalmia found, and though Dettmering wrote of 30 R., "this case suggests that the physiological level of tension is above normal in hydrophthalmia", these two cases can hardly be considered as instances of cured hydrophthalmia.

I. The following eyes showed evidence of hydrophthalmia, but had fair vision at a relatively late age without treatment:

Case	Cornea	Other evidence of H.	Onset	Vision	Tension
F. 2 R.	Large	None. Other eye H.	.	.	Normal
3 R.	12 mm.	,, ,, ,,	.	.	14 mm. Hg
5 L.	12·5 mm.	,, ,, ,,	.	.	21 ,,
Z. 7 R.	12·5 mm.	,, ,, ,,	.	6/4	Normal
17 L.	12 mm.	,, ,, ,,	.	.	,,
Q. 22 L.	12 mm.	Deep a.c. Other eye H.	.	6/9	Full
25 L.	13 mm.	Sl. a.c. ,, ,,	.	6/9	.

Case	Cornea	Other evidence of H.	Onset	Vision	Tension
S. 19 R.	Sl. + ? tear	None. Other eye H.	.	6/15 at 6	Normal
26 R.	12 mm.	Iris atrophy, cup, T. +	Birth	6/24 at 10	+ →N after 7 years
26 L.	12 mm.	,, ,, ,,	,,	6/60 at 10	+ →N after 7 years
St. 10 R.	13 mm.	Cup, T. +. Other eye H.	? 12½ yrs.	6/8 at 12½	? → + after 4 years
Q. 38 R.	Large	Deep a.c., T. +½. Two brothers and sisters H. Other eye H.	Birth	6/60 at 5 6/24 at 17	½
39 L.	Large	Deep a.c. Other eye H.	?	6/60 at 3½ 6/18 at 17	Normal
D. 1 L.	11 mm.	Glaucoma cup, corneal opacities, marked myopia Other eye H.	. <5/12	6/24 c–14.0 D.s	28→20 after 20 years
3 R.	.	Cloudy cornea, T.=60. Other eye H.	Birth	6/30 c–8 D.s	60→23 after 8 years
22 R.	14 mm.	Other eye H. and three others in family	3 yrs.	6/18	20 after 18 years
24 R.	14 mm.	Tears in Descemet's membrane	Youth	6/60 c–9.0 D.s	22 after 18 years
24 L.	14 mm.	,, ,,	,,	6/30 c–5.0 D.s	22 after 18 years

These are probably examples of spontaneously arrested hydrophthalmia.

Note. In these and the following tables:
F. = Fleischer, Z. = Zeeman, Q. = Questionnaire, S. = Seefelder, St. = Stölting, D. = Dettmering, H. = Hydrophthalmia.

II. The following retained good vision till the age of ten years or over, but required operation later:

Case	Cornea	Other evidence of H.	Onset	Vision	Tension	Treatment
Q. 26 L.	Large	Deep a.c., R.E.H. with cup	10 yrs.	6/18 at 10 6/12 at 24	56 mm.	3 Scl., 1 Cycl. at 10
33 L.	12·0 mm.	Cup and atrophy. R. eye and brother H.	?	6/18 at 15 6/12 at 19	? →17 after 4 years	T. at 15
51 L.	13·5 mm.	A.c. 7 mm., iris atrophy. R.E. H.	Birth	6/18 at 12 6/12 at 13	20–14 after 1 year	Cycl. at 12
F. 13 R.	Large	Cornea cloudy, cup. L.E., two brothers and cousin H.	,,	5/6 at 21 5/8 at 23	52 at 21	T. at 21
S. 38 L.	Large	Tears in D.'s M., cup, and other eye H.	?	6/6 at 9 6/100 at 15 C.F. at 18	High	I. at 15

Probably some of these are examples of a type of hydrophthalmia in which tension rises periodically. Another example is Q. 40 L., whose vision was 6/9 at fifteen, and whose cornea was 14·0 mm. A doubtful cup was present and tension became normal after trephine operations at six and eight years, and cyclodialyses at eight and fifteen. The onset was considered to be at birth. Probably the tension rose periodically and the first attack was early enough to produce the enlarged cornea.

The variable nature of the prognosis in hydrophthalmia is discussed elsewhere.

It is not out of place to mention a patient whose tension remained high while his vision remained good. Fleischer (13 R.) reported a young man of twenty-one years whose left eye had been removed elsewhere some years before, because it was enlarged and probably blind. The remaining eye had been enlarged since birth. At two years of age the cornea showed diffuse opacities. At twenty-one the tension was 52·0 mm. Hg, the vision was 6/5 with arcuate field loss and nasal step, and partial glaucomatous cupping of the optic disc. He was trephined and two years later the tension was 15·0 mm. and the vision 5/6. It is improbable that the tension had been high all his life, otherwise the vision would scarcely be 6/5. This is evidently an example of mild hydrophthalmia, with spontaneous arrest and a recurrence at the age of twenty-one years.

To show how slow the progress may be at times the following case may be recalled: D. 27 L. The patient was hydrophthalmic by the age of two years. Each eye at the age of fourteen showed a cupped atrophic disc, an enlarged cornea (14·0 mm.) with tears in Descemet's membrane. The right eye was excised a few months later following a vitreous loss at the time of trephining. The left eye at fourteen years with −5·0 D. read 6/18 and at 23½ still read the same with −6·0 D.

By the courtesy of Colonel R. E. Wright of Madras I had access to notes of twenty-nine patients who apparently had hydrophthalmia. This series differs from all the others in the extreme mildness of the majority of cases.

Of the twenty-eight cases diagnosed as congenital glaucoma in this series nineteen eyes of eleven patients can be considered as examples of mild hydrophthalmia if one takes good vision at a late age as the criterion. Were it not for the fact that the majority of these had large corneae one would prefer to consider "adolescent

glaucoma" as a more exact diagnosis. How then can one explain
these cases? Are we to consider that as a result of a certain amount
of stretching in the neighbourhood of the angle the channels of exit
are opened and the condition arrested? Or is there any evidence
to show that the corneae of Indian patients remain capable of distension until a relatively later age than in other countries and that
these cases are really examples of adolescent glaucoma.

Of the nineteen eyes under consideration

8 had 6/5 at from 15–37 years of age.
3 ,, 6/9 ,, 20–24 ,, ,,
5 ,, 6/12–6/18 at from 19–22 years of age.
3 ,, 6/24–6/36 ,, 19–26 ,, ,,

Of the eight with 6/5 vision (average age twenty-four) all had enlarged corneal diameters but only three had one of the following
signs: cup, raised tension, enlarged blind spot. Thirteen of these
cases were not operated on, ten of these were not followed and one
three years later had 6/5, one four years later had no P.L. and the
other five years later had 6/9. Six of these cases were trephined, two
were not followed, one three years later had 6/5, one two years later
had 6/12, one two years later had 6/36, and one four years later had
6/60.

Fresh exacerbations may occur at puberty or as a result of other
upsets. Therefore caution must be displayed regarding a prognosis
even after years of apparent arrest. Pflüger (1894) referred to a man
whose vision remained stationary till the age of sixty years when
blindness from glaucoma occurred. Zahn (1904) observed an outbreak of acute glaucoma at the age of forty-eight years after an
apparent cure of congenital glaucoma.

It appears certain, therefore, that some mild forms of hydrophthalmia may be arrested early and simply leave behind a myopic
eye with tell-tale tears in Descemet's membrane, and possibly 6/6
vision. In more severe cases no arrest occurs until some cupping of
the disc has appeared with permanent visual loss. In others the raised
tension may return to normal before visual loss, but at a later date
hypertension reappears and the condition may be mistaken then for
adolescent or adult glaucoma. In others no relief from hypertension
is experienced until the very last ray of light is wrung from the optic
nerve.

II. THE RESULTS OF OPERATIVE TREATMENT
IN DIFFERENT SERIES

Series	Total	6/6	6/9 to 6/12	Good	6/18 to 6/60	Fair	C.F. H.M.	P.L.	Blind	Xtn	No mention
Questionnaire	76	3	7	5	8	8	10	4	6	13 (2 burst)	10
Wright	8	3	.	.	2	.	2	.	.	.	1
Zeeman	33	2	1	.	9	.	9	1	5	6	.
Dettmering	39	1	.	2	8	4	8	4	6	4	2
Stölting	18	3	1	1	4	.	3	.	1	2	2
Seefelder	38	.	.	.	4	5	7	4	10	2	3
Fleischer	18	1	1	1	.	.	5	.	3	1	6
Lagrange and Poulard	25	.	.	.	5	7	10	2	1	.	.
Total	255	13	10	9	40	24	54	15	32	30	24
		8·6 %		19 %		9 %	21 %	6 %		24 %	

These patients were observed for at least two years after operation. Two of Seefelder's patients (three eyes) and one of Stölting's (one eye) died (1908).

III AND IV. VISION OF UNOPERATED AND OPERATED
PATIENTS IN LATER LIFE (APPROXIMATE FIGURES)

No. of cases	Age when last seen	6/4 to 6/6	6/8 to 6/12	6/15 to 6/60	<6/60	Blind (including P.L. and excision)
Operated cases						
159	12 years and under	0·6 %	8 %	26 %	32 %	33·4 %
62	Between 12–25 years	6 %	13 %	18 %	29 %	34 %
13	Between 25–50 years	0	0	31 %	46 %	23 %
Unoperated cases						
23	12 years and under	0	13 %	13 %	30·5 %	43·5 %
24	Between 12–25 years	8 %	17 %	21 %	17 %	37 %
10	Between 25–50 years	0	0	40 %	0	60 %

From III and IV the following visual expectations are justified:

(*a*) If operation is performed we may expect one patient in three to be blind, one to have less than 6/60 and one to have more than this by the age of twelve years. In the great majority there is no further serious visual loss until after the age of twenty-five years. After this age no patients were found with vision better than 6/36.

(*b*) If no operation is performed only one patient in four will retain 6/60 or better and two will be blind by the age of twelve. Little change will probably occur until after twenty-five. Sixty per cent. of patients examined between twenty-five and fifty were blind.

It must be remembered that the majority of adult patients with congenital glaucoma are in Blind Institutions and that therefore many of them do not attend hospital clinics. For this reason few of these patients are included in our figures, and we find that of 292 eyes only 7 % belong to patients over twenty-five years of age.

V. INFLUENCE OF AGE AT OPERATION ON VISION AND TENSION

250 cases from the combined series.

A. Vision

Of those operated

at 3/12 and under,	19 %	got 6/24 or better,	60 %	got < 6/60.
from 4/12 to 6/12,	21·6 %	,, ,,	38 %	,,
from 7/12 to 9/12,	30 %	,, ,,	41 %	,,
from 10/12 to 1 year,	11·8 %	,, ,,	77 %	,,
from 1 1/12 to 2 years,	2·6 %	,, ,,	80 %	,,
from 2 1/12 to 6 years,	6 %	,, ,,	90 %	,,
Over 6 years,	20 %	,, ,,	66 %	,,

Of those unoperated, 46 % got 6/24 or better, 44 % got < 6/60 (probably a considerable number were mild).

Of operated cases with final vision of 6/24 and better:
67·6 % had been operated at 1 year and under
(out of total of 113 operated at 1 year and under).
8·1 % had been operated between 1 and 6 years
(out of total of 69 operated between 1 and 6 years).
24·3 % had been operated over 6
(out of total of 41 operated over 6).

B. Vision and Tension

Age at operation	6/24 or better	Less than 6/60	Normal tension
6 months and under	21 % } 23 %	44 %	50 %
1 year ,, ,,	24 %	66 %	50 %
3 years and under	4·4 % } 4·3 %	82 %	36 %
6 ,, ,,	4 %	89 %	33 %
Over 6 years	22 %	66 %	60 %
No operation	46 %	43 %	41 %

Age at first operation	Vision										Tension			
	6/4 to 6/8	6/9 to 6/15	6/18 to 6/24	6/36 to 6/60	6/60 C.F. H.M.	P.L.	O.	Excision	?	Died under 1 yr.	Normal (up to 25 mm. Hg)	Full satisfactory 30 mm.	30 mm. and over	Soft
Under 3 mths.	.	1	2	3	3	.	2	5	1	.	2	5	2	2
4–6 mths.	2	4	2	15	8	2	2	2	8	1	18	8	9	1
7–9 mths.	3	1	8	12	7	4	4	2	2	.	17	8	6	2
10 mths.–1 yr.	2	.	.	2	3	1	6	4	4	3	8	.	9	.
13 mths.–2 yrs.	1	.	.	6	16	3	10	2	4	.	12	3	15	3
2¼–3 yrs.	.	.	1	.	1	1	3	1	1	.	1	.	4	.
3¼–6 yrs.	.	.	1	2	8	5	2	6	3	.	4	1	7	1
Over 6 yrs.	4	4	1	5	12	5	5	5	1	.	18	3	10	5
No operation	5	7	7	4	3	1	4	10	.	.	7	4	6	.

C. Tension

Of 90 operated at 1 year or under, 50 % developed normal tension.
Of 87   ,,   over 1 year,   40 %   ,,   ,,   ,,

VI. INFLUENCE OF SIZE OF CORNEA ON VISUAL PROGNOSIS

The visual loss and the corneal distension keep pace to a marked extent. This is shown by the following summary of cases with large corneae and an analysis of the vision present:

Corneal diameter		Vision
23 mm.	1 case	Excision
17 mm. and over.	6 cases	Blind, 2 eyes
		P.L., 1 eye
		H.M., 1 eye
		< 6/60, 2 eyes
16 mm. and over.	4 cases	Blind, 3 eyes
		P.L., 1 eye
15 mm. and over.	16 cases	Excision, 2 eyes
		C.F., 4 eyes
		6/36–6/60, 4 eyes (first operation at 6 months, 8 years, 18 years, 18 years)
		6/24, 1 eye (first operation 6 months) (onset childhood)

Of twenty-seven eyes with a corneal diameter of 16·0 mm. or over thirteen were either excised or quite blind.

An enlarged and prominent cornea is very exposed to serious trauma. Very frequently an injury has led to enucleation. A bump on a chair appears to be the commonest form of injury. The following eyes were removed after an injury: Q. 7 L., 22 L., 37 L., 48 R., 60 L., Seefelder 38 L.

Occasionally, if the period of corneo-scleral distensibility had passed, an early and marked cup was found with an almost normal cornea, and marked visual loss, e.g. case 35 L. questionnaire, reported by Verderame, onset one year, at 6½ years cornea 12·5 × 12·0 mm., but a deep cup in an atrophic disc. Without operative treatment the tension was normal and the vision with 16 D. 3/10 6½ years later. The other eye was enucleated at 6½ years.

The following summary compares results obtained from various operations, where the cornea was 13·0 mm. or less in diameter, with results in cases where the corneal diameter was over 13·0 mm.:

Operation	No. of eyes with final vision 6/24 or better		No. with final vision <6/60	
	13 mm. and under	Over 13 mm.	13 mm. and under	Over 13 mm.
Anterior sclerotomy	6 out of 9	2 out of 8	0 out of 9	5 out of 8
Trephine	4 ,, 6	6 ,, 34	1 ,, 34	19 ,, 34
Iridectomy	0 ,, 5	0 ,, 4	2 ,, 5	3 ,, 4
Total all operations	11/26 = 42 %	13/62 = 21 %	7/26 = 23 %	37/62 = 60 %

Optic disc

The following table shows the relationship between final vision and the state of the optic disc:

	Normal disc	Glaucoma cup	Atrophy
Total no. of cases	44	54	15
Final vision = 6/24 or better	22 = 50 %	7 = 13 %	1 = 7 %
Final vision = < 6/60	12 = 27 %	34 = 63 %	13 = 87 %

(NOTE. Cases where disc was described as "pale, without cupping" are included as normal, and "glaucoma cup" includes ones where disc was cupped and pale, but not white.) Total number of cases where state of disc was mentioned = 113. Of these, 39 % were normal, 48 % cupped, 13 % atrophic. In many cases the disc could not be seen owing to corneal opacities or cataract, and if these were included the percentage with a cupped disc would be greater.

VII. ANALYSIS OF CASES WITH FINAL VISION OF AT LEAST 6/12

There are thirty-seven cases in the combined series under consideration with vision of 6/12 and better at a relatively late age. They are:

Stölting 1 R., 1 L., 4 L., 10 R.
Fleischer 2 R., 3 R., 5 L., 8 R., 8 L., 13 R.
Seefelder nil.
Dettmering nil.
Questionnaire: General 9 R., 22 L., 25 L., 26 L., 29 R., 32 R., 32 L., 33 L., 34 L., 40 L., 51 L.
Wright 7 R., 7 L., 9 R., 10 R., 10 L., 19 R., 20 L., 23 R., 24 R., 24 L., 25 L.
Zeeman 1 L., 4 L., 7 R., 9 L., 17 L.

Of these cases fifteen received no operative treatment. Many of these have been classed as examples of mild glaucoma, *e.g.* Fleischer 2 R., 3 R., 5 L., questionnaire 22 L., 25 L., Zeeman 7 R., 17 L. Those which have been described as large normal eyes in unilateral hydrophthalmia, were Wright's cases 7 L., 10 R., 19 R. and L., 20 L., 24 R. and L. The remaining one, Stölting 10 R., had vision 6/8 at 12½ years, but the presence of a cornea of 13·0 mm., cupped disc, and raised tension, suggested that the hydrophthalmia had become spontaneously arrested, and had recurred by 12½.

In six of the twenty-two operated cases the good results could be attributed either to the condition being mild, or to early operation. They were:

Series	Vision	Cornea	Cup	Tension	Operation
St. 1 R.	6/4 at 18 years	Rather large	Normal	Became normal	Scl. at 7 mths.
1 L.	6/8 at 18 ,,	,, ,,	,,	,, ,,	,, ,,
4 L.	6/8 at 31 ,,	12·5 mm.	?	,, ,,	2 scl. at 10 mths.
Q. 32 R.	6/12 at 13 ,,	12 mm.	Normal	Full	T. at 5 mths.
32 L.	6/8 at 13 ,,	14 mm.	,,	Full	3 T., 1 cycl. at 5 mths.
34 L.	6/5 at 9½ ,,	12 mm.	?	Became normal	T. at 1½ yrs.

Early and correct operation was probably the only cause of good vision in seven eyes:

Series	Vision	Cornea	Cup	Tension	Operation
F. 8 R.	6/12 at 6½ years	14 mm.	Normal	40 normal	T. at 4 mths.
8 L.	6/9 at 6½ ,,	14 mm.	,,	40 ,,	,, ,,
Q. 9 R.	6/12 at 7¾ ,,	+	,,	Full	2 scl., at 3 and 6 mths.
29 R.	6/12 at 7 ,,	14 mm.	,,	?	T. at 7 mths.
Z. 9 L.	6/6 at 9 ,,	13 mm.	,,	Normal	T. at 8 ,,
1 L.	6/8 at 6 ,,	+	?	,,	T. at 6 ,,
4 L.	6/12 at 8 ,,	13·5 mm.	Normal	,,	T. at 5 ,,

The remaining nine cases include Wright, 7 R., 10 L., 12 R., 23 R., which were operated at the ages of fifteen, twenty, nineteen and twenty-seven years respectively, and Fleischer 13 R., questionnaire 26 L., 33 L., 51 L., and 40 L., which have already been discussed as examples of spontaneous arrest or periodic hydrophthalmia.

VIII. THE PROGNOSIS OF HYDROPHTHALMIA WHEN ASSOCIATED WITH NEUROFIBROMATOSIS AND FACIAL NAEVI

Of eighteen eyes with hydrophthalmia associated with neuro-fibromatosis:

27·7 % were blind or excised by 3 years of age.
44·4 %   ,,   ,,   ,,   6   ,,   ,,
72 %   ,,   ,,   ,,   12   ,,   ,,

Of the 5 remaining ones:

2 were blind by 16 years.
1 had H.M. at 7 years.
1 had 0·1 at 15 years.
1 was excised at 27 years.

So it appears that an eye is doomed when affected by neuro-fibromatosis. The outlook is less gloomy in the next group.

Of twenty-four eyes with hydrophthalmia associated with facial naevi:

8·3 % were blind or excised by 3 years of age.
16·6 %   ,,   ,,   ,,   6   ,,   ,,
37·5 %   ,,   ,,   ,,   12   ,,   ,,

Of the fifteen remaining

    1 was blind or excised by 20 years.

    4 were   ,,   ,,   28 ,,

    4 had very poor vision (1/60 at 21, H.M. at 28, 1/300 at 12, C.F. at 26 years).

    7 had relatively good vision (6/15 at 59, 5/20 at 6, "good" at 9, 6/21 at 21, 6/60 at 2, 6/24 at 8 years, 6/30 at 35 years).

Fortunately all the cases of neurofibromatosis had only unilateral facial and ocular lesions, whilst of the patients with facial naevi 34 % had bilateral naevi and 11 % had bilateral glaucoma.

When a naevus is present there is probably a greater tendency to haemorrhage and recurrence of hypertension after operation than in other cases. The only satisfactory result was that obtained by Knapp (1927). The right eye of Mehney's patient (1937) with bilateral adolescent glaucoma and naevi was trephined. A complete retinal detachment with a peripheral tear developed. This persisted in spite of two diathermy operations.

Further evidence of the different outlooks in these two forms of associated hydrophthalmia is found if we study the ages when excision of the affected eyes became necessary.

1. With neurofibromatosis (11 cases):

    4 removed at or under 2½ years.

    8   ,,   ,,   9   ,,

    10   ,,   ,,   16   ,,

    11   ,,   ,,   27   ,,

2. With facial naevi (5 cases):

    1 removed at 9 years.

    3   ,,   or under 21 years.

    5   ,,   ,,   28 ,,

In addition Arnold (1891) referred to two patients of sixteen years, who died a few weeks after sclerotomies. Jaensch's case I died under the anaesthetic for a trephine at the age of ten months: Zaun's one-year-old child (1924) died from heart failure the day after an anaesthetic for anterior sclerotomy; Kalt's patient died thirty-six hours after a slight ethyl-chloride anaesthetic: Magitot's two patients died a few hours after short chloroform anaesthesia at the ages of twelve and fourteen months.

IX. JUVENILE MORTALITY (UNDER 12)

Series	No of patients in series	No. of deaths	Percentage deaths	Average age at operation	Average age at death
Dettmering	30	0	0	·	·
Fleischer	13	1	7·5 %	16/12	3
Seefelder	38	3	8 %	13/12	2½
Stölting	11	1	9 %	11/12	2
Wright	20 (?)	0	0	·	·
Questionnaire	55	1	1·8 %	16/12	13
Zeeman	19	0	0	·	·
Lagrange and Poulard	18	0	0	·	·
Total	204	6	2·5 %	14/12	4¾

Delord considered a general anaesthetic to be unsafe and thought that this was an extra argument in favour of sclerotomy.

Magitot (1912) and Spielberg (1911) considered that death was due to an insufficiency of the antitoxic function of the liver.

Information regarding prognosis obtained from the Questionnaire

It is of interest to compare the state of the eyes in two extreme groups, viz. those that some years after operation, or first observation, had good (or fair) vision, that is from 6/5 to 6/60, and those that became quite blind. Of twenty-two affected eyes in the first group five (23 %) had a corneal diameter of 12·0 mm. The relative frequency of certain features can be studied in the following statement:

	GROUP A Good (or fair) vision	GROUP B Blind
Corneal diameter of 12 mm.	23 %	8 %
12–14 mm. and large	45 %	22 %
14–15 mm. and very large	32 %	54 %
16–18 mm.	0	16 %
Total	22 cases	13 cases
State of optic disc: Cup	36 %	44 %
Pale	0	12 %
Pale and cup	14 %	6 %
Not visible	9 %	38 %
No cup	41 %	0
Total	22 cases	16 cases

		Group A Good (or fair) vision	Group B Blind
Tension:	Normal	32 %	6 %
	Full	32 %	5 %
	+	26 %	50 %
	+2, +3	11 %	39 %
	Total	19 cases	18 cases

Approximate age at first operation		Group A Good (or fair) vision	Group B Blind
	under 6/12	35 %	19 %
	7/12 to 1 year	17 %	14 %
	13/12 to 3 years	4 %	5 %
	3¼ to 10 years	13 %	34 %
	Over 10 years	9 %	5 %
	No operation	22 %	23 %
	Total	21 cases	23 cases

Vision at first examination:	Good (or fair) vision		Blind	
	6/18	8 %	C.F.	5 %
	6/36	8 %	H.M. and ? H.M.	15 %
	6/60	8 %	P.L. and ? P.L.	40 %
	Good	4 %	No P.L.	15 %
	No note	16	Bad	10 %
	Total	23 cases	No note	4
			Total	21 cases

Operations used first:	Good (or fair) vision	Blind
Trephine	44 %	66 %
Herbert's Sclerotomy	11 %	0 %
Anterior Sclerotomy	22 %	7 %
Cyclodialysis	6 %	7 %
Paracentesis	11 %	13 %
Iridectomy	6 %	7 %
Total	18 cases	15 cases

SUMMARY

1. Of 255 cases treated by operation and followed for at least two years 8·6 % retained vision of 6/12 or better, 19 % retained vision that was good or not less than 6/60, and 51 % had the ability to count fingers or became blind. Of those with 6/12 or better 60 % had an operation performed before they were one year old, 16 % received no treatment and 21 % were over six years of age when first operated on (six, twelve, ten and fifteen years). These were probably examples of mild or periodic glaucoma.

2. 25 % of operated cases and 54 % of unoperated were blind by the age of twelve years. 45 % of operated cases and 60 % of unoperated were blind by the age of twenty-five years. 53 % of operated cases and 65 % of unoperated were blind by the age of fifty years. None of the operated cases and 7 % of the unoperated cases had 6/12 or better at the age of twenty-five years.

3. Of those operated at three months or under 19 % obtained 6/24 or better and 60 % less than 6/60. The best operative results were obtained between seven and nine months, of these cases 30 % obtained 6/24 or better and 41 % less than 6/60. From this period to six years of age the results are much worse. Of those over six years 20 % obtained 6/24 or better and 66 % less than 6/60. In this group there were probably a large proportion of mild or periodic cases of hydrophthalmia.

To emphasise further the presence of two periods that are less unfavourable than others it may be pointed out that of those with 6/24 and better 67·6 % had been operated on at or under one year of age, 3 % between one and six years and 24·3 % over six years.

4. Of those operated at or under one year 50 % obtained normal tension. Of those operated over this age 40 % developed normal tension.

5. The results obtained by operation were worse if the corneal diameter was over 14·0 mm., if the optic disc was pale or cupped, if the tension was very high and if the initial vision was less than 6/60.

6. When hydrophthalmia is associated with neurofibromatosis the outlook is particularly bad. In almost 75 % blindness or enucleation had occurred by the age of twelve years. When facial naevi are present the outlook is less grave. In 37·5 % blindness or enucleation had occurred by the age of twelve years.

7. The mortality under anaesthetics of young children with hydrophthalmia is sufficiently high to make extreme care essential.

REFERENCES

PROGNOSIS

1891 ARNOLD, TH. *Beitr. z. Augenheilk.* **3**, 16.
1894 PFLÜGER. Inaug. Dissert. Zürich. Quoted by Schmidt-Rimpler.
1896 COLLINS, E. T. *Researches into the Anatomy and Pathology of the Eye*, p. 105. London: Lewis.
1904 ZAHN, C. Inaug. Dissert. Tübingen. Quoted by Schmidt-Rimpler.
1908 STÖLTING. *Arch. f. Ophthal.* **67**, 171.

1911 Spielberg, C. *Klin. Monatsbl. f. Augenheilk.* **49**, 314.
1912 Magitot, A. *Ann. d'Ocul.* **147**, 1.
1916 Seefelder, R. *Klin. Monatsbl. f. Augenheilk.* **56**, 227.
1918 Fleischer, B. *Klin. Monatsbl. f. Augenheilk.* **61**, 152.
1918 Zeeman, W. P. C. *Klin. Monatsbl. f. Augenheilk.* **60**, 400.
1919 Snellen. *Amer. Jl. Ophthal.* **2**, 146.
1924 Axenfeld, Th. *Klin. Monatsbl. f. Augenheilk.* **73**, 403.
1924 Zaun, W. *Klin. Monatsbl. f. Augenheilk.* **72**, 58.
1927 Jaensch, P. A. *Arch. f. Ophthal.* **118**, 21.
1927 Knapp, A. *Trans. Amer. Ophthal. Soc.* **25**, 154.
1932 Mulock Houwer, A. W. *Geneesk tijdschr. v. Nederl.-Indië*, **72**, 1410.
1932 Dettmering, M. Inaug. Dissert. Göttingen.
1937 Mehney, G. H. *Arch. of Ophthal.* **17**, 1020.

CHAPTER VIII

GENERAL REFLECTIONS

Wisdom will repudiate thee, if thou think to enquire
WHY things are as they are or whence they came: thy task
is first to learn WHAT IS, and in pursuant knowledge
pure intellect will find pure pleasure and the only ground
for a philosophy conformable to truth.

ROBERT BRIDGES.

Uncertainty regarding the ultimate cause of Congenital Glaucoma persists and will persist as long as so much concerning the influence of heredity and the forces in prenatal life that make for maldevelopment continues to be wrapped in mystery.

We have concentrated on an investigation of the earliest specimens with this disease and we have sought for traces of pre-existing inflammation, and we have found little. Either such a state is far from being universal or its manifestations in foetal life are not recognised because they can rapidly disappear or because they differ from those so well known in adult tissues. If an attack of inflammation had been initiated early, its influence would be great enough to lead to grave and obvious malformation. One may ask, can such an attack commence prior to the development of an efficient blood-vascular system? If not, its onset must be restricted to the second half of pregnancy. If this attack be of any but the mildest degree, surely histological evidence of inflammation would be revealed in an examination of specimens obtained during the first few weeks of life.

Though the abnormal findings in the earliest specimens are varied and diverse yet they as a whole resemble defects in development. They suggest that growth has been retarded or has become aberrant. A study of human embryology and of comparative anatomy throws light on these anomalous states. Collateral evidence is supplied by the presence of other developmental defects in patients with congenital glaucoma. Not only do we find ocular defects but facial naevi or neurofibromatous changes on the same side of the face and head as the affected eye.

We cannot, however, assume that congenital glaucoma is due, as a rule, to defective development and nothing else, for one does not know what factors underlie errors in development in general. It is conceivable that a deficiency in some vitamin or some endocrine substance may exist, or that some upset in the maternal nervous system may so lower resistance that inflammation or some other dystrophic influence may be permitted to disturb the smoothness that characterises normal growth.

Without doubt hereditary disease plays a part and possibly a greater one than we think, for the arrival of a defective offspring often means that it is the last of the family. In addition, the obvious nature of its physical disability and the manner in which this excludes it from the labour market leads, as a rule, to a life of celibacy. In such ways the influence of inheritance may be obscured. Consanguinity may accentuate the dangers of inheritance if morbid tendencies are present in the parents. Ill health of either parent is not infrequent and the patients as a rule are born into conditions that are far from ideal. The majority of them live in communities where rickets, syphilis and tuberculosis are common. Not infrequently the patient or his mother bears unmistakable signs of spirochaetal infection. Two points must be borne in mind regarding such a state. Firstly, an attack of interstitial keratitis just before or immediately after birth may produce a condition that is indistinguishable from congenital glaucoma. Secondly, the origin of Schlemm's canal and the development of a vascular system sufficiently complete to permit the invasion of the eye by spirochaetes are approximately simultaneous.

From our studies there arises a clear conception of a grave and progressive disease with features so much its own that other diseases with which it was once confused can now be separated from it with ease. It is so characterised by hypertension and its effects that in their absence its diagnosis cannot be made. Such effects play no part in the appearance of myopia and megalocornea so these diseases can be recognised as separate entities. Difficulties may arise, however, in the very rare cases where inflammation has so weakened the sclero-corneal tunic that it cannot withstand the stretching power of even normal tension and where an innate corneal defect or possibly a prenatal perforation is associated with pupillary and peripheral synechiae that promote hypertension. Instances of these forms of infantile interstitial keratitis and congenital anterior synechiae are very uncommon. Even though glaucoma is not present at birth it may occasionally be wise to diagnose congenital glaucoma if, at birth, so defective a state existed that hypertension occurred later but sufficiently early to produce ocular distension. As a rule the clinical and the histological manifestations of congenital glaucoma are sufficiently typical to justify a definite diagnosis and only too certain a prognosis.

Though the precise manner in which the aqueous escapes at the angle of filtration is uncertain, the unrivalled importance of the canal of Schlemm is beyond doubt. The intra-ocular fluid may be secreted, dialysed, or it may filter into the chambers of the globe. There may or may not be a pump-like mechanism, or absorption by osmosis, and the living trabecular tissue may filter the aqueous as adequately as a multitude of grains of sand may filter water. Uncertainty may exist in these matters but not concerning the vital importance of Schlemm's canal. Any doubt concerning the importance of this canal vanishes when one studies its development in the animal world. In the lowest mammals it may be represented by two or three scleral capillaries that do not form an annular channel around the angle. They may have only isolated ostia that communicate with the anterior chamber. Coarse pillars of hyaline and other tissue, that stretch from the cornea to the iris may partially cover the entrance to such a canal. Profuse meshwork and even isolated strands of muscle-like tissue may separate such channels from the angle. These variations may exist but the utility of Schlemm's canal is constant. There is a significant development to protect the primitive canal of Schlemm once accommodation demands structural changes which jeopardise the integrity of its lumina. The forward movement of the canal and the development of an annular band of equatorial fibres—the scleral spur—provide means for firm fixation of the elaborated muscle of accommodation without obstruction to the channels for the escape of aqueous. We can regard glaucoma, at least when it arises early in life, as a price we pay for the power of accommodation. Adaptation to the needs of man's immediate ancestors has led to the development of a powerful ciliary muscle and the concentration of its insertion in the neighbourhood of those channels that are essential for the escape of intra-ocular fluid. These changes have narrowed the margin of safety between normal function and a state in which these channels may become embarrassed. Once again we see how phylogenetic youth has made for structural instability.

In the earliest specimens of congenital glaucoma the following defects are of frequent occurrence: absence or partial obliteration of the canal of Schlemm and its position far behind the angle of filtration; a scleral-like density of the trabeculae; an undue persistence of the uveal meshwork, and a process of iris-like tissue that fills the angle. Not only are all these defects errors in development, but they all interfere with the patency of the channels of exit.

A local patch of inflammation, due to some general infection, may be the underlying cause of what are apparently developmental defects. There may be considerable spoiling of the vessel walls and infiltration round them, interfering with the development of the tissues nourished by these vessels. Take, for example, the anterior ciliary veins; if an adjacent process of inflammation restricts their capacity, surely the canal of Schlemm, which drains into them, will also be affected. Its walls may be affected and its lumen obstructed, or its whole development and that of the scleral spur be arrested, and both structures may appear poorly developed and in a posterior or foetal position.

It is a striking fact that though peripheral synechiae are frequently found in specimens with advanced hydrophthalmia they are very rarely found in the early stages. When one realises how distended the globe and how wide the angle may become it appears remarkable that adhesions could form in this angle. Possibly they develop mainly in the type that has a process of iris-like tissue filling the angle.

Though degeneration may play a great part in producing glaucoma, yet our destiny regarding certain types of this disease is largely determined by the state of the angle at birth. If the characteristic defects be so extensive as to lead to complete obstruction, ocular distension may occur as soon as aqueous is ready to escape. They may, however, be less advanced and only constitute an obstruction when inflammation or another cause of congestion leads to the formation of excessive fluid and the channels that could cope with a normal quantity of fluid become embarrassed. This conception links the congenital form of glaucoma with the infantile and adolescent forms. Even in the simple so-called idiopathic form of adult life there may be some minimal lesion in these tissues that is the turning point in the development of glaucoma. The division of glaucoma into congenital, infantile and senile forms is largely arbitrary. Too much emphasis can be attached to the change of environment that occurs at birth.

When we consider the means at our disposal for the treatment of this disease it is essential to keep in mind the nature and the situation of the lesions that, in all probability, are present. Miotics are always worth a trial though results from their use are very disappointing. If tension is very high and for any reason it is not wise to attempt fistulisation immediately, it may be essential to reduce tension by one or more paracenteses. Two certain results will follow prolonged and unrelieved hypertension and they demand operation as soon as the patient's condition permits it. These results are the gradual distension that destroys the normal functioning of structures and the cupping of the optic disc that leads to atrophy of the optic nerve. The surgeon's experience will largely determine the exact operation he chooses. Some are more skilled and have more confidence in one of the following methods: sclero-corneal trephining, Lagrange's operation or a modification of it, or one of the many forms of sclerotomy.

Unfortunately there can be more decision about our opinions concerning the prognosis of congenital glaucoma than about any of its other aspects. It progresses, as a rule, in a relentless fashion until the best setting for the patient is some institution that caters for the blind. There is just sufficient hope from operation, provided it be performed early and skilfully, to bind the oculist to an endeavour to restore normal tension before distension of the globe has destroyed all hope of retaining any degree of visual function. In this endeavour the oculist must not be satisfied to regard a single operation as the end of his duty, unless, of course, hypertension is removed and distension has ceased. On the other hand, the surgeon may gravely err if in his ardour for a surgical triumph he neglects the general condition, and particularly the mental state of his patient. It is better for the patient to continue life relying on the compensations provided for the blind than be so maimed in mind that these compensations are of little avail. Occasionally the condition of ocular hypertension ceases spontaneously and a benign state commences which may persist for many years. Such an occurrence explains in some measure the presence of the second relatively satisfactory period for operative interference that lies over the age of six years. So variable are the responses to decompressive measures that the experience with one eye of an individual or with one member of a family throws little or no light on the prospects for the other eye or for other members of the family if such be affected.

The future of patients with hydrophthalmia is dark. Little hope of preserving sufficient sight to permit the earning of a livelihood can be held out to them. All that the surgeon can do is to adopt a method of treatment of proved value, and apply it to the best of his ability when the setting for the operation and the condition of the patient are as good as possible.

INDEX

rinted in the United States
y Bookmasters